POLYCYSTIC OVARIAN SYNDROME: AN ENIGMATIC ENDOCRINOLOGICAL DISORDER

OBSTETRICS AND GYNECOLOGY ADVANCES

Additional books in this series can be found on Nova's website
under the Series tab.

Additional E-books in this series can be found on Nova's website
under the E-books tab.

ENDOCRINOLOGY RESEARCH AND CLINICAL DEVELOPMENTS

Additional books in this series can be found on Nova's website
under the Series tab.

Additional E-books in this series can be found on Nova's website
under the E-books tab.

POLYCYSTIC OVARIAN SYNDROME: AN ENIGMATIC ENDOCRINOLOGICAL DISORDER

ROSA SABATINI
EDITOR

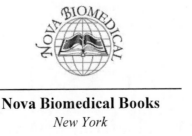

Nova Biomedical Books
New York

Copyright ©2011 by Nova Science Publishers, Inc.

All rights reserved. No part of this book may be reproduced, stored in a retrieval system or transmitted in any form or by any means: electronic, electrostatic, magnetic, tape, mechanical photocopying, recording or otherwise without the written permission of the Publisher.

For permission to use material from this book please contact us:
Telephone 631-231-7269; Fax 631-231-8175
Web Site: http://www.novapublishers.com

NOTICE TO THE READER

The Publisher has taken reasonable care in the preparation of this book, but makes no expressed or implied warranty of any kind and assumes no responsibility for any errors or omissions. No liability is assumed for incidental or consequential damages in connection with or arising out of information contained in this book. The Publisher shall not be liable for any special, consequential, or exemplary damages resulting, in whole or in part, from the readers' use of, or reliance upon, this material. Any parts of this book based on government reports are so indicated and copyright is claimed for those parts to the extent applicable to compilations of such works.

Independent verification should be sought for any data, advice or recommendations contained in this book. In addition, no responsibility is assumed by the publisher for any injury and/or damage to persons or property arising from any methods, products, instructions, ideas or otherwise contained in this publication.

. It is sold with the clear understanding that the Publisher is not engaged in rendering legal or any other professional services. If legal or any other expert assistance is required, the services of a competent person should be sought. FROM A DECLARATION OF PARTICIPANTS JOINTLY ADOPTED BY A COMMITTEE OF THE AMERICAN BAR ASSOCIATION AND A COMMITTEE OF PUBLISHERS.

Additional color graphics may be available in the e-book version of this book.

Library of Congress Cataloging-in-Publication Data

Polycystic ovarian syndrome : an enigmatic endrocrinological disorder /
editor, Rosa Sabatini.
    p. ; cm.
 Includes bibliographical references and index.
 ISBN 978-1-61761-853-6 (hardcover)
 1. Polycystic ovary syndrome. I. Sabatini, Rosa.
 [DNLM: 1. Polycystic Ovary Syndrome. WP 320]
 RG480.S7P645 2010
 618.11--dc22
                    2010036152

Published by Nova Science Publishers, Inc. + New York

Contents

Preface		7
Introduction		9
Chapter I	**Polycystic Ovarian Syndrome: Definition**	15
	Rosa Sabatini , Raffaele Cagiano and Francesca Scaramuzzi	
Chapter II	**Polycystic Ovarian Syndrome: Epidemiology, Aetiology and Pathogenesis**	35
	Rosa Sabatini and Raffaele Cagiano	
Chapter III	**Polycystic Ovarian Syndrome: Symptoms and Clinical Manifestations**	111
	Rosa Sabatini	
Chapter IV	**Metabolic Syndrome in PCOS Women**	179
	Rosa Sabatini and Raffaele Cagiano	
Conclusion		277
	Rosa Sabatini	
Index		283

Preface

Polycystic ovary syndrome (PCOS) is a very common endocrinopathy whose etiology is still uncertain. It is estimated that 5-12% of the female population of childbearing age, amongst all races and nationalities, experience this problem. Nonetheless, the heterogeneous clinical and biochemical presentation, the overproduction of ovarian androgens leading to symptoms as hirsutism, acne, and anovulation, may be considered the hallmark of this syndrome. However, the symptoms and the severity of this disorder greatly vary among affected women. This book presents current treatments and research regarding this particular syndrome.

Introduction

Polycystic ovary syndrome (PCOS) otherwise named Stein-Leventhal syndrome, polycystic ovary disease , ovarian hyperthecosis and sclerocystic ovary syndrome, is a very common endocrinopathy whose etiology is still uncertain. It is estimated that 5-12 % of the female population of childbearing age, amongst all races and nationalities, experience this problem [1,2,3]. Nonetheless the heterogeneous clinical and biochemical presentation, the overproduction of ovarian androgens leading to symptoms as hirsutism , acne, and anovulation , may be considered the hallmark of this syndrome [4]. However, the symptoms and the severity of this disorder greatly vary among affected women. Typically, PCOS symptoms first appear in adolescents around the start of menstruation; occasionally, some symptoms until even their 20s.The most common early problems of the sufferers are irregular periods and overweight or obesity. Today, it seems that the prevalence is increasing secondarily to the recent trend of the increasing obesity among teenagers. Currently, hyperinsulinemia, exacerbated by obesity, is considered the crucial point of this ambiguous syndrome. Obesity may unmask or amplify symptoms and endocrine-metabolic abnormalities [5,6,7] Really, the prevalence of obesity in PCOS women is increased when compared to the general female population, and conversely, the prevalence of PCOS is increased in overweight and obese women when compared to their lean counterparts. Obesity seems to occur in approximately 50% of hyperandrogenic anovulatory women, some of whom also have non-insulin dependent diabetes mellitus [8].Consequently, body mass index is a primary mediator in the relationship between PCOS and health-related quality of life in obese PCOS adolescents. Any intervention directed at reducing central obesity will not only improve quality of life, but also correct hyperinsulinaemia and improve fertility as well as lipid and androgen profiles [3].It is also the only currently available way that can have a lifelong impact on reducing possible long- term complications of the syndrome. The aetiology of PCOS is unclear but studies in the Rhesus monkey suggested that exposure to excess androgen, during intrauterine life, could result in many of the features of human PCOS, including ovarian dysfunction, abnormal LH secretion and insulin resistance. Therefore, it is possible to suppose that PCOS in adolescents arises as a result of a genetically determined disorder of ovarian function. This condition might induce hypersecretion of androgens, possibly during fetal life and also during physiological activation of the hypothalamic- pituitary-ovarian axis, in infancy and at the onset of puberty [9].There is plentiful evidence for a genetic basis for PCOS but gestational environment, and lifestyle factors as nutrition, or both could influence the clinical and biochemical phenotype [10,11,12]. Obesity exerts a major impact on the PCOS phenotype, particularly on the metabolic association and complications of this syndrome. In fact, the presence of obesity is clearly related to the infertility of PCOS women, and increases the risk of metabolic syndrome and its constellation of cardiovascular risk factors [11]. Furthermore, may be important to consider that the ethnic background of women with PCOS may affect the clinical, hormonal, and metabolic characteristics of this condition [12] Adolescents and young women often show hirsutism, irregular menses, and obesity [5].Other features of PCOS are insulin resistance, impaired glucose tolerance, dyslipidaemia, and obstructive sleep apnoea. PCOS is the major cause of anovulatory infertility but the reproductive problems are secondary to metabolic concerns associated with health long-term consequences [3]. In fact, the sufferers have a 7-fold increased risk for the development of non- insulin dependent diabetes mellitus (NIDDM) and may be considered as a group of women at high risk for the development of coronary heart disease (CHD) [12,13, 14, 15]. Until now, there has not been a common factor that identifies all women with polycystic ovary syndrome. Not surprisingly, therefore, the definition of, and diagnostic criteria for, the clinical heterogeneity of polycystic ovary syndrome remain controversial and the unceasing debate on the most appropriate diagnostic criteria continues [16]. Polycystic ovarian syndrome, then called Stein-Leventhal syndrome, was firstly described in 1935; originally, diagnosis required pathognomonic ovarian findings and the clinical triad of hirsutism, amenorrhea and obesity. In the last two decades, it was registered an unceasing debate about the most appropriate diagnostic criteria for this syndrome. Particularly, in 1990 a consensus workshop sponsored by the NIH/ NICHD, suggested that a patient has PCOS if she has signs of androgens excess(clinical and /or biochemical) and oligoovulation/anovulation. While, other entities that would cause polycystic ovaries have been excluded. In 2003 , a consensus workshop ,sponsored by ESHRE / ASRM in Rotterdam, indicated PCOS to be present if 2 out of 3 criteria are met: oligoovulation and/or anovulation,excess androgen activity and polycystic ovaries , while other endocrine disorders are excluded. The Rotterdam definition is wider, including many more patients, notably patients without androgen excess; whereas in the NIH/NICHD definition, androgen excess is a prerequisite [17].Therefore, it was considered the possibility that there may be forms of PCOS without overt evidence of hyperandrogenism, but it was recognized that more data are required before validating this supposition. Rotterdam definition has received much consensus but the debate continues. Finally, the Task Force recognized and fully expects that the definition of this syndrome will evolve over time to incorporate new research findings [18].PCO appearance is not a prerequisite for the diagnosis of this endocrinopathy [19]. Recent studies focused on the long-term metabolic and cardiovascular sequelae of PCOS (20). In addition, past and recent researches reported the potential risk of endometrial cancer [21,22] Early recognition and prompt treatment of PCOS in adolescents is important to prevent it [7].Efforts to diagnose and to treat these women in adolescence should be made to minimize the development of to prevent potentially the onset of cardiovascular, metabolic and neoplastic problems [5]. Treatment depends on the presenting symptoms, which may often be ameliorated by weight loss, where significant. Antiandrogen preparations are used for hyperandrogenic symptoms; while,clomiphene citrate(CC) seems to be the first-line treatment for anovulation and infertility. Aromatase inhibitors are being investigated as an alternative to clomiphene citrate. Failure to conceive with CC can be treated in a number of ways, including the addition of insulin-lowering agents ,mainly metformin, low-dose gonadotrophin therapy or surgically by laparoscopic ovarian drilling. Although the exact aetiology of PCOS is not known, the therapeutic alternatives provide reasonably successful symptomatic treatment [23]. Newer therapies, such as insulin-sensitizing agents, are beneficial in correcting the underlying metabolic disorder and, therefore, theoretically may have a more significant impact on reducing associated long-term mobility [5]. Adverse CHD risk profiles of women with PCOS have been demonstrated in several studies. However, actual health outcome studies have been inconclusive as to whether this translates into increased rates of cardiovascular disease in PCOS cases when compared to controls. Controversies still exist surrounding the potential relationship between cardiovascular disease outcomes and polycystic ovary syndrome [24]. While, the causes are unknown, insulin resistance, diabetes, and obesity are all strongly correlated with PCOS [3,25,26]. In conclusion, polycystic ovary syndrome is a heterogeneous condition, the pathophysiology of which appears to be both ,multifactorial and polygenic.The definition of the syndrome has been much debated. Key features include menstrual cycle disturbances, hyperandrogenism and obesity. There are many extra-ovarian aspects to the pathophysiology of PCOS, yet ovarian dysfunction seems to be central. According to the available literature, the distribution of follicles and a description of the stroma are not required in the diagnosis. Increased stromal echogenicity and/or stromal volume are specific to PCO, but it has been shown that the measurement of ovarian volume is a good surrogate for quantification of the stroma in clinical practice. A woman having PCO in the absence of an ovulation disorder or hyperandrogenism should not be considered as having PCOS, until more is known about this situation. On the other hand, the presence of a single PCO is sufficient to provide the diagnosis but PCO appearance is not a prerequisite for the diagnosis of PCOS [27,28,29]. Therefore, Polycystic ovary syndrome is a complex endocrinopathy characterized by a wide spectrum of phenotypes. A recent study estimated worldwide 1 out of 15 women suffering from PCOS [30]. Traditionally it was considered as a reproductive disorder showing hyperandrogenism, chronic anovulation and infertility. It is now well accepted that PCOS represents a "multifaceted" syndrome with substantial metabolic and cardiovascular long- term consequences. Although PCOS is heralded as one of the most common endocrine disorders occurring in women, its diagnosis, management, and associated long-term health risks remain controversial. Historically, the combination of androgen excess and anovulation has been considered the hallmark of PCOS. Today, these symptoms remain the most prevalent among PCOS patients, neither is considered an absolute requisite for the syndrome [31]. Many controversies still exist about the genetic background , the pathogenesis,the definition and the management of this intriguing syndrome [32,33,34]. On the other hand, the prevention of long-term sequelae is an absolute priority. Efforts should be made to early diagnosis and prompt treatment of adolescents with PCOS, in order to minimize the development of symptoms, and to prevent potentially the onset of cardiovascular, metabolic and neoplastic problems. In this light, it is important to remember that obesity exerts a major impact on the PCOS phenotype, particularly on the metabolic association and complications of this syndrome. Long-term prospective data are clearly needed to better delineate the nature and magnitude of disease risks associated with PCOS, with appropriate adjustment for associated obesity. Such information is a necessary background for understanding the role of established and emerging PCOS therapies, including oral contraceptives, intermittent progesterone, ovulation induction agents, and insulin sensitizers, in modifying such risks. In the meantime, close follow-up of women with PCOS and encouragement of lifestyle practices likely to reduce disease risks, such as regular exercise and weight control, should be standard practice [17]. High endocrinological competence and experience in this field are mandatory for the beneficial management of this complex disorder and for the prevention of potential long-term sequelae.

References

[1] Waterworth DM, Bennet S T ,Gharani N ,McCarthy MI, Hague S, Batty S, Conway GS, White D,Todd JA, Franks S, Williamson R. Linkage and association of insulin gene VNTR regulatory polymorphism with polycystic ovary syndrome. *Lancet* 1997; 349:986-902.

[2] Jakubowski L. Genetic aspects of polycystic ovary syndrome. *Endokrynol. Pol.* 2005;56(3):285-93.

[3] Stankiewicz M ,Norman R. Diagnosis and management of polycystic ovary syndrome :a practical guide. *Drugs* 2006;66(7): 903-12.

[4] Nisenblat V, Norman RJ. Androgens and polycystic ovary syndrome. *Curr. Opin. Endocrinol. Diabetes Obes*.2009;16(3): 224-31.

[5] Hassan A, Gordon CM. Polycystic ovary syndrome update in adolescence. *Curr. Opin. Pediatr.* 2007;19(4), 389-97.

[6] Franks S. Polycystic ovary syndrome in adolescents. *Int. J. Obes .(Lond),* 2008: 32(7): 1035-41.

[7] Creatas G, Deligeoroglou E. Polycystic ovarian syndrome in adolescents. *Curr. Opin. Obstet. Gynecol.*2007;19(5):420/6

[8] Goudas VT, Dumesic DA. Polycystic ovary syndrome. Endocrinol. *Metab. Clin. North Am.* 1997;26(4): 893-912.

[9] Norman RJ, Dewailly D ,Legro RS, Hickey TE. Polycystic ovary syndrome. *Lancet* 2007;370 (9588):685-97.

[10] Boomsma CM, Fauser BC, Macklon NS (2008). "Pregnancy complications in women with polycystic ovary syndrome". *Semin. Reprod. Med*. 26 (1): 72–84.

[11] Martinez- Bermejo E, Luque - Ramirez M, Escobar-Morreale HF. Obesity and polycystic ovary syndrome. *Minerva Endocrinol*. 2007; 32(3): 129-40.

[12] Yu Ng EH, Ho PC. Polycystic ovary syndrome in asian women. *Semin. Reprod. Med.* 2008; 26(1): 14-21.

[13] Weerakiet S,Srisombut C,Bunnaq P,Sanqtong S,Chuanqsoonqnoen N.Rojanasakul A.Prevalence of type 2 diabetes mellitus and impaired glucose tolerance in Asian women with polycystic ovary syndrome. *Int .J. Gynaecol. Obstet*. 2001;75(2): 177-84.

[14] Pelusi B, Gambineri A, Pasquali R .Type 2 diabetes and the polycystic ovary syndrome. *Minerva Ginecol*. 2004;56(1):41-51. 25.

[15] Orio F,Vuolo L,Palomba S,Lombardi G,Colao A.Metabolic and cardiovascular consequences of polycystic ovary syndrome. *Minerva Ginecol*. 2008; 60(1):39-51.

[16] Franks S. Controversy in clinical endocrinology: diagnosis of polycystic ovarian syndrome: in defense of the Rotterdam criteria. *J .Clin. Endocrinol. Metab*. 2006; 91(3): 786-9.

[17] Solomon C.G. The epidemiology of polycystic ovary syndrome. Prevalence and associated disease risks. *Endocrinol. Metab Clin North Am*. 1999 ;28(2):247-63.Review.

[18] Azziz R, Carmina E ,Dewailly D ,Diamanti- Kandarakus E, Escobar –Morreale HF, Futterweit W, Janssen OE, Legro R S, Norman R J, Taylor A E , Witchel SF. Task Force on the Phenotype of the Polycystic Ovary Syndrome of the Androgen Excess and PCOS Society. The Androgen Excess and PCOS Society criteria for the polycystic ovary syndrome: the complete task force report. *Fertil. Steril*. 2009;91(2):456-88.

[19] Nardo LG, Gelbaya TA. Evidence-based approach for the use of ultrasound in the management of polycystic ovary syndrome. *Mminerva Ginecol*. 2008;60(1): 83-9.

[20] Gutman G, Geva E, Lessing JB, Amster R. Long-term health consequences of polycystic ovaries syndrome: metabolic, cardiovascular and oncological aspects. *Harefuah* 2007;146(1): 889-93,908.

[21] Laszlo J,Gyoery G. Stein-Leventhal Syndrome and uterine carcinoma. *Zentralbl. Gynakol*. . 1963; 85: 1506-9-15

[22] Giudice LC. Endometrium in PCOS: Implantation and predisposition to endocrine CA. *Best Pract. Res. Endocrinol. Metab*. 2006; 20(2): 235-44-16.

[23] Homburg R. Polycystic ovary syndrome. *Best Pract. Res. Clin. Obstet. Gynaecol*. 2008:22(2): 261 74.

[24] Talbott EO, Zborowskii J V ,Boudraux MY. Do women with polycystic ovary syndrome have an increased risk of cardiovascular disease? Review of the evidence. *Minerva Ginecol*. 2004; 56(1):27-39.

[25] Yucel A, Noyan, Saqsoz The association of serum androgens and insulin resistance with fat distribution in polycystic ovary syndrome. *Eur.J. Obstet.Gynecol. Reprod.Biol*. 2006; 126(1):81-6.

[26] Li X, Lin JF.Clinical features, hormonal profile, and metabolic abnormalities of obese women with obese polycystic ovary syndrome] *Zhonghua Yi.Xue Za Zhi* 2005;85(46):3266-71.

[27] Nardo LG,Burkett WM, Orio F.Jr. Ultrasonography in polycystic ovary syndrome: an update. *J.Reprod. Med*. 2007; 52(5): 390-6.

[28] Lin JF,Li X,Zhu MW. Exploration of the classification of polycystic ovarian syndrome.*Zhonghua Fu Chan Ke Za Zhi* 2006;41(10):684-8.

[29] Balen A, Homburg R, Franks S. Defining polycystic ovary syndrome.*B.M.J.* 2009;338:2968.

[30] Orio F,Vuolo L,Palomba S,Lombardi G,Colao A.Metabolic and cardiovascular consequences of polycystic ovary syndrome. *Minerva Ginecol*. 2008; 60(1):39-51.

[31] Lujan ME,Chizen DR, Pierson RA.Diagnostic criteria for polycystic ovary syndrome: pitfalls and controversies. *J. Obstet. Gynaecol. Can*.2008;30(8):671-9.

[32] Legro RS,Kunselman AR,Dodson WC, Dunaif A. Prevalence and predictors of risk for type 2 diabetes mellitus and impaired glucose tolerance in polycystic ovary syndrome: a prospective, controlled study in 254 affected women. *J. Clin. Endocrinol. Metab.*1999; 84(1): 165-9.

[33] Hayden BJ, Balen AH.The role of the central nervous system in the pathogenesis of polycystic ovary syndrome. *Minerva Ginecol.* 2006; 58(1):41-54.

[34] Balen A, Raikowha M. Polycystic ovary syndrome--a systemic disorder? *Best Pract. Res.Clin.Obstet.Gynaecol*.2003;17(2):263-74.

In:Polycystic Ovarian Syndrome: An Enigmatic...
Editor: Rosa Sabatini

ISBN: 978-1-61761-853-6
©2011 Nova Science Publishers, Inc.

Chapter I

Polycystic Ovarian Syndrome: Definition

Rosa Sabatini, Raffaele Cagiano** and Francesca Scaramuzzi**

*Expert Family Planning Service. Department of Obstetrics and Gynecology **Department of Pharmacology and Human Physiology Policlinico-University of Bari. Piazza Giulio Cesare 11. 70124 Bari. Italy

Polycystic ovarian syndrome (PCOS) affecting 4-10% of women, is one of the most common causes of infertility, due to anovulation Nevertheless, its considerable phenotypic variability has led to proven difficulty in the development of a clinically applicable classification . Besides, endocrinological, biochemical ,morphological, and more recently molecular researches have identified an array of underlying abnormalities and added to the confusion concerning the pathophysiology of this disorder [1].Historically, the syndrome, then called Stein-Leventhal syndrome, was firstly diagnosed in 1935. In fact, in that time Stein and Leventhal described seven surgical cases presenting oligomenorrhea combined with the presence of bilateral polycystic ovaries (PCO). Three of these women also presented obesity, while five showed signs of hirsutism. Only one woman had both obesity and hirsutism. Originally, surgical findings of enlarged polycystic ovaries represented the hallmark of the syndrome but the diagnosis required, over the pathognomonic ovarian feature, the clinical triad of hirsutism, amenorrhea and obesity (Figure 1)[2].

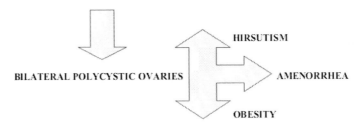

Figure 1. Stein - Leventhal Syndrome (1935)

Since 1990 the National Institute of Health-sponsored Conference on PCOS clearly established that the syndrome encompasses a broader spectrum of signs and symptoms of ovarian dysfunction than those defined by the original diagnostic criteria. Following, Polson and others reported that polycystic ovaries may be a common finding in normal women, and Franks began to consider PCOS as a challenge [3,4]. The first problem is the following: why the ovary or the ovaries of these women have polycystic feature? Polycystic ovaries are the expression of the hormonal dysregulation in PCOS women. In fact, in contrast to the characteristic picture of fluctuating hormone levels in the normal cycle, a "steady state" of gonadotropins and sex steroids in women with PCOS is due to the persistent anovulation in which the production of estrogens and androgens are both increased [5,6] Anovulatory women with PCOS also have a higher luteinizing hormone (LH) and gonadotropin-releasing hormone (GnRH) pulse frequency and amplitude when compared to the normal midfollicular phase [7].This enhanced pulsatile secretion of GnRH can be attributed to a reduction in hypothalamic opioid inhibition because of the chronic absence of progesterone [8]. The increased LH secretion, as expressed by the LH/FSH (follicle-stimulating hormone) ratio, is positively correlated with the increased free estradiol [9,10]. A sensitive assay for inhibin-B has detected high levels in women with PCO, suggesting that multiple small follicles can suppress FSH by increasing the circulating levels of inhibin-B[11].However; FSH levels are not totally depressed. Hence new follicular growth is continuously stimulated but not reaching full maturation and ovulation [12].Therefore, multiple follicular cysts develop 2-10 mm in diameter, which are theca cells often luteinized, in response to high LH levels.Hyperthecosis refers to patches of luteinized theca-like cells scattered throughout the ovarian stroma. It is characterized by the same histological findings as seen in polycystic syndrome [13] The clinical picture of more intense androgenization is a result of greater androgen production. This condition is associated with lower LH levels, which are a possible consequence of the higher testosterone levels blocking estrogens action at the hypothalamic pituitary level. It seems appropriate to view hyperthecosis as a manifestation of the same process of persistent anovulation, but with greater intensity. A greater degree of insulin resistance is correlated with the degree of hyperthecosis [14]. As insulin and insulin-like growth factor1(IGF-1)stimulate proliferation of thecal interstitial cells,hyperinsulinemia may be an important factor contributing to hyperthecosis[15]. However, recent evidence suggests that LH is not a major player in the hyperandrogenism of PCOS, and LH excess may be a consequence of the metabolic alterations in PCOS.

Ultimately, it is getting clearer that the LH dysregulation associated with PCOS is not primary but secondary to the peripheral events within the ovary. However, in contrast to what has been recently published, the mechanism of neuroendocrine dysfunction resulting in an elevated LH in PCOS may be an uncoupling of hypothalamic estradiol inhibition by elevated ovarian androstenedione. The abnormal secretion of ovarian androstenedione seems to be an intrinsic property of PCOS theca/ granulosa cells. At a particular threshold, this uncoupling is associated with an estradiol-related sensitization of pituitary LH release and hence an increase in LH secretion. Finally, a case has been made to support the view that in some hyperandrogenic women with PCOS, obesity leads to decreased androstenedione synthesis and/or to develop of insulin resistance, both of which seem to decrease LH secretion independently of each other [16].Today, despite the progressive improved knowledge, proved by the vast literature regarding the etiology and classification of PCOS, no general consensus was reached about the validity of the different proposed criteria. Anyway, three major diagnostic criteria for PCOS have been proposed by the National Institute of Health (NIH 1990), the Rotterdam European Society for Human Reproduction and Embryology/American Society for Reproductive Medicine sponsored PCOS Consensus Workshop Group (ESHRE/ASRM 2003) and recently by the Task force of the Androgen Excess Society (AES 2006).

Definitions commonly used for Polycystic Ovary Syndrome

1. In 1990 a consensus workshop sponsored by the NIH/NICHD _ suggested that a patient has PCOS if she has all of :

- o Sign of androgen excess (clinical or biochemical)
- o oligoovulation
- o other entities that would cause polycystic ovaries are excluded

2.In 2003 a consensus workshop sponsored by ESHRE / ASRM in Rotterdam indicated PCOS to be present if 2 out of 3 criteria are met

- o Oligoovulation and/or anovulation,
- o excess androgen activity,
- o polycystic ovaries (by gynecologic ultrasound),while other endocrine disorders are excluded.

3.In 2006 the Androgen Excess Society Task Force (AES-PCOS 2006)proposed that PCOS should be defined by the presence of:

- o Hyperandrogenism (clinical and/or biochemical),
- o ovarian dysfunction (oligo-anovulation and/or polycystic ovaries),
- o exclusion of other endocrine disorders

Polycystic ovary syndrome (PCOS) is defined most commonly according to the proceedings of an expert conference sponsored by the National Institutes of Health (NIH) in April 1990, which noted the disorder as having 1) hyperandrogenism and/or hyperandrogenemia, 2) oligoovulation, and 3) exclusion of other known disorders. The appearance of the polycystic ovary on ultrasound was firstly described in 1985 [17]. Nevertheless, a 1990 National Institutes of Health (NIH) Conference suggested diagnostic criteria for PCOS that did not include ultrasound evidence of polycystic ovarian morphology (PCOM) [18] . These criteria were revised in 2003 at the Rotterdam European Society of Human Reproduction and Embryology/American Society of Reproductive Medicine Consensus Workshop to include ultrasound polycystic ovarian morphology (PCOM) as one of the two of three criteria necessary for establishing the diagnosis of PCOS [19]. The inclusion of PCOM sparked a controversy as it broadens the population of women who meet the criteria for PCOS and allows for the creation of two phenotypically different patient populations who previously would have been excluded. Hence, the expert conference held in Rotterdam in May 2003 defined PCOS, after the exclusion of related disorders, by two of the following three features: oligo-or anovulation,clinical and/or biochemical signs of hyperandrogenism , or polycystic ovaries [20]. In essence, the Rotterdam 2003 expanded the NIH 1990 definition creating two new phenotypes:

- ovulatory women with polycystic ovaries and hyperandrogenism
- oligoanovulatory women with polycystic ovaries, but without hyperandrogenism.

This commentary on the European Society of Human Reproduction and Embryology/American Society for Reproductive Medicine (ESHRE/ASRM) consensus on diagnosis, nomenclature and long-term health risks of the polycystic ovarian syndrome (PCOS) (Conference in Rotterdam, Netherlands, March 2003) questions whether the preservation of the term PCOS sufficiently considers the modern aspects of the aetiology and pathogenesis of this complex syndrome. The misleading and simplified term PCOS, which comprises a variety of different entities, carries with it the risk of misinterpretation and under- and overestimation of symptoms as well as of overlooking contraindications [21]. Several studies led to ascertain the validity of using the Rotterdam 2003 criteria rather than the NIH 1990 criteria for the diagnosis of PCOS. Interventions included the use of the Rotterdam 2003 criteria for diagnosing PCOS and, in particular, the proposal to define the two new phenotypes of PCOS. Broekmans clearly showed that with the new Rotterdam consensus criteria, oligo/anovulatory women with less severe metabolic derangement would be added to the heterogeneous group of women with PCOS [22].The Rotterdam European Society of Human Reproduction and Embryology (ESHRE)/ American Society of Reproductive Medicine (ASRM)-sponsored PCOS consensus workshop group reemphasized the importance of polycystic ovarian morphology (PCOM) in the diagnostic criteria .However, the inclusion of PCOM in the definition of PCOS remains controversial [23,24]. In fact, PCOM is found consistently in women with PCOS defined by oligomenorrhea and hyperandrogenism but an identical ovarian morphology has been documented in 16–25% of normal women [3, 25, 26,27,28]. Available data suggest that hyperandrogenic ovulatory women with polycystic ovaries tend to have mild insulin resistance and mild evidence of ovarian dysfunction, in any case, significantly less than women with anovulatory PCOS. However, whether these women will have an increased risk of infertility or metabolic complications, such as type 2 diabetes, remains to be determined. Alternatively, the risk of insulin resistance and long-term metabolic risks of oligoovulatory women with polycystic ovaries is even less well characterized.

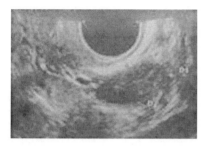

Additional research on the two new phenotypes, their long-term implications and the potential negative impact on research, clinical practice, and patient insurability, led to consider the adoption of the Rotterdam 2003 criteria for defining PCOS to be premature (Aziz 2006).

Figure 2. Normal ovary in a fertile woman

As polycystic ovaries are a frequent feature of PCOS, a modification of the NIH 1990 criteria was proposed. Additional researches characterizing the phenotypes and associated morbidities of PCOS were urgently required [24]. Based on the available data, the point of view of the AES Task Force on the Phenotype of PCOS was that there should be an acceptance of the original 1990 National Institutes of Health criteria with some modifications, taking into consideration the concerns expressed in the proceedings of the 2003 Rotterdam Conference. A principal conclusion was that PCOS should be first considered a disorder of androgen excess or hyperandrogenism, although a minority considered the possibility that there may be forms of PCOS without overt evidence of hyperandrogenism but recognizing that more data are required before validating this supposition. Hence, the task force recognized, and fully expects, that the definition of this syndrome will evolve over time to incorporate new research findings [29]. The criteria for diagnosis and definition of polycystic ovary syndrome used by clinicians and investigators are almost as heterogeneous as the syndrome itself.

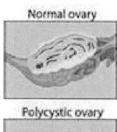
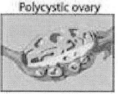

This condition has confused and seriously hindered the clarification of the genetics, aetiology, clinical associations and, the assessment of treatment and later sequelae of the syndrome. For a long time there was the debate between the predominately American biochemical marker-based diagnosis and predominately European reliance on ultrasound as a sine qua non for diagnosis. In 2002 Homburg proposed a consensus for a unifying balanced and pratical working definition for use as a standard.

Figure 3.

The proposal incorporated the confirmation of the diagnosis suggested by clinical symptoms and ultrasound and the use of hormonal estimations if typical ultrasound features are not seen, and for the purpose of defining subsets of the syndrome [30]. However, sometimes may be difficult to clearly distinguish a patient with PCOS from a normal woman only by transvaginal ultrasound criteria using the ovarian volume and /or the number of follicles, but these parameters could be clinically useful for the screening of PCOS [31]. In the meantime, it is suggested that 12 or more follicles 2–9 mm in size per ovary is a critical threshold for identifying women with metabolic abnormalities and in 2003 the International consensus criteria for the ultrasound diagnosis of the polycystic ovary had been published it [32,33]. Anyway, it is important to consider that the PCO appearance is not a prerequisite for the diagnosis of PCOS [34]. On the other hand, it has been proved that PCO appearance has no significant impact on fertility in women without symptoms; whereas, obesity, menstrual irregularities, and /or hyperandrogenism are factors associated with subfertility in women with polycystic ovaries [35]. Current concepts include the use of high-resolution, three-dimensional ultrasound instead of conventional two-dimensional ultrasound; formulaic methods of measuring ovarian volume; and correlation between ultrasonographic features, biochemical indices and ovarian stromal changes, such as enhanced echogenicity and increased blood flow [36]. Particularly, the gynecologists consider very important the ultrasound ovarian feature and several investigators outline evidence for the current ultrasound definition of the polycystic ovary and technical specification. The mean number per ovary of follicles (FNPO) 2-5 mm in size seems significantly higher in polycystic ovaries than in controls, while it seems similar within the 6-9 mm range. Setting the threshold at 12 for the 2-5 mm, FNPO offers the best compromise between specificity (99%) and sensitivity (75%). Considering the 2-5 mm follicular range, Jonard found significant positive relationships between the FNPO and androgens.levels.

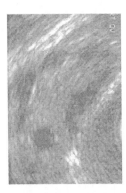

According to the available literature data, the criteria fulfilling sufficient specificity and sensitivity to define the PCO should have at least one of the following: either 12 or more follicles measuring 2-9 mm in diameter, or increased ovarian volume (> 10 cm³). If there is a follicle > 10 mm in diameter, the scan should be repeated at a time of ovarian quiescence (early follicular phase) in order to calculate volume and area. The presence of a single PCO is sufficient to provide the diagnosis (Balen 2003).

Figure 4. Polycystic ovary.

The FNPO within the 6-9 mm range was considered significantly and negatively related to body mass index and fasting insulin level. These observations seem to support the theory that the intraovarian hyperandrogenism promotes excessive early follicular growth and that further progression cannot proceed normally because of hyperinsulinism and/or other metabolic influence linked to obesity [32]. A multivariate statistical analysis applied retrospectively to clinical,biological and ultrasound data collected during 5 years in 457 patients with polycystic ovaries and in 188 age-matched non-hyperandrogenic and regularly cycling controls without PCO at ultrasound, showed in PCOS that the 2-5 mm follicle number gave the strongest relationship to severity of the follicular arrest, followed by age and then by fasting insulin level. Therefore, this investigation showed as the size of the 2-5 mm may be an independent and important contributor to the follicular arrest in PCOS ovaries [37]. Nevertheless, the distribution of follicles and a description of the stroma are not required in the diagnosis. Increased stromal echogenicity and/or stromal volume are specific to PCO, but it has been shown that the measurement of ovarian volume (or area) is a good surrogate for quantification of the stroma in clinical practice. Three- dimensional and Doppler ultrasound studies may be useful research tools but are not required in the definition of PCO (33). Ovarian size is obtained by measuring the largest plane of the ovary in two dimensions and then turning the vaginal probe 90 degrees and obtaining a third measurement. Volume of the ovary is calculated using the formula for an ellipsoid [length x height x width x (/6)] [38]. In all subjects both ovaries are visualized on ultrasound, allowing for the calculation of total ovarian volume (right + left ovarian volume). Polycystic ovary volume (PCOV or non-PCOV) is determined by the criteria of Balen et al. which are defined as at least one ovary having a volume greater than 10 cm^3 with no cysts or follicles greater than 10 mm as mean diameter [33].Endometrial thickness was determined as the largest anterior-posterior measurement of the endometrium in the sagittal plane. Obesity is a significant confounder in visualizing ovaries trans abdominally; whereas, there is less literature to support that this is a confounder with transvaginal scans; nonetheless, it merits mention [39].A stronger correlation between ultrasound features of the ovary and other circulating androgens.has been found in the clinical trials considering testosterone because it is still the largest contributor in terms of bioactivity to the circulating androgen pool and also because it has been used to identify women with PCOS [40,41]. Another androgen of lower bioactivity but with a greater ovarian contribution, such as androstenedione, may have had more association with the polycystic ovary morphology or volume [42,43]. Ultrasound technologies,such as Doppler flow studies or three-dimensional ultrasonography, to further qualify and quantify polycystic ovary morphology have not received again widespread clinical application [44,45,46]. 3D ultrasound is a relatively new imaging modality that it seems to permit improved spatial awareness, true volumetric calculation and quantitative assessment of the vascularity within a defined volume of tissue. Studies on the 3D ultrasound features of PCO have consistently demonstrated the intrinsic characteristics of a polycystic ovary confirming an increased antral follicle population and larger ovarian volume [47]. However, conflicting results on the degree of vascularity within a polycystic ovary as a whole or within its stroma have been observed and the study with the most scientifically robust design did not demonstrate the widely held belief that stromal vascularity is increased [48].The study by Ng et al. included only anovulatory Chinese women with ultrasound appearances of PCO, and did not consider the degree of clinical or biochemical hyperandrogenism. Another study has shown that there are no differences in women with anovulatory and ovulatory PCO and that the apparent differences relate more to body weight and clinical hyperandrogenism with ovarian vascularity being more prominent in women with PCOS who are of normal weight, or who have hyperandrogenism. In keeping with this, Ng et al. did observe significantly higher ovarian blood flow in women with PCOS and a BMI <25 kg/m^2 than in their overweight counterparts..These findings support that ovarian vascularity is influenced by the phenotypic expression of PCOS [48]. It has been suggested that the variation between studies may relate to different characteristics of the study population, the use of inappropriate controls and inconsistent criteria for the diagnosis of PCOS [49]. PCOS is a complex heterogeneous endocrine disorder. Furthermore, ovarian volume calculations based on 2D measurements are less accurate and less reproducible than those made with 3D ultrasound [50].The 2003 Rotterdam consensus represents an important first step in defining uniform diagnostic criteria for PCOS and specific ultrasound features of a polycystic ovary. The new Rotterdam criteria allow a diagnosis of PCOS to be made when two of three clinico-pathological features are present: oligomenorrhoea or anovulation, clinical or biochemical hyperandrogenism and clearly defined polycystic ovaries (PCOs) on ultrasound. This revised classification supports the objective role of ultrasound in the diagnosis of PCOS which should include either 12 or more follicles measuring 2–9 mm in diameter or an increased ovarian volume >10 cm^3 in either ovary [33]. However, there are certain limitations in these ultrasound criteria [49].

Ultrasonographic criteria used for the diagnosis of PCO

External morphological signs	Internal morphological signs
Increased ovarian area or volume	Number of small, echoless regions < 10 mm in size per ovary
Increased roundness index (ovarian width /ovarian length ratio)	Peripheral position of microcysts
Decreased uterine width /ovarian length ratio (U/O)	Increased echogenicity of ovarian stroma
	Increased surface of ovarian stroma on a cross-sectional cut, (computerized measure)

While an objective measurable increase in the number of antral follicles is possible, the real-time interpretation of two-dimensional (2D) ultrasonography may underestimate the absolute number of follicles compared with three-dimensional (3D) ultrasound [51]. Furthermore, ovarian volume calculations based on 2D measurements are less accurate and less reproducible than those made with 3D ultrasound [50]. Several other ultrasound features that were previously considered important, such as an increase in ovarian stromal echogenicity and vascularity, have not been included in the new diagnostic criteria..This probably relates to the inherent subjectivity in the objective or semi-quantitative assessment of these parameters and to a resultant inability to standardize the measurements [33]. 3D ultrasound provides a new method for the objective quantitative assessment of all of these parameters as well as blood flow within the ovary as a whole [50,52]. The first study using 3D ultrasound technique on women with PCOS according to the revised Rotterdam consensus criteria and consistent with previous observations confirmed the intrinsic characteristics of a polycystic ovary with more antral follicles and a larger ovarian volume. This study has also shown that women with PCOS have ovaries with a larger stromal volume and a more pronounced blood supply, but are of comparable echogenicity with normal ovaries. Differences do exist within the different subgroups of women with PCO according to their phenotypic expression of the disease. However, body weight and clinical hyperandrogenism appear important and anovulation does not seem to modify the ultrasound findings. Any differences in vascularity between the groups were only apparent with 3D ultrasound and were not identified through the application of pulsed wave Doppler. 3D ultrasound allows the calculation of stromal volume, either manually or automatically using the inversion mode and thresholding. The Authors showed as stromal volume is significantly increased in women with PCO and more so in women with PCO who are clinically hirsute [52]. This would support the hypothesis that the probable source of excessive androgen production in these groups of patients is the thecal cell in the ovarian stroma which undergo to hypertrophy. Kyei-Mensah et al. also showed as stromal volume was significantly higher in women with PCOS and PCO than in controls (16.7 and 15.0 ml versus 9.6 ml, all $P < 0.05$)[42]. They examined 26 women with PCOS, 24 women with regular menstrual cycles but PCO on ultrasound scan and 50 subfertile women with regular menstrual cycles and normal ovarian morphology.

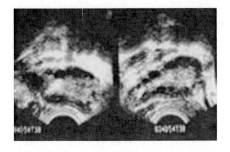

> Initially, the researchers calculated the stromal volume through the subtraction of total follicular volume from total ovarian volume both of which were measured manually. Such measurements are time-consuming and more open to measurement error as a result.

Figure 5 .3D image of polycystic ovaries.

The fact that both techniques, manual and automated, have shown a significant increase in stromal volume suggests some degree of compatibility, but when we directly compare the time needed for the calculation of stromal volume by either technique, one must assume that the automated technique is quicker. The study of Kyei-Mensah et al revealed important differences between women with PCOS who are of normal weight or hyperandrogenic and their counterparts, supporting the concept that ovarian characteristics may influence, or be influenced by the phenotypic expression of the disease. Increased stromal vascularity in women with PCOS who are of normal weight, or who are hirsute, suggests that ovarian stroma may play an important role in the development of hyperandrogenism. This study highlights the potential importance of the objective quantification of stromal echogenicity, ovarian and stromal volume and ovarian vascularity by 3D ultrasonography [53]. The original diagnosis defined by Adams et al included reference to an 'increased stromal echogenicity', but this was assessed subjectively and this may explain its absence from the diagnostic criteria set by the Rotterdam consensus [17]. 3D ultrasound allows for an objective measure of ovarian echogenicity through the calculation of the MG value which reflects the average intensity of the grey voxels within the VOI. Jarvela et al. have objectively examined stromal echogenicity as measured by the 3D calculation of the MG value of the whole ovary. They showed no differences in stromal echogenicity between 14 women with PCO and 28 women with ultrasonographically normal ovaries [54]. On the other hand, an objective measurable increase in the number of antral follicles is possible; the real-time interpretation of two-dimensional(2D) ultrasonography may underestimate the absolute number of follicles compared with three-dimensional (3D) ultrasound [51]. The ovarian morphology at two-dimensional ultrasound and that at three dimensional ultrasound were compared in 45 women with regular menstrual cycles and proven fertility and 38 women with oligo-anovulation, clinical and/or biochemical features of hyperandrogenism, and polycystic ovary morphology.The parameters studied in both groups were follicle number per ovary (FNPO), ovarian volume (OV), mean gray value (MG) and three vascular indices: vascularization index (VI), flow index (FI) and vascularization flow index (VFI). The results showed a higher mean OV as well as FNPO in PCO group. No differences in MG, VI, FI and VFI were found between the groups [55]. Previous studies have shown very low intra- and interobserver variation for the measurement of ovarian volume by ultrasound and this parameter has been used in a number of settings in women's health in addition to identifying polycystic ovaries [25,56.57] The observer variation for the assessment of polycystic ovaries is a more subjective measure and may be higher [58,59] .This suggests the need for evidence-based guidelines during the recognition of polycystic ovaries. In a population of control women, who were carefully screened to exclude those with hirsutism, hyperandrogenemia, and glucose intolerance, polycystic ovaries were an infrequent finding (<10%). It is plausible to suppose that earlier prevalence studies based on polycystic ovary morphology in women with unrecognized reproductive or metabolic abnormalities may be inconsistent and, many of the women with polycystic ovary morphology may have evidence, however subtle, of androgen excess and/or insulin resistance with more detailed testing [27,60,61,62,63,64]. The low prevalence of polycystic ovary morphology in the reproductively and metabolically normal women supports the hypothesis that polycystic ovaries are intrinsically abnormal and may be the ovarian morphologic consequence of intrinsic defects in follicular development and steroidogenesis [42,65]. However, these issues together with the Rotterdam 2003 European Society of Human Reproduction and Embryology (ESHRE)/American Society for Reproductive Medicine (ASRM)-sponsored consensus criteria for the diagnosis of PCOS, are again object of discussion among clinicians and investigators.To highlight differences between NIH and ESHR/ASRM criteria, 375 women with oligo/amenorrhea and signs of hyperandrogenism were studied. In this sample, 273 women with PCOS were identified according to NIH definition, whereas 345 were identifies according to ESHR/ASRM definition .The 72 patients exhibiting a lower expression of clinical signs ,represented the gap between the two classifications. To the whole group was applied the ESHRE/ASRM criteria modified to include a reproducible ultrasound examination of the ovarian stroma, (UCSC criteria). This procedure permitted to identify 30 healthy women according to all criteria, 37 affected by PCOS according to ESHRE/ASRM Consensus , 35 affected according to UCSC and ESHRE/ASRM criteria and 273 who have PCOS by all criteria.Therefore, the sonography support can permit the identification of a subgroup of women missed by NIH definition and with more pronounced stigmas than those identified by ESHRE/ ASRM criteria [66], An agreement was found on the new guidelines at a joint meeting of ESHRE and ASRM in 2004. At the same meeting new criteria for sonographic diagnosis were suggested. The new guidelines for diagnosis of polycystic ovary syndrome have represented a reasonable compromise between different opinions and because of it ,they have got a great success. During 2005, a consensus conference and a special expert committee have evaluated the new guidelines and reached some conclusion. However,only a better understanding of the pathogenesis of polycystic ovary syndrome can definitely establish the diagnostic criteria.[67] New diagnostic criteria for polycystic ovary syndrome were proposed in Rotterdam in 2003, which expanded the previous definition that arose from an expert conference sponsored by the National Institutes of Health (NIH) in 1990. However, these newer criteria give rise to phenotypes that may not actually represent PCOS, and a simple modification of the 1990 NIH/National Institute of Child Health and Human Disease diagnostic criteria may be more consistent with currently available data [68]. Woman having PCO in the absence of an ovulation disorder or hyperandrogenism ('asymptomatic PCO') should not be considered as having PCOS, until more will be known about this situation. It is important to take into account that polycystic ovaries may be found in 16-25% of apparently normal women with regular menses [69]. Some Authors suggested that these features may be associated with other abnormalities common in PCOS women as abnormal gonadotropin levels,lower levels of IGF-binding protein-1,increased insulin resistance and increased ovarian 17hydroxyprogesterone and androgen responses to GnRH agonists[70,71]. However, these conditions have not been proved. Anyway,elevated levels of gonadotropin have been reported in women with this feature and normal cycle but were not seen in an apparently similar population [3,4,47,51,58,59] .On the other hand, this situation is supported by the presence of polycystic ovaries during normal childhood,when gonadotropin levels are low and occasionally in women with amenorrhea due to idiopathic hypogonadotropic hypogonadism in which gonadotropins are virtually absent [72,73].Several other ultrasound features that were previously considered important, such as an increase in ovarian stromal echogenicity and vascularity, have not been included in the new diagnostic criteria..This probably relates to the inherent subjectivity in the objective or semi-quantitative assessment of these parameters and a resultant inability to standardize measurements [33].3D ultrasound provides a new method for the objective quantitative assessment of all of these parameters as well as blood flow within the ovary as a whole [50,52].

Advantages of three-dimensional ultrasonography

An objective measurable increase in the number of antral follicles is possible. The real-time interpretation of two-dimensional (2D) ultrasonography may underestimate the absolute number of follicles compared with three-dimensional (3D) ultrasound (Allemand 2006)

Ovarian volume calculations based on 2D measurements are less accurate and less reproducible than those made with 3D ultrasound (Raine-Fenning 2003)

3D ultrasound provides a new method for the objective quantitative assessment of all of these parameters as well as blood flow within the ovary as a whole (Raine-Fenning 2003, Po 2007)

Several other ultrasound features that were previously considered important, such as an increase in ovarian stromal echogenicity and vascularity, have not been included in the new diagnostic criteria.

Finally, the quantification of the vascular flow, including the VI, FI, and VFI of the entire ovarian stroma using 3D power Doppler, is more accurate than the previously reported quantification analysis using 2D imaging, and may be a new parameter to assist in the ultrasound diagnosis of PCOS [47]

Ultrasound Evaluation in Virgin PCOS Patients

PCOS is the most frequent cause of hyperandrogenism in adolescent girls[74].Generally, the diagnosis of PCOS has rested primarily on the typical appearance of bilateral PCO in women showing signs of hyperandrogenism [74,75]. In virgin patients, a transvaginal ultrasonographic examination is seldom possible, and transabdominal ultrasonography (TAS) has been the preferred method for pelvic examination. Nonetheless, it is difficult to get precise imaging of the ovaries transabdominally. Magnetic resonance imaging (MRI) is useful as an adjunct. Although MRI is more sensitive than ultrasonography, its findings are less specific. Timor-Tritsch et al suggested transrectal sonography to be an effective diagnostic tool for pelvic exploration when transvaginal sonography cannot be performed. [76]. Particularly,it seems that high-frequency 3D-TRS combined with TAS results superior to transvaginal sonography in the diagnosis of PCOS [49]. Atiomo et al suggested that stromal brightness was the most specific criteria in the diagnosis of PCOS, and Fulghesu proposed as objective and easily reproducible diagnostic criterion, the S/A ratio, for the ultrasonographic determination of PCOS [77,78]. Three-dimensional imaging improves spatial awareness, stores information for later use, and provides a better record of the ovarian anatomy [79].Thus, it is the method to use for the objective,quantitatively assessment of follicle size, ovarian volume, ovarian stromal area, total ovarian area, and S/A ratio [49,52, 80].

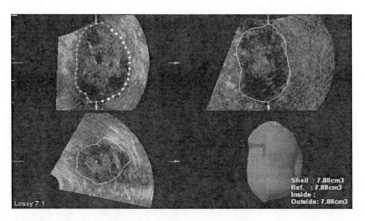

3D-TRS ultrasonographic evaluation of ovarian area and stromal area in PCOS.

When all parameters were analyzed, the S/A ratio was found to be the parameter the most closely related with androgen levels Assessing the delicate structure of the ovary in virgin patients, 3D-TRS seems to be convenient, accurate, specific, sensitive, and more reliable overall than transabdominal ultrasonography. Ovarian stromal area and stromal area to total area ratio(S/A) were significantly greater in patients with PCOS than in controls.These findings indicated that, in adolescent patients, 3D-TRS combined with transabdominal ultrasonography can improve the precision of the diagnosis of PCOS. The S/A ratio may become the ultrasonographic diagnostic marker for PCOS [49,81]. Finally, 3D-TRS combined with TAS can supersede transvaginal sonography and significantly improve the detection of PCOS in virgin adolescent girls and women.In conclusion,the precision of the diagnosis of PCOS seems to be greater with 3D-TRS. However, a follow-up study of asymptomatic adolescent girls with PCO is recommended to estimate their risk of developing the syndrome and the long-term effect of PCO on fertility [82].

Conclusion

The three dimensional ultrasonography offers many advantages to diagnose polycystic ovaries in the PCOS women but until now its use is limited in many countries. The recent introduction of 3D Transrectal Sonography(3D-TRS) may be an effective diagnostic tool for the evaluation of virgin girls with PCO but its use is until now limited. However, 3D-TRS seems to be convenient, accurate, specific, sensitive, and more reliable overall than transabdominal ultrasonography. Furthermore,3D-TRS combined with TAS can supersede transvaginal sonography and significantly improve the detection of PCOS in virgin adolescent girls and women The S/A ratio may become the ultrasonographic diagnostic marker for PCOS The appearance of the polycystic ovary ,on ultrasound, was firstly described in 1985 [17]. In spite of this long history , the comparisons of many studies and clinical experiences cannot be performed because of the different criteria used for the diagnosis It is well known that woman having PCO in the absence of an ovulation disorder or hyperandrogenism ('asymptomatic PCO') should not be considered as having PCOS, until more is known about this situation. Nonetheless, these women were often considered as having PCOS. On the contrary, many women with polycystic ovaries who present hyperandrogenic features are treated only for the specific complaint without to assess their endocrinological and metabolic profiles. It is important to take into account that polycystic ovaries may be found in 16-25% of apparently normal women with regular menses [69] In conclusion, only a good understanding of the pathogenesis of polycystic ovary syndrome can definitely help to exact diagnosis and consequent treatment.[67]

References

[1] Laven JS,Imani B,Eijkemans MJ,Fauser BC. New approach to polycystic ovary syndrome and other forms of anovulatory infertility. *Obstet. Gynecol.Surv.* 2002;57(11):755-67.

[2]   Laven JS,Imani B,Eijkemans MJ,Fauser BC. New approach to polycystic ovary syndrome and other forms of anovulatory infertility. *Obstet. Gynecol.Surv.* 2002;57(11):755-67.

[3]   Stein IF, Leventhal MI. Amenorrhea associated with bilateral polycystic ovaries .*Am. J. Obstet Gynecol.*1995; 29:181-191.

[4]   Polson DW,Adams J,Wadsworth J,Franks S. Polycystic ovaries: a common finding in normal women *Lancet* 1988;1: 870-872

[5]   Franks S.Polycystic ovary syndrome :a changing perspective. *Clin. Endocrinol.* (Oxf.) 1989; 31:87-120.

[6]   Chang RJ. Ovarian steroid secretion in polycystic ovarian disease. *Semi Reprod. Endocrinol.* 1984;2:244.

[7]   Calogero AE, Macchi M, Montanini V, Mongioi A, Maugeri G, Vicari E, et al . Dynamics of plasma gonadotropin and sex steroid release in polycystic ovarian disease after pituitary-ovarian inhibition with an analog of gonadotropin-releasing hormone. *J. Clin. Endocrinol. Metab.* 1987;64: 980-5.

[8]   Burger CW, Korsen TJ, van Kessel H, van Dop PA, Caron FJ, Schoemaker J. Pulsatile luteinizing hormone patterns in the follicular phase of the menstrual cycle, polycystic ovarian disease (PCOD) and non-PCOD secondary amenorrhea. *J. Clin. Endocrinol. Metab.* 1985;61:1126-32.

[9]   Berga Sl, Yen SS. Opioidergic regulation of LH pulsality in women with polycystic ovary syndrome. *Clin. Endocrinol.* 1989;30:177-84.

[10]   Lobo RA, Granger L, Goehelsmann U, Mishell DR Jr. Elevations in unbound serum estradiol as a possible mechanism for inappropriate gonadotropin secretion in women with PCO. *J. Clin. Endocrinol. Metab.* 1981; 52:156-8.

[11]   Taylor AE, McCourt B, Martin KA, Anderson EJ, Adams JM, Schoenfeld DA, Hall JE Determinants of abnormal gonadotropin secretion in clinically defined women with polycystic ovary syndrome. *J. Clin. Endocrinol. Metab.* 1997 ;82:48–2256

[12]   Lockwood GM, Muttukrishna S, Groome NP, Mathews DR, Ledger WL. Mid follicular phase pulses of inhibits B are absent in PCOS and are initiated by successful laparoscopic ovarian diathermy: A possible mechanism regulating emergence of the dominant follicle. *J. Clin. Endocrinol. Metab.* 1998;83:1730-5

[13]   Fauser BC. Observations in favour of normal early follicle development and disturbed dominant follicle selection in polycystic ovary syndrome. *Gynecol. Endocrinol.* 1994;8:75-82.

[14]   Judd HL, Scully RE, Herbst AL, Yen SS, Ingersol FM, Kleman B. Familial hyperthecosis: Comparison of endocrinologic and histologic findings with PCOD. *Am. J. Obstet. Gynecol.* 1973;117:979-82.

[15]   Nagamani M, Vam Dinh T, Kelver ME. Hyperinsulinemia in hyperthecosis of the ovaries. *Am. J. Obstet. Gynecol.* 1986;154:384-9.

[16]   Duleba AJ, Spaczynski RZ, Olive DL. Insulin and insulin like growth factor-I stimulate the proliferation of human ovarian theca-interstitial cells. *Fertil Steril* 1998;69:335-40.

[17]   Russell A.Foulk The Relationship Between Luteinizing Hormone (LH) and Hyperandrogenism *Clinical Medicine and Research* 2008;6, 2 : 47 -53.(15)

[18]   Adams J, Franks S, Polson DW, Mason HD, Abdulwahid N, Tucker M, Morris DV, Price J, Jacobs HS Multifollicular ovaries: clinical and endocrine features and response to pulsatile gonadotropin releasing hormone. *Lancet* 1985;2:1375–1379

[19] Zawadski JK, Dunaif A. Diagnostic criteria for polycystic ovary syndrome: Towards a rational approach. In : Dunaif A, Givens JR, Haseltine F, editors. Polycystic Ovary Syndrome. Blackwell Scientific: Boston; 1992. p. 377-84.

[20] Porter MB.Polycystic ovary syndrome:the controversy of diagnosis by ultrasound. Semin. *Reprod. Med.* 2008;26(3):241-51-3 .

[21] Rotterdam ESHRE/ASRM-Sponsored PCOS Consensus Workshop Group. Revised 2003 consensus on diagnostic criteria and long-term health risks related to polycystic ovary syndrome. *Fertil Steril* 2004;81:19-25.

[22] Geisthovel F. A comment on the European Society of Human Reproduction and Embryology/American Society for Reproductive Medicine consensus of the polycystic ovarian syndrome. *Reprod. Biomed.Online* 2003;7(6):602-5.

[23] Broekmans FJ,Knauff EA,Valkenburg O,Laven JS,Eijkemans MJ,Fauser BC.PCOS according to the Rotterdam consensus criteria: Change in prevalence among WHO-II anovulation and association with metabolic factors. *BJOG* 2006;113(10):1210-7.

[24] Franks S . Controversy in clinical endocrinology: diagnosis of polycystic ovarian syndrome: in defense of the Rotterdam criteria. *J. Clin. Endocrinol. Metab.* 2006;91:786–789.

[25] AzizR.Controversy in clinical endocrinology: diagnosis of polycystic ovarian syndrome: the Rotterdam criteria are premature. *J.Clin.Endocrinol. Metab.* 2006 ;91(3):781-5.

[26] Legro RS, Chiu P, Kunselman AR, Bentley CM, Dodson WC, Dunaif A Polycystic ovaries are common in women with hyperandrogenic chronic anovulation but do not predict metabolic or reproductive phenotype. *J. Clin. Endocrinol. Metab.* 2005;90:2571–2579

[27] Farquhar CM, Birdsall M, Manning P, Mitchell JM, France JT The prevalence of polycystic ovaries on ultrasound scanning in a population of randomly selected women. *Aust. NZ. J. Obstet. Gynaecol.* 1994;34:67–72

[28] Clayton RN, Ogden V, Hodgkinson J, Worswick L, Rodin DA, Dyer S, Meade TW How common are polycystic ovaries in normal women and what is their significance for the fertility of the population? *Clin. Endocrinol.* (Oxf) 1992;37:127–134

[29] Murphy MK., Hall JE, Adams JM, Lee H ,Welt CK Polycystic Ovarian Morphology in Normal Women Does Not Predict the Development of Polycystic Ovary Syndrome The *Journal of Clinical Endocrinology and Metabolism* 2006; 91, 10 3878-3884

[30] Azziz R, Carmina E, Dewailly D, Diamanti-Kandarakis E, Escobar-Morreale HF, Futterweit W, Janssen OE, Legro RS, Norman RJ, Taylor AE, Witchel SF; Task Force on the Phenotype of the Polycystic Ovary Syndrome of The Androgen Excess and PCOS Society The Androgen Excess and PCOS Society criteria for the polycystic ovary syndrome: the complete task force report. *Fertil Steril.* 2009 ;91(2):456-88.

[31] Homburg R. What is polycystic ovarian syndrome? A proposal for a consensus on the definition and diagnosis of polycystic ovarian syndrome. *Hum.Reprod.* 2002;17(10):2495-9.

[32] Takahashi K,Okada M,Ozaki T,Uchida A,Yamasaki H,Kitao M. Transvaginal ultrasonographic morphology in polycystic ovarian syndrome. *Gynecol. Obstet. Invest.* 1995;39(3):201-6

[33] Jonard S, Robert Y, Cortet-Rudelli C, Pigny P, Decanter C, Dewailly D Ultrasound examination of polycystic ovaries: is it worth counting the follicles? *Hum. Reprod.* 2003;18:598–603

[34] Balen AH,Laven JS,Tan SL,Dewailly D. Ultrasound assessment ot he polycystic ovary: international consensus definitions. *Hum. Reprod. Update* 2003;9(6):505-14.

[35] Nardo LG,Gelbaya TA.Evidence-based approach for the use of ultrasound in the management of polycystic ovary syndrome. *Minerva Ginecol.* 2008;60(1):83-9.

[36] Hassan MA,Killick SR.Ultrasound diagnosis of polycystic ovaries in women who have no symptoms of polycystic ovary syndrome is not associated with subfecundity or subfertility. *Fertil Steril.* 2003;80(4):966-75.

[37] Nardo LG,Buckett WM,Orio F Jr.Ultrasonography in polycystic ovary syndrome:an update. *J. Reprod. Med.* 2007;52(5):390-6.

[38] Dewailly D, Catteau-Jonard S,Reyss AC,Maunoury-Lefebvre C,Poncelet E,Pigny P. The excess in 2-5 mm follicles seen at ovarian ultrasonography is tightly associated to the follicular arrest of the polycystic ovary syndrome. *Hum. Reprod.* 2007;22(6):1562-6.

[39] Pache TD, Hop WC, Wladimiroff JW, Schipper J, Fauser BC Transvaginal sonography and abnormal ovarian appearance in menstrual cycle disturbances. *Ultrasound Med. Biol.* 1991;17:589–593.

[40] Ardaens Y, Robert Y, Lemaitre L, Fossati P, Dewailly D Polycystic ovarian disease: contribution of vaginal endosonography and reassessment of ultrasonic diagnosis. *Fertil Steril.* 1991; 55:1062–1068

[41] Azziz R, Ehrmann D, Legro RS Whitcomb RW, Hanley R, Fereshetian AG, O'Keefe M, Ghazzi MN Troglitazone improves ovulation and hirsutism in the polycystic ovary syndrome: a multicenter double blind, placebo-controlled trial. *J. Clin. Endocrinol. Metab.* 2001;86:1626–3245

[42] Nestler JE, Jakubowicz DJ, Evans WS, Pasquali R Effects of metformin on spontaneous and clomiphene-induced ovulation in the polycystic ovary syndrome. *N. Engl. J. Med.* 1998;338:1876 1880

[43] Kyei-Mensah AA, LinTan S, Zaidi J. Jacobs. HS. Relationship. of ovarian stromal volume to serum androgen concentrations in patients with polycystic ovary syndrome. *Hum. Reprod.* 1998;13: 1437–1441

[44] Dewailly D, Robert Y, Helin I, Ardaens Y, Thomas-Desrousseaux P, Fossati P Ovarian stromal hypertrophy in hyperandrogenic women. *Clin. Endocrinol.* (Oxf)1994; 41:557–562

[45] Al-Took S, Watkin K, Tulandi T, Tan SL Ovarian stromal echogenicity in women with clomiphene citrate-sensitive and clomiphene citrate-resistant polycystic ovary syndrome. *Fertil. Steril.* 1999;71:952–954

[46] Nardo LG, Buckett WM, White D, Digesu AG, Franks S, Khullar V Three-dimensional assessment of ultrasound features in women with clomiphene citrate-resistant polycystic ovarian syndrome (PCOS): ovarian stromal volume does not correlate with biochemical indices. *Hum. Reprod.* 2002; 17:1052–1055

[47] Laurel, MD American Institute of Ultrasound Medicine 1995 Guidelines for performance of the ultrasound examination of the female pelvis.

[48] Pan HA, Wu MH, Cheng YC, Li CH, Chang FM. Quantification of Doppler signal in polycystic ovary syndrome using three-dimensional power Doppler ultrasonography: a possible new marker for diagnosis. *Hum. Reprod.* 2002; 17:.201–206.

[49] Ng EH, Chan CC, Yeung WS, Ho PC. Comparison of ovarian stromal blood flow between fertile women with normal ovaries and infertile women with polycystic ovary syndrome. *Hum. Reprod.* 2005; 20:1881–1886

[50] Lam PM, Raine-Fenning N. The role of three-dimensional ultrasonography in polycystic ovary syndrome. *Hum. Reprod.* 2006; 21:2209–2215.

[51] Raine-Fenning NJ, Lam PM. Assessment of ovarian reserve using the inversion mode. *Ultrasound Obstet. Gynecol.* 2006; 27:104–106.

[52] Raine-Fenning NJ, Campbell BK, Clewes JS, Johnson IR. The interobserver reliability of ovarian volume measurement is improved with three-dimensional ultrasound, but dependent upon technique. *Ultrasound. Med. Biol.* 2003; 29:.1685–1690

[53] Allemand MC, Tummon IS, Phy JL, Foong SC, Dumesic DA, Session DR. Diagnosis of polycystic ovaries by three-dimensional transvaginal ultrasound. *Fertil. Steril.* 2006; 85:214–219

[54] Po M. Lam, Ian R. Johnson and Nick J. Raine-Fenning..Three-dimensional ultrasound features of the polycystic ovary and the effect of different phenotypic expressions on these parameters *Human. Reproduction.* 2007; 22(12):3116-3123

[55] Zaidi J, Campbell S, Pittrof R, Kyei-Mensah A, Shaker A, Jacobs HS, Tan SL. Ovarian stromal blood flow in women with polycystic ovaries—a possible new marker for diagnosis? *Hum. Reprod.* 1995; 10:1992–1996.

[56] Pascual MA, Graupera B, Hereter L, Tresserra F, Rodriguez I,AlcázarJA Assessment of ovarian vascularization in the polycystic ovary by three-dimensional power Doppler ultrasonography. *Gynaecological Endocrinology* 2008; 24 (11): 631-636 .

[57] Jarvela IY, Mason HD, Sladkevicius P, Kelly S, Ojha K, Campbell S, Nargund G. Characterization of normal and polycystic ovaries using three-dimensional power Doppler ultrasonography. *J. Assist. Reprod. Genet.* 2002; 19:582–590.

[58] Higgins RV, van Nagell JRJ, Woods CH, Thompson EA, Kryscio RJ Interobserver variation in ovarian measurements using transvaginal sonography. *Gynecol. Oncol.* 1990;39:69–71

[59] Kyei-Mensah A, Maconochie N, Zaidi J, Pittrof R, Campbell S, Tan SL Transvaginal three-dimensional ultrasound: reproducibility of ovarian and endometrial volume measurements. *Fertil. Steril.* 1996 ;66:718–722

[60] Lass A, Brinsden P The role of ovarian volume in reproductive medicine. *Hum. Reprod. Update.* 1999;5:256–266

[61] Amer SA, Li TC, Bygrave C, Sprigg A, Saravelos H, Cooke ID An evaluation of the inter-observer and intra-observer variability of the ultrasound diagnosis of polycystic ovaries. *Hum. Reprod.* 2002;17:1616–1622

[62] Scheffer GJ, Broekmans FJ, Bancsi LF, Habbema JD, Looman CW, Te Velde ER Quantitative transvaginal two- and three-dimensional sonography of the ovaries: reproducibility of antral follicle counts. *Ultrasound. Obstet. Gynecol.* 2002; 20:270–275

[63] Knochenhauer ES, Key TJ, Kahsar-Miller M, Waggoner W, Boots LR, Azziz R Prevalence of the polycystic ovary syndrome in unselected black and white women of the southeastern United States: a prospective study. *J. Clin. Endocrinol. Metab.* 1998;83:3078–3082

[64] Carmina E, Lobo RA Polycystic ovaries in hirsute women with normal menses. *Am. J. Med.* 2001;111:602–606

[65] Adams JM, Taylor AE, Crowley Jr WF, Hall JE Polycystic ovarian morphology with regular ovulatory cycles: insights into the pathophysiology of polycystic ovarian syndrome. *J. Clin. Endocrinol. Metab.* 2004;89:4343–4350

[66] Webber LJ, Stubbs S, Stark J, Trew GH, Margara R, Hardy K, Franks S Formation and early development of follicles in the polycystic ovary. *Lancet.* 2003; 362:1017–1021

[67] Belosi C,Selvaggi L,Apa R,Guido M,Romualdi D,Fulghesu AM,Lanzone A.Is the PCOS diagnosis solved by ESHRE/ASRM 2003 consensus or could it include ultrasound examination of the ovarian stroma? *Hum. Reprod.* 2006;21(12):3108-15.

[68] Carmina E.Polycystic ovary syndrome: an update on diagnostic evaluation. *J. Indian. Med. Assoc.* 2006 ;104(8):439-40, 442, 444

[69] Azziz R.Diagnostic criteria for polycystic ovary syndrome: a reappraisal. *Fertil. Steril.* 2005; 83 (5):1343-6

[70] Carmina E,Wong L,Chang L, Paulson RJ,Sauer M.V,Stankzyk FZ,Lobo RA. Endocrine abnormalities in ovulatory women with polycystic ovaries on ultrasound.*Hum. Reprod.* 1997;12:905-909.

[71] Norman RJ,Hague WM,Masters SC,Wang XJ.Subjects with polycystic ovaries without hyperandrogenaemia exhibit similar disturbances in insulin and lipid profiles as those with polycystic ovary syndrome. *Hum. Reprod.* 1995;10:2258-2261

[72] Chang PL,Lindheim SR,Lowre C,Ferin M,.Gonzales F,Berglund L,Carmina E,Sauer MV,Lobo RA.Normal ovulatory women with polycystic ovaries have hyperandrogenic pituitary-ovarian responses to gonadotropin-releasing hormone-agonist testing.*J. Clin. Endocrinol. Metab.* 2000; 85:995-1000.

[73] Bridges NA, Cooke A, Healy MJ, Hindmarsh PC, Brook CG, Standards for ovarian volume in childhood and puberty. *Fertil, Steril,* 1993;60:456-460.

[74] Stanhope R,Adams J, Pringle JP ,Jacobs HS, Brook CG. The evolution of polycystic ovaries ina girl with hypogonadotropic hypogonadism before puberty and during puberty induced with pulsatile gonadotropin-releasing hormone. *Fertil. Steril.* 1987;47:872-875

[75] Sultan C, Paris F.Clinical expression of polycystic ovary syndrome in adolescent girls, *Fertil. Steril.* 2006; 86 (suppl 1): 6.

[76] [17] R.S. Legro, Diagnostic criteria in polycystic ovary syndrome*, Semin. Reprod. Med.* 21 (3) (2003), pp. 267–275. View Record in Scopus Cited By in Scopus (18)Legro RS. Diagnostic criteria in polycystic ovary syndrome, *Semin. Reprod. Med.* 2003; 21 (3): 267–275.

[77] Timor-Tritsch IE, A. Monteaqudo A, Rebarber A, Goldstein SR, Tsymbal T. Transrectal scanning: an alternative when transvaginal scanning is not feasible, *Ultrasound Obstet Gynecol* 2003; 21 (5) : 473–479.

[78] Atiomo W.U, Pearson S, Shaw S., Prentice A,.Dubbins P.Ultrasound criteria in the diagnosis of polycystic ovary syndrome (PCOS), *Ultrasound. Med. Biol.* 2000; 26 (6): 977–980.

[79] Fulghesu AM, Ciampelli M, Belosi C, Apa R., Pavone V, Lanzone A. A new ultrasound criterion for the diagnosis of polycystic ovary syndrome: the ovarian stroma/total area ratio, *Fertil. Steril.* 2001;76 (2) :326–331.

[80] Nardo L.G., Buckett W.M, Khullar V. Determination of the best-fitting ultrasound formulaic method for ovarian volume measurement in women with polycystic ovary syndrome, *Fertil. Steril.* 2003; 79 (3): 632–633.

[81] Sun L, Fu Q. Three-dimensional transrectal ultrasonography in adolescent patients with polycystic ovarian syndrome. Int. *J. Gynecol. Obstet.* 2007; 98(1): 34-38..

[82] Crequat J, Teboul-Faure L , Fortin A, Batallan A, Madelenat P. Endorectal sonography in gynecology: usefulness and diagnostic accuracy, *Gynecol. Obstet. Fertil.* 2004; 32 (11) : 950–953.

Polycystic Ovarian Syndrome: Epidemiology, Aetiology and Pathogenesis

Rosa Sabatini and Raffaele Cagiano**

*Expert Family Planning Service. Department of Obstetrics and Gynecology
**Department of Pharmacology and Human Physiology Policlinico-University of Bari.
Piazza Giulio Cesare 11.70124 Bari. Italy

PCOS : Epidemiology

The prevalence of PCOS is variable due to the lack of a universal definition linked to the variability of the phenotype [1].In fact, the different possible association of hyperandrogenism and/or polycystic ovaries with oligo-anovulation leads to different PCOS phenotypes (Table1).

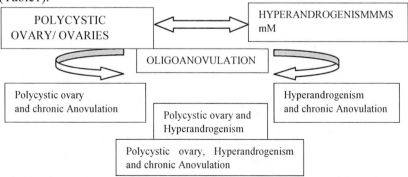

Table 1

Furthermore, if PCOS is defined by the ultrasonographic appearance of PCO, the prevalence varies depending on the study settings used. Polycystic ovaries are seen in 92% of women with idiopathic hirsutism, 87% of women with oligomenorrhea, 21-23% of randomly selected women , 23 % of women who consider themselves normal and who report regular menstrual cycles and in 17% of women participating in routine PAP smear [2,3,4,5,6]. Up to 25% of patients with this sonographic picture may be entirely asymptomatic , however, not all the patients with hyperandrogenism demonstrate PCO [7,8,9,10].When, biochemical parameters have been used as diagnostic criteria,the prevalence of PCOS varies from 2.5 to 7.5% [11,12].It has recently been observed in an unselected , minimally-biased population of women, that the overall prevalence of PCOS appears to be approximately 4.6%, although it could be as low as 3.5% and as high as 11.2% [13]. It is accepted, however, PCOS is one of the most common reproductive endocrinological disorders in women. Population studies of randomly selected normal white European women in reproductive age, report the prevalence of PCO to be 20 to 22% , and 33% in the post-menarcheal group [3,14] Using the USA criteria, the prevalence of PCOS in population based studies was 5% to 11.2% in Alabama, 9% in Greece and 6.5% in Spain.[13,15,16].The highest reported prevalence of PCO in a community survey was 52% in South Asian immigrants in Britain, of whom 49% had menstrual irregularity [17].There is a paucity of data on the prevalence of PCO and PCOS in South Asian women.[16,17,18].At the moment,ethnic differences in the prevalence of PCOS have not been explored [1]. An increased rate of PCOS was reported among Caribbean Hispanics , but is similar between black and white women (3.4% versus 4.7%) [19].There may be ethnic variation in overt features of PCOS despite similar biochemical manifestations across races ; for example, affected Japanese women are less obese and hirsute than Caucasians although with similar androgen excess and insulin resistance [18,19]. The majority of the studies on PCOS are conducted in Caucasian populations suggesting that it is an extremely prevalent syndrome, which varies from 5% in the USA to as high as 33% in the UK [3,4]. The prevalence rate of PCOS for black and white women in USA is not significantly different [20].

Table 2. Environmental factors

Familial history of PCOS	Thyroid disease
Early adrenarche	Familial history of diabetes
Early menarche	Familial history of obesity
Lifestyle	Familial history of dyslipidemia
Overweight or Obesity	Depression and/or anxiety
Dyslipidemia	Sexual behaviour
Diabetes	Helicobacter Pilory ?

Evidence suggests that PCOS is neither population-specific nor restricted to any particular region. In fact, European and Maori are more likely to present hirsutism than other ethnic groups, whereas Maori and Pacific Island women are more obese and have the highest insulin resistance and lipid abnormalities [21]. The ethnic difference seems to be less pronounced in obese women [22].Furthermore, South Asian women residing in the UK report higher prevalence of PCOS than the native Caucasian [23].These observations seem to underline the role of environmental mechanisms in the etiology of the syndrome (Table 2).It was reported that the prevalence of PCOS in women with epilepsy exceeds that in women without epilepsy [24]. A recent study focused the attention on the higher prevalence of PCO and PCOS in lesbian women. Six hundred eighteen women undergoing ovarian stimulation, with or without IUI treatment, were considered. 254 of these were self-identified as lesbians and 364 were heterosexual. Baseline pelvic ultrasound and blood tests revealed that 80% of lesbian women, compared with 32% of the heterosexual women,had PCO on pelvic ultrasound examination [25].

References

[1]   Solomons CG. The epidemiology of polycystic ovary syndrome ; prevalence and associated disease risks. *Endocrinology and Metabolism Clinics of North America* 1999; 28: 247-63.

[2]   Adams J,Polson DW,Franks S.Prevalence of polycystic ovaries in women with anovulation and idiopathic hirsutism. *Br. Med. J. (Clin. Res. Ed.)* 1986 Aug 9;293(6543):355-9.

[3]   Clayton RN, Hogkinson J, Worswick L, Rodin DA, Dyser S, Meade TW. How common are polycystic ovaries in normal women and what is their significance for the fertility of the population? *Clinical Endocrinology* 1992; 37: 127-34.

[4]   Farquhar CM, Birdsall M, Manning P, Mitchell JM, France JT. The prevalence of polycystic ovaries on ultrasound scanning in a population of randomly selected women. *Aust. N. Z. J. Obstet. Gynaecol.* 1994 Feb;34(1):67-72.

[5]   Polson DW, Adams J, Wadsworth J, Franks S. Polycystic ovaries--a common finding in normal women. *Lancet.* 1988 Apr 16;1(8590):870-2.

[6]   Botsis D, Kassanos D, Pyrgiotis E, Zourlas PA.Sonographic incidence of polycystic ovaries in a gynecological population.*Ultrasound Obstet.Gynecol.* 1995 Sep;6(3):182-5.

[7]   Swanson M, Sauerbrei EE, Cooperberg PL.Medical implications of ultrasonically detected polycystic ovaries. *J. Clin. Ultrasound.* 1981 May-Jun;9(5):219-22.

[8]   Orsini LF, Venturoli S, Lorusso R, Pluchinotta V, Paradisi R, Bovicelli L. Ultrasonic findings in polycystic ovarian disease. *Fertil. Steril.* 1985 May;43(5):709-14.

[9]   El Tabbakh GH, Lotfy I, Azab I, Rahman HA, Southren AL, Aleem FA Correlation of the ultrasonic appearance of the ovaries in polycystic ovarian disease and the clinical, hormonal, and laparoscopic findings. *Am. J. Obstet. Gynecol.* 1986 Apr;154(4):892-5.

[10]   Carmina E, Lobo RA.Adrenal hyperandrogenism in the pathophysiology of polycystic ovary syndrome. *J. Endocrinol. Invest.* 1998 Oct;21(9):580-8. Review.

[11]   Mechanick J, Dunaif A 1990 Masculinization: a clinical approach to the diagnosis and treatment of hyperandrogenic women. In: Mazzaferri E (ed) Advances in Endocrinology and Metabolism. Mosley Year Book, Inc, Chicago, IL, 1990 pp 129–173.

[12]   Futterweit W, Dunaif A, Yeh H, Kingsley P 1988 The prevalence of hyperandrogenism in 109 consecutive women presenting with diffuse alopecia. *J. Am. Acad. Dermatol.* 1988 ;19:831–836.

[13] Knochenhauer ES, Key TJ, Kahsar Miller M et al. Prevalence of the polycystic ovary syndrome in unselected black and white women of the South eastern United States: A prospective study. *Journal of Clinical Endocrinology and Metabolism* 1998; 83: 3078-82. 38.

[14] Michelmore KF, Balen AH, Dunger DB, Vessey MP. Polycystic ovaries and associates; clinical and biochemical features in young women. *Clinical Endocrinology* 1999; 51: 779-86.

[15] Diamanti-Kandarakis E, Kouli C, Tsianateli T, et al. A survey of PCOS in Greek population. 79th Annual Meeting of the Endocrine Society,Minneapolis, MN, 1997. 39.

[16] Asunction M, Calvo RM, San Millan JL, Sancho J, Avila S, Escoar-Morreale HF. A prospective study of the prevalence of the polycystic ovary syndrome in unselected Caucasian women in Spain. *Journal of Clinical Endocrinology and Metabolism* 2000; 85: 2434-38. 40.

[17] Rodin DA, Bano G, Bland JM, Taylor K, Nussey SS. Polycystic ovaries and associated metabolic abnormalities in Asian women. Clinical Endocrinology 1998; 49: 91-99.

[18] Dunaif A, Sorbara L, Delson R et al. Ethnicity and polycystic ovary syndrome are associated with independent and additive decreases in insulin action in Caribbean Hispanic women. *Diabetes* 1993; 42: 4162-68. 42.

[19] Carmina E, Koyama T, Chang L, Stanczyk FZ, Lobo RA. Does ethnicity influence the prevalence of adrenal hyperandrogenism and insulin resistance in polycystic ovary syndrome? *American Journal of Obstetrics and Gynaecology* 1992; 167: 1807-12 .

[20] Homburg R. What is polycystic ovary syndrome? *Hum.Reprod.* 2002; 17: 2495-9.

[21] Williamson K, Gunn AJ,Johnson N,Milson SR. The impact of ethnicity on the presentation of polycystic ovarian syndrome.*Aust. NZJ.Obstet.Gynecol*.2001; 41: 202-6.

[22] Norman RJ,Mahabeer S,Master S, Ethnic differences in insulin and glucose response to glucose between white and Indian women with polycystic ovary syndrome. *Fertil. Steril.* 1995;63:58-62.

[23] Wijeyaratne CN,Balen AH,Barth JH,Belchetz PE. Clinical manifestations and insulin resistance(IR) in polycystic ovary syndrome (PCOS) among South Asian and Caucasian :Is there a difference? *Clin. Endocrinol.* 2002;57:343-50.

[24] Isojarvi JT,Laatikainen TI, Pakarinen AI,Juntunen KT,Myllyla W.Polycystic ovaries and hyperandrogenism in women taking valproate for epilepsy. *N. Engl. J. Med.* 1993;329: 1383-88.

[25] Agrawal R,Sharma S,Bekir J,Conway G,Bailey J,Balen AH,Prelevic G.Prevalence of PCOS in lesbian women compared with heterosexual women. *Fertil. Steril.* 2004; 82(5):1352-7.

PCOS: Aetiology and Pathogenesis

Despite polycystic ovary syndrome is the most common endocrine disorder found in reproductive-age women, a comprehensive explanation of pathophysiology is still lacking [1]. In contrast to the characteristic picture of fluctuating hormone levels in the normal cycle , women with PCOS exhibit an abnormal gonadotropin secretion with high LH and relatively low FSH [2,3] Consequently,the production of estrogen and androgens are both increased [4,5].The resulting imbalance of estrogenic and androgenic steroids in turn accentuates the hypersecretion of LH by anterior pituitary. Estradiol levels may not fall low enough to allow sufficient FSH response for initial growth stimulus and levels of estradiol may be inadequate to produce the positive stimulatory effects necessary to induce the ovulatory surge of LH. The mechanism of the disturbed folliculogenesis includes relative FSH deficiency and loss of LH stimulation, deficiency of certain local growth factors and abnormal ovarian steroidogenesis.The LH stimulates the theca cells to produce androgens witch are the precursor for estrogen synthesis. Besides, insulin resistance and abdominal obesity are frequent metabolic traits of this multifactorial nosologic entity.The heterogeneity of PCOS may well reflect multiple pathophysiological mechanisms, but the definition of each contributing mechanism has been slow to emerge. Controversial definitions of the disorder and different phenotypic subgroups present a challenge for clinical and basic research.In fact , the phenotypic variability and the different definitions hamper the efforts towards understanding the aetiology and pathogenesis of PCOS. We adopted the Revised Definition of the ESHRE / ASRM -2004 (6).

The Rotterdam ESHRE/ ASRM revised diagnosis of PCOS

PCOS can be diagnosed, after the exclusion of other possible causes of hyperandrogenism, when at least two of the following criteria are present:

- *Hyperandrogenism or clinical manifestations of androgen excess (hirsutism,acne or androgenetic alopecia).*
- *Oligoovulation or Anovulation (oligomenorrhea or amenorrhea)*
- *Polycystic ovaries defined by ultrasound examination*

Despite the past and current research, is still impossible to determine the primary etiologic factor of the Polycystic ovary syndrome. The natural course of PCOS appears to originate in fetal life and factors of the intrauterine environment have been incriminated in the early pathogenesis of the syndrome. However,the endocrinopathy becomes manifest in the peripubertal years and unfolds as patients enter later stages of life and may change over time [7,8,9,10]. In adolescence, PCOS may masquerade itself as physiological adolescent anovulation. Asymptomatic adolescents with a polycystic ovary occasionally (8%) have subclinical PCO but often (42%) have a subclinical PCOS type of ovarian dysfunction [11].

Aetiopathogenetic history of PCOS

Animal studies

The long history of the PCOS begins in 1961 when Barraclough and Gorski hypothesized that the hypothalamus may be responsible for androgen induced sterility ,in the female rat [12,13]. After several years, Vom Saal and Bronson demonstrated that the sexual characteristics of adult female mice are related with their blood testosterone levels, during prenatal development, and that their exposure to androgen excess can induce the development of anovulatory sterility and polycystic ovaries [14].These experimental studies established the basis for the research around a prenatal origin of polycystic ovary syndrome. Later, some studies showed that the androgen prenatal exposure of the female rhesus monkeys induced all features of PCOS: ovarian hyperandrogenism, adrenal hyperandrogenism, ovulatory dysfunction and oligomenorrhea .However, in nonhuman primate the LH excess was found exclusively in the female monkey exposed to androgens in early gestation. Furthermore, it was also showed that the menstrual dysfunction was greatest in those female rhesus monkeys with high body mass index, and this data suggested that hyperinsulinemia can also contribute to anovulation [15,16]. Other studies revealed that female monkeys exposed in utero to androgen excess tend to develop visceral fat in adulthood independently from obesity [17]. Early gestation exposure resulted in insulin resistance, impaired pancreatic beta-cell function and type 2 diabetes; while, late gestation exposure resulted in abnormal insulin sensitivity that decreased with increasing body mass index [18,19]. Therefore, it seems that prenatal androgenization in early gestation , might induce adiposity-dependent visceral fat accumulation and hypeinsulinemia and, in late gestation might .increase total body and non visceral fat mass.

Human Studies

The results of nonhuman primate experimental studies led to consider some human models like the women with congenital adrenal hyperplasia or with congenital adrenal virilizing tumors.These subjects,despite the normalization of the androgen excess, with the treatment or the tumour removal after birth, showed the PCOS features [20,21]. Another field of this research draw attention to offspring of human-PCOS mothers. The apparent influence of intrauterine milieu in poorly controlled diabetics who end with stillborn fetuses, showed ovarian changes similar to those seen in PCOS. Pregnant women with PCOS exhibit higher androgen levels than normal pregnant women. Female born from androgenized women have a low birth weight and high insulin resistance that start at an early age [22].

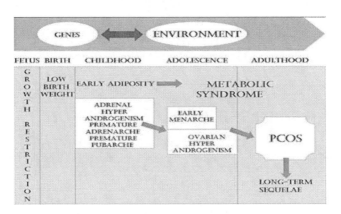

Figure 1

The prevalence of small infants for gestational age (SGA) seems significantly higher in the offspring of PCOS mothers compared to the SGA infants of normal women (12.8% > 2.8% p<.0.02); while, the prevalence of large infants for gestational age (LGA) seems similar in both groups ,but birth length of LGA newborns is greater in PCOS women than in the controls (P<0-05) [23]. A study assessed adrenal function during childhood and pubertal development in daughters of women with PCOS (PCOSd). Ninety-eigth PCOSd [64 during childhood (ages 4-8 yr) and 34 during the peripubertal period (ages 9-13 yr)] and 51 daughters of control women (Cd)[30 during childhood and 21 during the peripubertal period] were included. PCOSd and Cd were similar in age and body mass index. During the peripubertal period, basal and post-stimulated DHEAS concentrations were higher in PCOSd compared to Cd. Among PCOSd, 12.5% of girls in childhood and 32.4% in peripuberty presented biochemical evidence of exaggerated adrenarche. Stimulated insulin was higher in PCOSd compared to Cd during childhood (P = 0.03)and peripuberty (P = 0.03). An advancement of 8 months between bone and chronological age was observed in peripubertal PCOSd compared to Cd [24]. Despite these observations, a current prospective cohort study evaluating the relationship between maternal and umbilical cord androgen levels and Polycystic Ovary Syndrome in adolescence, did not support the hypothesis that maternal androgens, within the normal range for pregnancy, directly program PCOS in the offspring [25]. In any case , it may be of interest to know at which stage of pubertal development the hormonal and metabolic abnormalities may ensue in PCOS. With this aim ,the reproductive and metabolic profiles of daughters of women with PCOS (PCOSd) were assessed ,during the peripubertal period. Ninety-nine PCOSd [30 prepubertal and 69 pubertal (Tanner II-V)] and 84 daughters of control women (Cd) (20 prepubertal and 64 pubertal) were studied. An oral glucose tolerance test, a GnRH agonist test (leuprolide acetate, 10 microg/kg sc), and a transabdominal ultrasound were performed. Gonadotropins, sex steroids, SHBG, glucose, insulin, and lipids were determined. Ovarian volume and 2-h insulin were significantly higher in PCOSd compared to Cd at all Tanner stages. In Tanner stages IV and V, basal testosterone and post-stimulated LH, testosterone and 17hydroxyprogesterone concentrations were significantly higher in PCOSd compared to Cd. Hyperinsulinemia and an increased ovarian volume were present in PCOSd before the onset of puberty and remained constant during pubertal development [26].Therefore, the biochemical abnormalities of PCOS seem to appear during late puberty. The apparent influence of intrauterine milieu in poorly controlled diabetics who end with stillborn fetuses, showed ovarian changes similar to those seen in PCOS. Aerts et al have shown that maternal diabetes induces insulin resistance in her offspring and this defect seems to be acquired and not hereditary [27,28]. Considering the early onset and the nature of these alterations, they may constitute a high-risk for metabolic and reproductive future of PCOS daughters.Polycystic ovary syndrome is a familial endocrine-metabolic dysfunction, increasingly recognized in adolescent girls with hyperandrogenism.However, it is difficult to establish whether the metabolic abnormalities, described in PCOS, are present before the onset of hyperandrogenism.In children a strong association of the adiponectin levels with the metabolic parameters of insulin resistance has been described. A study evaluated fifty-three prepubertal and 22 pubertal (Tanner stages II-V) daughters of PCOS women (PCOSd) and 32 prepubertal and 17 pubertal daughters of control women (Cd) .In the prepubertal girls, 2-h insulin was higher and adiponectin levels were lower in the PCOSd group, compared with the Cd group. In the pubertal girls, triglycerides, 2-h insulin, and serum testosterone concentrations were higher and SHBG lower in PCOSd, compared with Cd, but adiponectin levels were similar in both groups. Therefore, it seems that some of the metabolic features of PCOS are present in daughters of PCOS women before the onset of hyperandrogenism. Adiponectin appears to be one of the early markers of metabolic derangement in these girls [29]. Another important part of these researches regards the role played by anti-Mullerian hormone (AMH) in peripubertal daughters of PCOS mothers. It was observed an increase of AMH levels in prepubertal daughters of polycystic ovary syndrome women, suggesting that these girls may have an altered follicular development.However, it is not known whether AMH levels remain increased during puberty. From this point of view, it seems important to establish whether the increased AMH levels, observed in prepubertal daughters of PCOS women, persist during the peripubertal period, a stage during which the gonadal axis is activated and PCOS may become clinically manifested. A study evaluating 28 daughters (8-16 yr old) of PCOS women (PCOSd) and 33 daughters (8-16 yr old) of control women (Cd), comparable in age, body mass index, and breast Tanner stage, showed that free androgen index, testosterone, AMH, and 2-h insulin levels were significantly higher in the PCOSd group compared with the control group; likewise, the average ovarian volume was significantly higher in the PCOSd group. In both groups a positive correlation between 2-h insulin levels and AMH concentrations was observed [30]. Therefore, AMH concentrations are increased in peripubertal PCOSd. These findings, along with the results of previous studies, suggest that PCOSd appear to show an increased follicular mass that is established during early development,and persists during puberty .

In conclusion,growing evidence suggests that prenatal exposure to steroids, either of fetal or maternal origin,could be a source of prenatal programming with detrimental consequences during adult life.

Premature Pubarche

PCOS often emerge during the peri-pubertal years with premature pubarche (PP) being the earliest manifestation for some girls.The term of premature or precocious pubarche indicates the appearance of pubic hair,which may be associated with axillary hair, in early or mid childhood (before the age of 8 yr in girls and 9 yr in boys).In girls with a history of a low birth weight, puberty tends to start earlier and to have a faster course, so that final height may be moderately reduced.Girls born small for gestational age (SGA), with a birth weight < 1.5 SDS, are at increased risk of early onset and rapid progression of puberty, with reduced final height. In contrast, idiopathic precocious pubarche (PP) does not seems to have negative effects on the onset of puberty or final height. In addition , the prevalence of ovarian hyperandrogenism, hyperinsulinism and dyslipidemia is increased among adolescent girls when premature pubarche is preceded by reduced fetal growth [31] During puberty, insulin resistance develops probably because of the increase in sex steroids and growth hormone, resulting in secondary increase in insulin and IGF-1, which leads to a decrease in the sex hormone binding globulin (SHBG) and would allow greater sex steroid activity for pubertal development. Thus,PCOS can be considered as a state of exaggerated puberty or hyperpuberty. After puberty, the insulin and IGF-1 levels progressively decline in most patients, resulting in normalization of the clinical and morphological picture. In subjects with PCOS, the higher levels persist either because hyperinsulinemia persists or because another pathogenic factor has taken over its role in the meantime. In the latter instance, hyperinsulinemia probably only served as an inducing event.

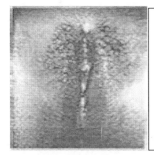

The female to male ratio is approximately 10:1. In female children dark and curly hair is limited initially to the labia majora and gradually extends in the pubic region. A transient acceleration of growth is common but final height is usually not affected. The onset of puberty usually occurs at the normal age (Leung 2008) (32).Pubarche is one of the physical changes of puberty but should not be adequated with it, since it may occur independentely of complete puberty.

Figure 2

Pubarche usually results from rising levels of androgens from the adrenal glands but may also result from exposure of a child to an anabolic steroid. Rarer causes leading to precocious puberty are congenital adrenal hyperplasia and androgen producing tumors of the adrenals or gonads.Premature adrenarche is the most common cause of premature pubarche. The ovarian hyperandrogenism is characterized by clinical signs of androgen excess and by an exaggerated ovarian 17hydroxy progesterone response to GnRH agonist stimulation.In girls, premature pubarche,hyperinsulinism, low IGFBP-1, dyslipidemia,anovulation, hyperan-drogenism and some combinations of these have been related to reduced fetal growth, indicating that these associations or sequences may have a prenatal origin [33].In fact, this sequence seems to occur more frequently when premature pubarche was preceded by reduced fetal growth and followed by excessive postnatal catch-up in height and particularly in weight.

Classification of the precocious puberty
Gonadotropin dependent precocious puberty (GDPP)
Gonadotropin independent precocious puberty (GIPP)
Variants of the normal pubertal development: isolated precocious thelarche isolated precocious pubarche isolated precocious menarche

Table 4

Therefore, hyperinsulinemia appears to play a crucial role in the development of this constellation of events. It was evaluated the relationship between birth weight, the onset and progression of puberty and final height in girls with PP. A retrospective study considered girls at the onset of puberty with a history of PP. A total of 124 girls (37 SGA) were investigated; 61 had presented menarche and 44 had reached final height. The mean age was 6.8 (0.8) years at pubarche, 9.5 (0.9) at the onset of puberty and 11.7 (0.9) at menarche. No significant differences were found in the correlation between birth weight and age at presentation of pubarche, bone age at presentation of pubarche, age at telarche or age at menarche. A positive correlation was found between birth weight and height at pubarche, telarche, and menarche and final height. These data suggest that pubertal progression is faster in SGA girls.All patients reached the familial target height but only those with an appropriate birthweight were taller than their mothers[34].Therefore,PP does not seem to modify age of onset or progression of puberty or final height in girls with adequate birth weight. In contrast, in SGA girls, PP is associated with faster puberal development and shorter final height. In girls with premature pubarche and a history of a low birth weight, metformin therapy may reverse the progression to clinical ovarian hyperandrogenism, normalize body composition and excess visceral fat, and delay pubertal progression without attenuating linear growth and bone mineralization, suggesting that adult height may be improved. However, long-term follow-up of these patients is needed to fully determine the maintenance of these benefits after discontinuation of therapy [35] .Perinatal stress is thought to underlie the Barker sequelae of low birth weight, of which precocious pubarche may be a manifestation. To explore whether prematurity as well as smallness for gestational age (SGA) predisposes to precocious pubarche, and the potential role of excess weight gain during childhood. a retrospective chart review of 89 children (79 girls) with precocious pubarche was performed. Sixty five per cent were overweight/obese at diagnosis, compared with 19-24% of control children. Thirty five per cent had a history of SGA and 24% of prematurity. The mean change in weight from birth to diagnosis was greater in those who were SGA versus AGA , with no difference in the incidence of overweight/obesity. The latter was lower among children born premature (40% versus 72%) but was associated with a mean increase in weight of 1.3 SDS during childhood.Nine out of ten girls and boys with precocious pubarche had at least one of the three mentioned risk factors.Therefore, both prematurity and SGA were associated with precocious pubarche, as was overweight/obesity, irrespective of size or gestation at birth. In any case, it seems that excess weight gain in childhood may predispose to precocious pubarche in susceptible individuals [36]

Functional Adrenal Hyperandrogenism

Adrenarche is the puberty of the adrenal gland.The key hormonal products of adrenarche are DHEA and DHEAS.Premature adrenarche has no adverse effects on the onset and progression of gonadarche and/or final height.Mechanisms for initiation of adrenal androgen secretion at adrenarche are still not well understood. Maturational increases in 17-hydroxylase and 17,20-lyase are seen together with a lower activity of 3beta-hydroxysteroid dehydrogenase (3beta-HSD). There is good evidence that the reticularis area is the source of adrenal androgens. Adrenarche and gonadarche are differently regulated.Although, premature adrenarche has been thought to be a benign normal variant of puberty, some findings indicate that, for certain girls,premature adrenarche represents an early clinical feature of the metabolic syndrome (obesity, hypertension, dyslipidemia, insulin resistance).Perhaps, the early identification of these patients will permit early therapy, such as lifestyle changes, including interventions on dietary and activity levels . As insulin resistance is an underlying feature of premature adrenarche, it seems rational to assess the efficacy and safety of using insulin-sensitizing agents to treat these individuals. Considering the paucity of controlled longitudinal studies, the available cross-sectional data suggest that premature pubarche , driven by premature adrenarche and hyperinsulinemia, may precede the development of ovarian hyperandrogenism, and this sequence may have an early origin with low birth weight serving as a marker. Premature adrenarche may thus be a forerunner of syndrome X in some girls [37,38]. However, it is not known whether PP girls still have adrenal hyperandrogenism after puberty and if so, which fraction of PP girls develops so-called functional adrenal hyperandrogenism (FAH), an entity characterized by ACTH-dependent 17-ketosteroid excess.

Both extra- and intraadrenal factors regulate adrenal androgen secretion. Recent studies have shown that premature adrenarche in childhood may have consequences such as functional ovarian hyperandrogenism, polycystic ovarian syndrome, and insulin resistance in later life, sometimes already recognizable in childhood or adolescence [31].A longitudinal study investigated the endocrine pattern of 47 girls with PP: at birth(weight for GA),at diagnosis of PP and in adolescence.Serum dehydroepiandrosterone sulphate (DHEAS) and androstenedione were measured at diagnosis as well as the 17 hydroxyprogesterone (17-OHP) response to ACTH. Postpubertal evaluation included assessment of adrenal and ovarian function, and of insulin responses to a glucose load.. PP girls were considered to have FAH in adolescence if both DHEA and androstenedione responses to ACTH were excessive (>1500 ng/dl and > 350 ng/dl,respectively). At diagnosis of PP,girls had high DHEAS and androstenedione levels, as well as high 17-OHP responses to ACTH. In adolescence, PP girls had a normal BMI, presented with mild hirsutism and had high baseline and post-ACTH concentrations of most adrenal androgens, low SHBG levels and tended to have hyperinsulinemia and to present biological signs of ovarian hyperandrogenism. More than a third of the PP cohort developed FAH in adolescence. Neither baseline DHEAS, A, nor post-ACTH 17-OHP values at diagnosis of PP predicted the development of FAH in adolescence.In PP girls,only a low weight at birth was found to be significantly associated with subsequent FAH. These longitudinal findings in girls with PP point to the possibility of an endocrine sequence of prenatal onset: low weight at birth, PP in childhood and adrenal hyperandrogenism in adolescence. The pathophysiological mechanisms underpinning this recognized sequence remain to be identified [39].Adolescent hyperandrogenemia is believed to be a precursor to adult PCOS.In addition to increased LH concentrations and pulse frequency, some girls with elevated androgen levels also demonstrate reduced hypothalamic sensitivity to progesterone feedback. It was hypothesized that excess peripubertal androgens may reduce the sensitivity of the GnRH pulse generator to sex steroid inhibition in susceptible individuals, resulting in increased GnRH pulse frequency and subsequent abnormalities in gonadotropin secretion, ovarian androgen production, and ovulatory function. Over time, these abnormalities may progress to the clinical hyperandrogenism and chronic oligo-ovulation typical of adult PCOS [40]. Corticotropin-releasing hormone (CRH) is an adrenal androgen secretagogue in men and has been proposed as a candidate regulator of adrenarche. CRH also affects androgen production by theca cells and may be involved in the pathogenesis of ovarian hyperandrogenism (OH). Precocious pubarche in girls can precede adolescent OH, a condition characterized by a high ovarian 17-hydroxyprogesterone (17-OHP) response 24 h after GnRH agonist challenge.In adolescent girls with a history of PP, it was assessed the early androgen response to CRH,as well as the CRH effect on the late ovarian response to GnRH agonist. Within a randomized cross-over design, saline or CRH (human CRH 1 microg/kg x h in saline) was infused over 3-h (1100-1400 h) into 12 adolescent girls (age 17 ± 2 yr; body mass index 21.4 ± 0.9 Kg/m2) who had been pretreated with dexamethasone (1 mg at 0 h) and GnRH agonist (leuprolide acetate 500 microg sc at 0800 h = time 0).All adolescents had hirsutism,irregular menses,hyperandrogenemia and hyperinsulinemia after PP. Serum LH, FSH, androstenedione, DHEA and DHEAS were measured at time 0, 3, 6, and 24 h, and ACTH and 17-OHP at time 0, 6, and 24 h. ACTH concentrations at the end of saline or CRH infusions were less than 45 pg/mL; neither saline nor CRH infusions evoked early changes in 17-OHP levels. Within 3 h of CRH infusion, DHEAS increased by 46%, on average; androstenedione increased 2.5-fold and DHEA increased 5-fold during CRH infusion (all $P < 0.0001$ compared with saline). There was no detectable CRH effect on the responses of LH, FSH, DHEA, DHEAS, 17-OHP, androstenedione, testosterone, and estradiol 24 h after GnRH agonist administration; five of 12 girls had elevated 17-OHP response suggestive of OH.

Functional adrenal hyperandrogenism (FAH)
In PP girls, a low weight at birth was found to be significantly associated with subsequent FAH
More than a third of the PP girls develop FAH in adolescence.
FAH may be diagnosed if: - both DHEA and androstenedione responses to ACTH were excessive (>1500ng/dl and > 350 ng/dl, respectively); - there is a high 17OH-P response to ACTH

In conclusion, CRH was found to be a potent adrenal androgen secretagogue in adolescent girls with hyperandrogenism after PP. In this study, CRH failed to detectably affect the ovarian androgen response to gonadotropins [41].

Functional Ovarian Hyperandrogenism

Evidence suggests that adolescent girls with premature pubarche will have an increased incidence of functional ovarian hyperandrogenism (FOH) at adolescence, which is usually associated with hyperinsulinemia and dyslipidemia. Functional ovarian hyperandrogenism is defined as abnormal ovarian 17OHP response to challenge with GnRH analog over 2 ng/ml , after exclusion of adrenal dysfunction. The hyperinsulinemia and lipid disturbances can often be detected in the prepubertal period and throughout puberty, and are associated with an exaggerated ovarian androgen synthesis.. Birth weight scores are lower in premature pubarche girls than in control girls, and particularly so in those girls who show hyperinsulinemia and subsequently develop ovarian hyperandrogenism. Therefore, although the mechanisms interlinking the triad of premature pubarche, hyperinsulinism and ovarian hyperandrogenism remain still elusive, these observations indicate that the triad may result, at least in part, from a common early origin, rather than from a direct interrelationship later in life [42]. FOH is considered to be a form of polycystic ovary syndrome (PCOS) at adolescence. Prepubertal girls with obesity or insulin resistance are at risk to develop the full PCOS phenotype after puberty. A study evaluated for PCOS or FOH.twenty-seven prepubertal girls, aged > 6 years, with premature pubarche and/or obesity. Sixteen patients had premature pubarche, seven were obese, and four had both premature pubarche and obesity. Eleven of 27 patients (40.7%) showed high (>2 ng/ml) 17OHP response to GnRH challenge. Three patients (11%) with FOH also showed PCO morphology on pelvic ultrasound examination. Therefore, in prepubertal girls who carry risk factors, including genetic polymorphisms and/or particular environmental factors, FOH/ PCOS could develop at a high rate [43]. Another study considered the postpubertal outcome of 35 girls diagnosed of premature pubarche during childhood. Sixteen of these girls showed baseline hirsutism, oligomenorrhea and high levels of testosterone and/or androstenedione.After leuprolide acetate subcutaneous administration (500 micrograms), similar increases in gonadotropin levels were found in oligomenorrheic girls, regularly menstruating women(19 girls) and controls (12 girls) , when tested at 6 h. While, 17-hydroxyprogesterone and androstenedione levels, at 24 h after the leuprolide stimulation, were significantly higher in oligomenorrheic patients rather than in the other two groups (P < 0.0001).These results show a distinct leuprolide acetate challenge response in 45% of the postpubertal premature pubarche girls studied, suggesting an increased incidence of FOH, and supporting the need for a continued routine of postmenarcheal evaluation of this group of patients [44]. Responses of 17-OHP to leuprolide acetate challenge facilitate the identification of FOH patients, indicating this test as a reliable diagnostic tool in FOH diagnosis, and confirming the ovaries as the source of hyperandrogenemia in most patients with androgen excess. Although, increased 17-OHP responses after leuprolide acetate stimulation seem to occur more frequently in girls with elevated dehydroepiandrosterone sulfate(DHEAS) and/or androstenedione (A), at the diagnosis of premature pubarche. Hence, specific biochemical markers predictive of FOH are still lacking. A Chinese study investigated whether the association between low birth weight and increased risk of developing premature adrenarche, adrenal hyperandrogenism, hyperinsulinism and insulin resistance is apparent in prepubertal girls born small for their gestational age (SGA) and analyzed when adrenarche occurs in SGA infants and normal birth weight girls. The study was performed in 39 prepubertal SGA girls with a mean age of 7.4 ± 1.7 years and 42 prepubertal, appropriate for gestational age (AGA), girls with the same mean age served as controls. There was no premature adrenarche in SGA and AGA groups. Birth weight was significantly lower in SGA group (P < 0.001).At the time of the study, the age, body mass index (BMI), fasting glucose, cortisol and estradiol did not significantly differ between the two groups,but body height and weight were significantly lower in the SGA group.The fasting plasma insulin in the SGA group was higher than that in AGA group .The insulin sensitivity index was not significantly different between the two groups The serum DHEAS was significantly higher in SGA children than in AGA children (P < 0.05). From about age 7, the concentration of DHEAS had a gradual rise in AGA children. The time of DHEAS rise tended to be earlier in SGA children compared with AGA children.Hence, adrenarche commences at approximately 7 years of age in AGA girls.There were adrenal hyperandrogenism and hyperinsulinism in prepubertal girls born small for gestational age. But there was no insulin resistance as assessed by insulin sensitivity index [45]. Previous studies have documented the association of insulin resistance and hyperandrogenism in adult women with functional ovarian hyperandrogenism (FOH) or polycystic ovary syndrome. However, the possible impact of adrenal hyperandrogenism development during childhood ,in premature pubarche (PP) patients, on postpubertal insulin secretion patterns remains unclear. The fasting insulin to glucose ratio, C peptide, early insulin response to glucose (IRG), mean blood glucose, mean serum insulin (MSI), glucose uptake rate in peripheral tissues (M), and insulin sensitivity indexes (SI) in response to a standard oral glucose tolerance test were evaluated in 13 PP girls with FOH (group A; age, 17.2 ± 0.5 yr), 11 eumenorrheic non hirsute PP girls (group B; age, 16.6 ± 0.5 yr), and 21 age-matched controls (group C). Body mass indexes (BMI) were similar in all 3 groups (group A, 23.3 ± 0.8; group B, 22.5 ± 0.6; group C, 20.6 ± 0.5 kg/m2); while, MSI values were significantly higher in FOH patients than in controls (74.7 ± 17.6 vs. 45.7 ± 4.1 mU/L; P < 0.01), but were not different from those in group B (63.3 ± 11.1 mU/L). Thirty-eight percent of FOH patients (group A) and 27% of non-FOH patients (group B), all of whom had normal BMI, showed MSI levels well above the upper normal limit for controls (> 83.3 mU/L). MSI well correlated with the degree of ovarian hyperandrogenism and with the free androgen index [testosterone (nanomoles per L)/sex hormone-binding globulin (nanomoles per L) x 100; groups A and B)]. Although IRG, glucose uptake rate in peripheral tissues,mean blood glucose,and SI values were not significantly different in the 3 groups. Only 3 patients in group A and 1 patient in group B showed decreased insulin sensitivity and/ or an enhanced early IRG. Among others, significant correlations between MSI and free androgen index values and between BMI and SI were found. Peak 17-hydroxyprogesterone responses to ACTH at PP diagnosis correlated positively with SI in both groups of patients. Hence, hyperinsulinemia is a common feature in adolescent PP patients with FOH and appears to be directly related to the degree of androgen excess [46].Luteinizing hormone responsiveness significantly increased during puberty in all subjects; whereas FSH levels changed less consistently.

Peaks of estradiol levels seem to differ among pubertal stages and were significantly higher in premature pubarche girls than in controls at B4 and at B5. Both peak and incremental increases of 17-Preg and DHEA throughout puberty and of 17-OHP and A(androstenedione) at B4 were significantly higher in premature pubarche girls than in controls. This pattern of ovarian steroidogenic response was most evident during mid and late puberty and seems similar to adrenal hyper-response to ACTH of exaggerated adrenarche, suggestive of increased ovarian activity of both the 17 alpha-hydroxylase and the 17,20 lyase, functions of cytochrome P450c17 alpha.Therefore, pubertal girls with a history of premature pubarche show a distinct pattern of ovarian maturation characterized by an exaggerated ovarian androgen synthesis throughout puberty [47] .

Functional ovarian hyperandrogenism (FOH)

Functional ovarian hyperandrogenism is defined as abnormal ovarian 17OHP response to challenge with GnRH analog of >2 ng/ml , after exclusion of adrenal dysfunction. This pattern of ovarian-steroidogenic response was most evident during mid and late puberty and seems similar to adrenal hyper-response to ACTH of exaggerated adrenarche , suggestive of increased ovarian activity of both the 17 alpha-hydroxylase and the 17,20 lyase , functions of cytochrome P450c17 alpha (Ibanez 1997,Pasquali 2007)(47,48). Hyperinsulinemia and lipid disturbances can often be detected in the prepubertal period and throughout puberty and are associated with an exaggerated ovarian androgen synthesis. Birth weight scores are lower in premature pubarche girls than in control and particularly so in those girls who show hyperinsulinemia and subsequently develop ovarian hyperandrogenism (Ibanez 1998)(42). FOH is considered to be a form of polycystic ovary syndrome (PCOS) at adolescence. Prepubertal girls with obesity or insulin resistance are at risk to develop the full PCOS phenotype after puberty. In prepubertal girls who carry risk factors, including genetic polymorphisms and/or particular environmental factors, FOH/PCOS could develop at a high rate (40%) (Siklar 2007)(43)..

These data may be consistent with the hypothesis that insulin excess may represent a candidate factor responsible for FOH in these women, through the overactivation of the cytochrome P450 17alpha-hydroxylase/17,20-lyase (CYP17) enzyme pathway [48]. A recent study indicated as the paradigm that FOH is a specific feature of the PCOS status cannot longer be sustained. It was showed that women with an exaggerated 17-hydroxyprogesterone response to a GnRH agonist, buserelin, are characterized by more severe hyperandrogenemia, glucose-stimulated beta-cell insulin secretion, and worse insulin resistance than those without evidence of FOH. Furthermore, these findings suggest that premature pubarche in girls should be considered the hallmark of the increased risk for a polyendocrine and metabolic disorder in adult life [33].

Pubertal Tanner' Stages

The onset of age puberty has dramatically decreased over the past 150 years ,at a rate of 2-3 months for decade. This has been attributed to a decline in the incidence of infection diseases and improvements in health care,vaccination programs, socioeconomic conditions, nutrition and physical activity. It has been showed that the percent body fat at age 5 might predict earlier pubertal development among girls. Furthermore, the influence of genetic factors on pubertal development has clearly been demonstrated [49,50, 51, 52, 53]. Existing data on girls, particularly for menarche, indicate that the trend for earlier sexual maturation has continued and that racial differences are significant, with African-American girls developing earlier than white girls[53].Non- Hispanic black girls mature early, but US children completed their sexual development at approximately the same ages. The reference data for the timing of sexual maturation are recommended for the interpretation of the assessments of sexual maturity in US children [54,55]. In the USA the prevalence of childhood overweight tripled between 1980 and 2000 and an association between overweight and PP has been reported.In fact, a study showed that 20/38 considered children (52.6%) with PP had a BMI >85th percentile. Furthermore, increased weight was more common among females (62%) and particularly in Hispanics (80%).It was also found that when the bone age was advanced >1.5 years, the predicted adult height was affected [56].The early onset of puberty may be related to obesity,so there is a need to know the prevalence of early pubertal milestones in non overweight children. Pubertal signs occur before 8.0 years of age in < 5% of the normal-BMI non-Hispanic white female population. However, pubertal milestones generally appear earlier in normal-BMI non-Hispanic black and Mexican American girls; thelarche occur before age 8.0 in 12% to 19% of these groups, and menarche in 5% of non-Hispanic black ,0.8 years earlier than non-Hispanic white subjects.Pubarche is found in ≤ 3% of 8.0-year-old girls with normal BMI of all of these ethnic groups but is significantly earlier in minority groups.Black women are particularly vulnerable to obesity, with a prevalence rate over 50%[57]. In recent years, a particular public health concern is the increasing secular trend in obesity with an even greater racial disparity, especially in girls and women. Between the early 1960s and late 1980s, the prevalence of obesity tripled in young black girls 6 to 11 years of age, while it doubled in white girls.Similarly, both overweight and obesity in adolescent girls 12 to 17 years of age also increased,with a greater increase again in young black girls 6 to 11 years of age, while it doubled in white girls.This secular trend in obesity with a greater increase in black girls signals a potential future chronic disease burden on black women, which is already higher than in white women The higher mortality and morbidity from cardiovascular disease, stroke, and diabetes have been attributed, in part, to the obesity.The increasing occurrence in children and adolescents of non insulin-dependent diabetes, traditionally viewed as an adult-onset condition,may be a consequence of the currently high prevalence of obesity in American youth.   Not surprisingly, this condition is more frequently seen among black than in white women [55]. Two epidemiological studies (PROS and NHANES III) from the USA noted earlier sexual maturation in girls, leading to increased attention internationally to the age at onset of puberty. However, a study evaluating the timing of puberty in a large cohort of healthy Danish children obtained different results.Girls with body mass index above the median had significantly earlier puberty (age at B2 10.42 years) compared with girls with BMI below the median (age at B2 11.24 years). Similarly, menarcheal age was significantly lower in girls with BMI above the median compared with girls with   BMI below the median: 13 vs.13.70 years. It was found that the age at breast development (B2) was 10.88 years, and the mean menarcheal age was 13.42 years. Both sexes were significantly taller compared with data from 1964, but timing of pubertal maturation seemed unaltered.

On the contrary, puberty occurred much later in Denmark compared with data from USA. We could not detect any downwards secular trend in the timing of puberty in Denmark between 1964 and 1991-1993 as seen in the US .Obesity certainly plays a role in the timing of puberty, but the marked differences between Denmark and USA cannot be exclusively attributed to differences in BMI.A possible role of other factors like genetic polymorphisms, nutrition, physical activity or endocrine disrupting chemicals must therefore also be considered [58].Therefore, these data underline the importance to monitor the pubertal development monitor the pubertal development.

It was hypothesized that this earlier presentation of PCOS may relate to an ncreased androgen sensitivity, indicated by androgen receptor geneCAG repeat length.This polymorphism was genotyped in 181 Barcelona girls (age, 10.9 yr; range, 4-19 yr) who had presented with PP, and in 124 Barcelona control girls. PP girls had shorter mean CAG number than Barcelona controls (PP vs. controls: P = 0.003) and greater proportion of short alleles 20 repeats or less (37.0% vs. 24.6%, P = 0.002). Among post-menarcheal PP girls (n = 69),shorter CAG number was associated with higher 17-hydroxyprogesterone levels post-leuprolide (P = 0.009), indicative of ovarian hyperandrogenism, higher testosterone levels, acne and hirsutism scores, and more menstrual cycle irregularities. It was suggested that ovarian hyperandrogenism risk was related to both low birth weight and shorter mean CAG number. In summary, shorter androgen receptor gene CAG number, indicative of increased androgen sensitivity, could increase risks for PP and subsequent ovarian hyperandrogenism [59].

P. stage	Pubic hair	Axillary hair	Breast
B1	None	None	Pre-adolescent
B2	Scanty, long, slightly pigmented	Scanty, long slightly pigmented	Breast and papilla elevated as small mound, areolar diameter increased
B3	Darker, starts to curl, small amount	Darker, curly, adult pattern	Breast and areola enlarged, no contour separation; increased breast contour
B4	Resembles adult type, but less in quantity, coarse, curly		Areola and papilla form secondary mound
B5	Adult distribution, spread to the medial surface of the thighs		Mature; nipple project areola part of general breast contour

B1=prepuberty; B2 = early pubertal,. B3 = midpubertal, B4 = late pubertal, B5 = post-pubertal

References

[1] Balen A. Pathogenesis of polycystic ovary syndrome : the enigma unravels? *Lancet* 1999; 354: 966-77.

[2] Yen SS, Vela P,Rankin J. Inappropriate secretion of follicle-stimulating hormone and luteinizing hormone in polycystic ovarian disease. *J. Clin. Endocrinol. Metab.* 1970;30(4):435-42.

[3] Franks S. Polycystic ovary syndrome: a changing perspective. *Clin. Endocrinol.* 1989; 31:87-120.

[4] Chang RJ.Ovarian steroid secretion in polycystic ovarian disease. *Semi. Reprod. Endocrinol.* 1984; 2: 244.

[5] Calogero AE,Macchi M,Montanini V,Mongioi A,Maugeri G,Vicari E et al. Dynamic of plasma gonadotropin and sex steroid release after pituitari-ovarian inhibition with an analog of gonadotropin- releasing hormone. *J. Clin. Endocrinol.* 1987; 64: 980-5.

[6] Rotterdam ESHRE/ASRM-Sponsored PCOS Consensus Workshop Group. Revised 2003 consensus on diagnostic criteria and long-term health risks related to polycystic ovary syndrome. *Fertil. Steril.* 2004;81:19-25 .

[7] Diamanti-Kandarakis E,Christakou C,Palioura E, Kandaraki E,Livadas S. Does polycystic ovary syndrome start in childhood ? Pediatr. *Endocrinol. Rev.*2008; 5(4): 904-11.

[8] Diamanti-Kandarakis E, Piperi C.Genetics of polycystic ovary syndrome: searching for the way out of the labyrinth. *Hum. Reprod. Update.* 2005 ;11(6):631-43.

[9] Franks S. Adult polycystic ovary syndrome begins in childhood .*Best Pract. Res. Clin. Endocrinol. Metab.* 2002; 16:263-272.

[10] Jablonski K. The influence of male sex hormone on the ovary of women. *Arch. Gynakol.* 1959; 57(1): 141-8).

[11] Rosenfield RL.Clinical review: identifying children at risk of polycystic ovary syndrome. *J. Clin. Endocrinol. Metab.* 2007; 92(3): 787-96

[12] Barraclough CA ,Gorski RA. Evidence that the hypothalamus may be responsible for androgen - induced sterility in the female rat. *Endocrinology* 1961; 68: 68-79

[13] Gorski RA, Barraclough CA. Effects of low dosages of androgen on the differentiation of hypothalamic regulatory control of ovulation in the rat. *Endocrinology* 1963; 73:210-6.

[14] Vom Saal FS, Bronson FH Sexual characteristics of adult female mice are correlated with their blood testosterone levels during prenatal development. *Science* 1980;208: 597-599.

[15] Abbott DH,Dumesic DA,Eisner JR, Colman RJ , Kemnitz JW. Insights into the development of PCOS from studies of prenatally androgenised female rhesus monkeys. *Trends Endocrinol. Metab.* 1998; 9:62-67.

[16] Dumesic DA, Abbott DH, Eisner JR, Goy RW.Prenatal exposure of female rhesus monkeys to testosterone propionate increases serum luteinizing hormone levels in adulthood. *Fertil. Steril.* 1997 Jan;67(1):155-63.

[17] Eisner JR,Dumesic DA,Kenmitz JW, Weindruch R,Abbott DA .Increased adiposity in female rhesus monkeys exposed to androgen excess during early gestation. *Obes. Res.* 2003; 11:279-86

[18] Bruns CM,Baum ST,Colman RJ,Dumesic DA,Eisner JR,Jensen MD,Whigham LD,Abbott DH. Prenatal androgen excess negatively impacts body fat distribution in a nonhuman primate model of polycystic ovary syndrome. *Int. J. Obes.* (London) 2007;31(10):1579-85.

Polycystic Ovarian Syndrome: Epidemiology, Aetiology and Pathogenesis   53

[19] Eisner JR,Dumesic DA, Kenmitz JW, Abbott DA. Timing of prenatal androgen excess determines differential impairment in insulin secretion and action in adulte female rhesus monkeys. *J. Clin. Endocrinol. Metab*. 2000: 85: 1206-1210.

[20] Hague WM,Adams J,Rodda C,Brook CG,DeBruyn R,Grant DB,Jacobs HS.The prevalence of polycystic ovaries in patients with congenital adrenal hyperplasia and their close relatives. *Clin. Endocrinol.*(Oxf) 1990;33:501-510.

[21] Barnes RB, Rosenfield RL, Ehrmann DA,Cara JF,Cuttler L,Levitsky LL,Rosenthal IM. Ovarian hyperandrogenism as result of congenital adrenal virilizing disorders: evidence for perinatal masculinization of neuroendocrine function in women. *J. Clin. Endocrinol. Metab*. 1994;79:1328-33.

[22] Recabarren SE,Sir-Petermann T, Maliqueo M,Lobos A,Rojas-Garcia P.Prenatal exposure to androgen as a factor of fetal programming. *Rev. Med. Chil.* 2006;134(1):101-8.

[23] Sir-Petermann T, Hitchsfeld C,Maliqueo M,Codner E,Echiburu B, Gazitua R,Recabarren SE,Cassoria F.Birth weight in offspring of mothers with polycystic ovary syndrome. Hum. Reprod. 2005;20(8):2122-6.

[24] Maliqueo M,Sir-Petermann T, Perez V,Echiburu B,de Guevara AL, Galvez C,Crisosto N,Azziz R Adrenal function during childhood and puberty in daughters of women with polycystic ovary syndrome. *J. Clin. Endocrinol. Metab*. 2009 Sep;94(9):3282-8

[25] Hickey M, Sloboda DM, Atkinson HC, Doherty DA, Franks S., Norman RJ, Newnham JP, Hart R. The relationship between maternal and umbilical cord androgen levels and Polycystic Ovary Syndrome in adolescence: A prospective cohort study. *J. Clin. Endocrinol. Metab*. 2009; 94(10): 3714-20

[26] Sir-PetermannT, Codner E,Pérez , Echiburu B, Maliqueo M, Ladròn de Guevara A, Preisler J, Crisosto N, Sànchez F, Cassorla F, Bhasin S.Metabolic and reproductive features before and during puberty in daughters of women with polycystic ovary syndrome. *J. Clin. Endocrinol. Metab*. 2009; 94(6):1923-30.

[27] Aerts L, Van Assche FA.Animal evidence for the transgenerational development of diabetes mellitus. Int J Biochem Cell Biol. 2006;38(5-6):894-903.Review

[28] Van Assche FA, Aerts L, Holemans K.Maternal diabetes and the effect for the offspring. *Verh. K. Acad. Geneeskd. Belg.* 1992;54(2):95-106

[29] Sir-PetermannT, Maliqueo M Codner E, Echiburu B, Crisosto N ,Pérez V, Pérez-Bravo F,Cassorla F. Early metabolic derangements in daughters of women with polycystic ovary syndrome. *J. Clin. Endocrinol. Metab*. 2007; 92(12): 4637-42.

[30] Crisosto N, Codner E,Maliqueo M, Echiburù B, Sànchez F, Cassorla F,Sir-Petermann T. Anti-Müllerian hormone levels in peripubertal daughters of women with polycystic ovary syndrome. *J. Clin. Endocrinol. Metab*. 2007;92(7): 2739-43.

[31] Ibanez L,Potau N,Marcos MV,de Zegher F. Adrenal hyperandrogenism in adolescent girls with a history of low birthweight and precocious pubarche. *Clin. Endocrinol.* (Oxf) 2000; 53(4): 523-7.

[32] Leung AK,Robson WL.Premature pubarche . *J. Pediatr. Health Care* 2008; 22(4):230-3.

[33] Ibanez L,Poteau N,Dunger D,de Zegher F. Precocious pubarche in girls and the development of androgens excess. *J. Pediatr. Endocrinol. Metab*. 2000; 13 Suppl. 5: 1261-3 Review.

[34] Curcoy Barcenilla AT, Trenchs Sainz de la Maza V, Ibanez Toda L., Rodriguez Hierro F. Influence of birthweight on the onset and progression of puberty and final height in precocious pubarche .*An. Pediatr(Barc)*.2004; 60(5) : 436-9.

[35] Ibáñez L, Díaz R, López-Bermejo A, Marcos MV.Clinical spectrum of premature pubarche: links to metabolic syndrome and ovarian hyperandrogenism. *Rev. Endocr. Metab. Disord*. 2009 Mar;10(1):63-76. Review.

[36] Neville KA,Walker JL.Precocious pubarche is associated with SGA, prematurity ,weight gain, and obesity. *Arch. Dis. Child.*2005; 90(3): 258-61

[37] Saenger P, Dimartino-Nardi J.Premature adrenarche. *J. Endocrinol. Invest.* 2001; 24(9): 724-33.

[38] Ibanez L, Dimartino –Nardi J, Potau N, Saenger P. Premature adrenarche--normal variant or forerunner of adult disease? *Endocr. Rev*. 2000; 21(6) : 671- 96.

[39] Blank SK, Mc Cartney CR, Helm KD, Marshall JC. Neuroendocrine effects of androgens in adult polycystic ovary syndrome and female puberty. *Semin. Reprod. Med.* 2007; 25(5): 352-9.

[40] Ibanez L, Potau N, Marcos MV, de Zegher F. Corticotropin-releasing hormone: a potent androgen secretagogue in girls with hyperandrogenism after precocious pubarche. *J. Clin. Endocrinol. Metab*. 1999; 84(12): 4602- 6.

[41] Ibanez L, de Zegher F, Poteau N. Premature pubarche, ovarian hyperandrogenism and the polycystic ovary syndrome: from a complex constellation to a simple sequence of prenatal onset. *J. Endocrinol. Invest*. 1998; 21(9): 558-66.

[42] Siklar Z,Ocal G, Adivaman P,Erour A,Berberoolu M. Functional ovarian hyperandrogenism and polycystic ovary syndrome in prepubertal girls with obesity and/or premature pubarche. J.Pediatr. Endocrinol. Metab. 2007; 20(4): 475-81.

[43] Ibanez L,Potau N,Virdis R,Zampolli M, Terzi C,Gussinvè M, Carrascosa A,Vicens-Calvet E. Postpubertal outcome in girls diagnosed of premature pubarche during childhood: increased frequency of functional ovarian hyperandrogenism. *J, Clin. Endocrinol. Metab*. 1993; 76(6): 1599-603.

[44] Jang YZ,Zhu M,Xiong F, Deng LL, Luo YH. Dehydroepiandrosterone sulfate and insulin of prepubertal girls born small for gestational age. *Zhonghua Er Ke Za Zhi* 2006; 44(1): 37-40

[45] Ibanez L, Potau N, Zampolli M, Prat N, Virdis R, Vicens/Calvet E,Carrascosa A. Hyperinsulinemia in postpubertal girls with a history of premature pubarche and functional ovarian hyperandrogenism. *J. Clin. Endocrinol. Metab*. 1996; 81(3): 237/43.

[46] Ibanez L,Potau N,Zampolli M,Street ME,Carrascosa A. Girls diagnosed with premature pubarche show an exaggerated ovarian androgen synthesis from the early stages of puberty: evidenced from gonadotropin-releasing hormone agonist testing. *Fertil. Steril*. 1997; 67(5): 849-55.

[47] Pasquali R, Patton L, Pocognoli P, Cognigni GE, Gambineri A.17-hydroxyprogesterone responses to gonadotropin-releasing hormone disclose distinct phenotypes of functional ovarian hyperandrogenism and polycystic ovary syndrome. *J. Clin. Endocrinol. Metab*. 2007 ; 2(11):4208-17.

[48] Arroyo A, Laughlin GA, Morales AJ, Yen SS.Inappropriate gonadotropin secretion in polycystic ovary syndrome: influence of adiposity. J Clin Endocrinol Metab. 1997 Nov;82(11):3728-33.hyperandrogenism and polycystic ovary syndrome. *J. Clin. Endocrinol. Metab*. 2007 ; 2(11):4208-17.

[49] Kalberg J. Secular trends in pubertal development. *Hormone research,* 2002, 57(Suppl. 2):19–30.

[50] Plamert MR, Boepple PA. Variation in the timing of puberty: clinical spectrum and genetic investigation. *Journal of clinical endocrinology and metabolism,* 2001, 86:2364–8.

[51] Braithwaite D,Moore DH,Lustig RH,Epel ES,Ong KK,Rehkopf DH,Wang MC,Miller SM,Hiatt RA.Socioeconomic status in relation to early menarche among black and white girls. *Cancer Causes Control* 2009; 20(5): 713-20.

[52] Davidson KK, Susman EJ, Birch LL. Percent body fat at age 5 predicts earlier pubertal development among girls at age 5. *Pediatrics,* 2003, 111(4):815–21.

[53] Herman- Giddens ME. Recent data on pubertal milestones in United States children:the secular trend toward earlier development. *Int. J. Androl.* 2006; 29(1): 241-6.

[54] Sun SS, Schubert CM, Chumlea WC, Roche AF, Kulin HE, Lee PA, Himes JH, Ryan AS. National estimates of the timing of sexual maturation and racial differences among US children. *Pediatrics* 2004; 113(1pt 1): 177-8.

[55] Rosenfield RTL, Bachrach LK, Chernausek SD. Current age of onset of puberty. Pediatrics, 2000, 106 :622–3Diaz A,Bhandari S, Sison C, Vogiatzi M.Characteristics of children with premature pubarche in the new york metropolitan area. *Horm. Res.* 2008; 70(3): 150-4

[56] Rosenfield RL, Lipton RB, Drum ML. Thelarche, pubarche, and menarche attainment in children with normal and elevated body mass index. *Pediatrics* 2009; 123(1) : 84-8.

[57] Kimm SY,Barton BA, Obarzanek E,McMahon RP, Sabry ZI, Waclawiw MA, Schreiber GB, Morrison JA, Similo S, Daniels SR.Racial divergence in adiposity during adolescence:NHLBI Growth and Health Study. *Pediatrics* 2001; 107(3): E34

[58] Juul A, Teilmann G, Scheike T,Hertel NT,Holm K, Laursen EM, Main KM, Skakkebaek NE,.Pubertal development in Danish children: comparison of recent European and US data. *Int. J. Androl.* 2006;29(1); 247-55. .

[59] Ibanez L,Ong KK,Mongan N,Jaaskelamen J, Marcos MV, Hughes IA,De Zegher F. Dunger DB. Androgen receptor gene CAG repeat polymorphism in the development of ovarian hyperandrogenism. *J. Clin. Endocrinol. Metab.* 2003; 88(7): 3333-8. .

PCOS Aetiology: Hypotheses

The heterogeneity of PCOS may reflect multiple pathophysiological mechanisms but the definition of each contributing mechanism has been slow to emerge. However the growing knowledge on the mechanisms leading to PCOS, induced to select four major hypothesis:

1) A primary neuroendocrine defect leading to an exaggerated LH pulse frequency and amplitude
2) A defect of androgen synthesis that results in enhanced ovarian androgen production
3) A defect in insulin action and secretion that leads to hyperinsulinaemia and insulin resistance
4) An alteration in cortisol metabolism resulting in enhanced adrenal androgen production

It must be accepted, however, that each of these ways are artificial stating points to our understanding of the metabolic-ovarian-pituitary circuit being closely interrelated. Clearly, the pathophysiology of this disease is complex, and much remains to be learned about it.

Primary Neuroendocrine Defect: LH Hypothesis

Primary LH excess has long been considered the cause of the increased ovarian androgen secretion in PCOS. Luteinizing hormone (LH) hypersecretion, both basically and in response to GnRH administration, is a characteristic hallmark of the syndrome [1,2].Really,the affected women exhibit an exaggerated high LH secretion with relatively constant low follicle stimulating hormone (FSH) secretion. Consequently, a LH/ FSH ratio of 2-3: 1 is generally considered the main indicator of PCOS [3,4]. Current studies have established that 94% of women meeting the broad criteria for PCOS have an increased LH/FSH ratio. Several lines of evidences suggest that the mechanisms underlying the increased LH/FSH ratio in PCOS, are partly due to an increased sensitivity of the pituitary to GnRH stimulation, manifested by an increase in LH pulse amplitude and frequency, but mainly amplitude . It is likely that this increased activity is taking place at both hypothalamic and pituitary levels [5]. This is consistent with an abnormal diurnal pattern of LH secretion that has been reported both in adolescent girls with PCOS and in adults with PCOS , with the highest LH values occurring in late afternoon rather than at night [3]. Finally, there is evidence that bioactive LH is elevated in many patients with PCOS, in whom immunoactive LH is normal [6,7]. Decreased sensitivity to progesterone and negative feedback on the GnRH pulse generator may play a role in this neuroendocrine defect.Additional factors which may contribute to the low and to the normal FSH levels in the face of increased LH levels, include chronic mild estrogen increases and possibly inhibin [8]. In addition to these effects on the differential control of FSH, there is increased pituitary sensitivity of LH secretion to GnRH. Both estrogen and androgens have been proposed as candidates mediating these effects [9]. Marshall and Eagleson have focused on pulsatile patterns of LH secretion as an indicator of altered hypothalamic secretion of GnRH. It is believed that although a pulsatile GnRH stimulus is required to maintain gonadotropin synthesis and secretion, are the frequency and amplitude of GnRH pulses that determine gonadotrophin subunit gene expression and secretion of pituitary LH and FSH [10].Thus, in ovulatory cycles, an increase in GnRH frequency during follicular phase favors LH synthesis prior to the LH surge, while following ovulation, luteal steroids slow GnRH pulses to favor FSH synthesis. In PCOS, LH / GnRH pulses are persistently rapid and favor LH synthesis, hyperandrogenaemia and impaired follicular maturation. Christman et al.(1991) showed that the administration of progesterone in anovulatory women with PCOS can slow GnRH pulse secretion,favor FSH secretion and induce follicular maturation [11].Furthermore, in another study, these authors reported an insensitivity of the GnRH pulse generator to the suppression by oestradiol and progesterone in PCOS women [12].Taken together, these data suggest that the increased plasma LH and GnRH/LH pulsatile secretion in PCOS are not simply a consequence of the low levels of progesterone due to anovulation, but reflect an underlying insensitivity of the hypothalamic GnRH pulse generator to oestrogen/ progesterone inhibition. Superimposed on these underlying abnormalities in gonadotropin secretion, there is a marked inhibitory effect of obesity on LH secretion which may be mediated at either a pituitary or hypothalamic level[6].Finally, it was suggested that such insensitivity during pubertal maturation could be a potential mechanism for the perimenarchal abnormalities seen in hyperandrogenaemic adolescents who appear to exhibit early manifestations of PCOS [10].

Prenatal Androgen Exposure

Rumsby et al in 1988 postulated that the intrauterine environment has a role in the pathogenesis of PCOS, and suggested that hyperandrogenism during fetal life may be the determining fact factor [13].

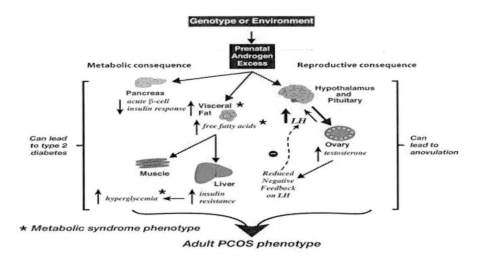

Figure 3

The hypothesis of a prenatal androgen exposure and adolescent studies suggest early in life androgen excess as the initiating factor of PCOS, but insufficient evidence is available to confirm this [6]. However,it was hypothesized that the peripubertal excess of androgens may reduce the sensitivity of the GnRH pulse generator to sex steroid inhibition in susceptible individuals, resulting in increased GnRH pulse frequency and subsequent abnormalities in gonadotropins secretion, ovarian androgen secretion and ovulation [14]A neuroendocrine hallmark of PCOS is the persistent rapid LH pulsatility, which favors pituitary synthesis of LH over that of FSH and contributes to the increased LH concentrations and LH /FSH ratios typical of PCOS.Inadequate FSH levels contribute to impaired follicular development,whereas elevated LH levels increase ovarian androgen production. On the contrary, luteal phase elevations in progesterone normally slow GnRH pulse frequency but women with PCOS do not experience normal progesterone-mediated slowing,due in part to impaired hypothalamic progesterone sensitivity.This reduction in hypothalamic progesterone sensitivity appears to be mediated by elevated androgens because sensitivity can be restored with the androgen receptor blocker flutamide. The ovulatory and hormonal abnormalities associated with PCOS, generally occur during puberty and are typically associated with hyperandrogenaemia. In addition to hyperandrogenism and ovulatory dysfunction, PCOS is characterized by neuroendocrine abnormalities including a persistently rapid gonadotropin-releasing hormone pulse frequency.Rapid GnRH pulsatility favors pituitary secretion of luteinizing hormone over that of FSH. Excess LH stimulates ovarian androgen production,whereas relative deficits in FSH impair follicular development. The rapid GnRH pulse frequency is a result of reduced progesterone-mediated feedback inhibition of the GnRH pulse generator secondary to infrequent luteal phase increases in progesterone, as well as reduced hypothalamic sensitivity to progesterone feedback. As such, hyperandrogenemia appears to play an important pathophysiologic role in PCOS [15].Along with elevated LH concentration and pulsatility, some girls with hyperandrogenaemia have impaired hypothalamic progesterone sensitivity similar to that seen in adult women with PCOS. It was supposed that peripubertal hyperandrogenaemia may lead to persistently rapid GnRH pulse frequency through impaired hypothalamic feedback inhibition. The subsequent abnormalities in gonadotropin secretion, androgen production and ovulatory function might support progression towards the adult PCOS phenotype [16].Growing evidence shows the primary role of androgens in pathophysiology of PCOS and metabolic derangement. The hypothesis suggested by Abbott states that PCOS is a genetically determined ovarian disorder characterized by excessive androgen production and that the heterogeneity can be explained on the basis of the interaction of this disorder with other genes and with the environment [17].

The theory that PCOS represent the common end point of several genetic and environmental, aetiological factors, was largely supported [17]. Therefore, the exposure to androgens excess , in human females, at any stage from foetal development of the ovary to the onset of puberty, could lead to many of the characteristic features of PCOS including abnormalities of LH secretion and insulin resistance (IR). A study on a sample of 235 middle-aged women whose size at birth was recorded in detail led to conclude that the two common forms of PCOS have different origins in intrauterine life: obese, hirsute women with polycystic ovaries have higher than normal ovarian secretion of androgens that are associated with high birth weight and maternal obesity, while the thin women with polycystic ovaries have altered hypothalamic control of LH release resulting from prolonged gestation [18]. A strong association between polycystic ovaries and large birth weight has also been described by Michelmore et al in a population-based study. In this study there were no differences in birth weight between women with polycystic ovaries alone and those with features of PCOS [19].However,the nature of the association between high birth weight and polycystic ovaries/ PCOS is uncertain and contrasts with recent reports of low birth weight in girls with precocious pubarche,hyperinsulinaemia and hyperandrogenism [20,21].Although it is unlikely that a fetal origin of PCOS in humans is based on exogenous ,environmental or maternal hyperandrogenism. Androgen excess originating from the fetal ovary or adrenal cortex, which are steroidogenically active during the second trimester of prenatal life could well explain many of the manifestations that present as PCOS. Finally, exposure of the foetal hypothalamic-pituitary-ovarian axis to androgen excess, influences the dynamics of early follicular development and can set up a train of events, which result in both the reproductive and metabolic sequences of PCOS [22].In conclusion, the LH hypothesis supposes a primary neuro- endocrine defect leading to exaggerated LH pulse frequency and amplitude resulting in ovarian hyperandrogenism;.the mechanisms underlying the reduced hypothalamic sensitivity, however, remain unclear. The potential roles of hyperinsulinaemia and hyperandrogenaemia often present in women with PCOS, in modifying ovarian steroid regulation of GnRH pulse generator have to be clarified, although an intrinsic abnormality could not also be excluded.

Ovarian-Pituitary Feedback

Classic studies in primates have demonstrated that pulsatile secretion of GnRH is an important prerequisite for normal pituitary function and that the regulation of gonadotrophin levels is controlled by ovarian steroid feedback on the anterior pituitary cells [23].

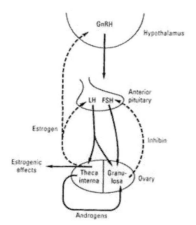

The theca cells provide androgens to the granulosa cells and produce the circulating estrogens that inhibit the secretion of GnRH, LH and FSH. Inhibin from the granulosa cells inhibits FSH secretion.

Figure 4

Thus, low levels of oestrogen inhibit LH and FSH at the pituitary level; FSH more than LH [24]. High levels of oestrogen exhibit a positive stimulatory feedback with LH, inducing the LH surge at midcycle, whereas high steady levels of oestrogen lead to sustained elevated LH secretion [25]. In addition, low levels of progesterone acting at the level of the pituitary gland enhance the LH response to GnRH and are responsible for the FSH surge at midcycle. As a consequence, the question of whether the gonadotropin abnormalities seen in PCOS might be secondary to an oestrogenic effect on the pituitary or even more to an effect of androgens, independent of their aromatization to oestrogens, at the level of the hypothalamus and/or the pituitary, has been considered. Although the data are inconsistent, they mainly suggest that if a primary abnormality of serum sex steroids concentrations has a stimulatory effect on LH secretion in PCOS, this effect must be minimal [26]. In addition, raising serum androgen concentrations in normal women or women with the PCOS does not stimulate the secretion of luteinizing hormone [27,28]. Although many hypotheses have been proposed for the aetiology of pituitary hypersecretion of LH, none of these fully explains the underlying neuroendocrine abnormality that leads to exaggerated LH pulse frequency. On the other hand, it is also clear that an elevated LH concentration is not necessary for ovarian dysregulation [29]. Indeed, hypersecretion of LH occurs only in approximately one-third of women with PCOS, particularly in nonobese patients [30]. Furthermore, there is a subgroup of hypogonadotropic patients with ultrasound finding of polycystic ovaries, in which the ovarian response to ovulation induction with pulsatile GHRH, is similar to patients with PCOS. Particularly, some observations not only found much higher serum LH concentrations following ovulation induction with GnRH in this group of patients, compared to hypogonadotropic patients with ultrasonographically normal ovaries, but also found that this difference preceded any observed changes in oestradiol levels [30]. This could suggest that the primary lesion in PCOS is in the ovary, with pituitary hypersecretion of LH secondary to disturbed ovarian feedback signaling.

References

[1] Yen SS, Vela P,Rankin J. Inappropriate secretion of follicle-stimulating hormone and luteinizing hormone in polycystic ovarian disease. *J. Clin. Endocrinol. Metab.* 1970;30(4):435-42.

[2] Barnes RB, Rosenfield RL, Ehrmann DA,Cara JF,Cuttler L,Levitsky LL,Rosenthal IMOvarian hyperandrogenism as result of congenital adrenal virilizing disorders: evidence for perinatal masculinization of neuroendocrine function in women. *J. Clin. Endocrinol. Metab.* 1994;79:1328-1333.

[3] Apter D, Bützow T, Laughlin GA, Yen SS. Accelerated 24-hour luteinizing hormone pulsatile activity in adolescent girls with ovarian hyperandrogenism: relevance to the developmental phase of polycystic ovarian syndrome. *J. Clin. Endocrinol. Metab.* 1994 Jul;79(1):119-25.

[4] Taylor AE. The gonadotropic axis in hyperandrogenic adolescents. *J. Pediatr. Endocrinol. Metab.* 2000;13 Suppl 5:1281-4.

[5] Venturoli S, Porcu E, Fabbri R, Magrini O, Gammi L, Paradisi R, Forcacci M, Bolzani R, Flamigni C. Episodic pulsatile secretion of FSH, LH, prolactin, oestradiol, oestrone, and LH circadian variations in polycystic ovary syndrome. *Clin. Endocrinol.* (Oxf). 1988 ;28(1):93-107.

[6] Hall JE, Taylor AE, Hayes FJ, Crowley WF Jr.Insights into hypothalamic-pituitary dysfunction in polycystic ovary syndrome. *J. Endocrinol. Invest.* 1998 ;21(9):602-11

[7] Yen SS, Apter D, Bützow T, Laughlin GA.Gonadotrophin releasing hormone pulse generator activity before and during sexual maturation in girls: new insights. *Hum. Reprod.* 1993 Nov;8 Suppl 2:66-71.

[8] Fauser BC, Pache TD, Hop WC, de Jong FH, Dahl KD.The significance of a single serum LH measurement in women with cycle disturbances: discrepancies between immunoreactive and bioactive hormone estimates. *Clin. Endocrinol. (Oxf).* 1992 Nov;37(5):445-52.

[9] Imse V, Holzapfel G, Hinney B, Kuhn W, Wuttke W. Comparison of luteinizing hormone pulsatility in the serum of women suffering from polycystic ovarian disease using a bioassay and five different immunoassays. *J. Clin. Endocrinol. Metab.* 1992 May;74(5):1053-61.

[10] Marshall JC, Eagleson CA.Neuroendocrine aspects of polycystic ovary syndrome. *Endocrinol. Metab. Clin. North Am.* 1999 Jun;28(2):295-324. Review.

[11] Christman GM, Randolph JF, Kelch RP, Marshall JC. Reduction of gonadotropin-releasing hormone pulse frequency is associated with subsequent selective follicle-stimulating hormone secretion in women with polycystic ovarian disease. *J. Clin. Endocrinol Metab.* 1991 ;72(6):1278-85

[12] Pastor CL, Griffin-Korf ML, Aloi JA, Evans WS, Marshall JC.Polycystic ovary syndrome: evidence for reduced sensitivity of the gonadotropin-releasing hormone

pulse generator to inhibition by estradiol and progesterone. *J. Clin. Endocrinol. Metab.* 1998 Feb;83(2):582-90.

[13] Rumsby G, Fielder AH, Hague WM, Honour JW.Heterogeneity in the gene locus for steroid 21-hydroxylase deficiency. *J. Med. Genet.* 1988 Sep;25(9):596-9

[14] Blank SK, McCartney CR, Helm KD, Marshall JC.Neuroendocrine effects of androgens in adult polycystic ovary syndrome and female puberty. *Semin. Reprod. Med.* 2007 Sep;25(5):352-9. Review

[15] Blank SK, McCartney CR, Marshall JC.The origins and sequelae of abnormal neuroendocrine function in polycystic ovary syndrome. *Hum. Reprod. Update.* 2006 Jul-Aug;12(4):351-61. Review.

[16] Abbott DH, Barnett DK, Bruns CM, Dumesic DA. Androgen excess fetal programming of female reproduction: a developmental aetiology for polycystic ovary syndrome? *Hum. Reprod. Update.* 2005 ;11(4):357-74. Review.

[17] Franks S,Mc Carthy MI,Hardy K.Development of polycystic ovarian syndrome:Involvement of genetic and environmental factors. *Int. J. Androl.* 2006;29:278-85.

[18] Cresswell JL, Barker DJ, Osmond C, Egger P, Phillips DI, Fraser RB. Fetal growth, length of gestation, and polycystic ovaries in adult life. *Lancet* 1997; 350: 1131-5

[19] Michelmore K, Ong K, Mason S, Bennett S, Perry L, Vessey M, Balen A, Dunger D.Clinical features in women with polycystic ovaries: relationships to insulin sensitivity, insulin gene VNTR and birth weight. *Clin. Endocrinol. (Oxf).* 2001 Oct;55(4):439-46.

[20] Ibáñez L, Jaramillo A, Enríquez G, Miró E, López-Bermejo A, Dunger D, de Zegher F.Polycystic ovaries after precocious pubarche: relation to prenatal growth. *Hum. Reprod.* 2007 Feb;22(2):395-400.

[21] 21. .Ibáñez L, de Zegher F, Potau N.Premature pubarche, ovarian hyperandrogenism, hyperinsulinism and the polycystic ovary syndrome: from a complex constellation to a simple sequence of prenatal onset. *J. Endocrinol. Invest.* 1998 Oct;21(9):558-66. Review.

[22] Abbott DH, Dumesic DA, Franks S.Developmental origin of polycystic ovary syndrome - a hypothesis. *J. Endocrinol.* 2002 Jul;174(1):1-5. Review.

[23] Mais V, Kazer RR, Cetel NS, Rivier J, Vale W, Yen SS. The dependency of folliculogenesis and corpus luteum function on pulsatile gonadotropin secretion in cycling women using a gonadotropin-releasing hormone antagonist as a probe. *J. Clin. Endocrinol. Metab.* 1986 Jun;62(6):1250-5.

[24] Gharib SD, Wierman ME, Shupnik MA, Chin WW. Molecular biology of the pituitary gonadotropins. *Endocr. Rev.* 1990 Feb;11(1):177-99. Review.

[25] Keye WR Jr, Jaffe RB.Strength-duration characteristics of estrogen effects on gonadotropin response to gonadotropin-releasing hormone in women. I. Effects of varying duration of estradiol administration. *J. Clin. Endocrinol. Metab.* 1975 Dec;41(06):1003-8 30.

[26] Ehrmann DA, Barnes RB, Rosenfield RL. Polycystic ovary syndrome as a form of functional ovarian hyperandrogenism due to dysregulation of androgen secretion. *Endocr. Rev.* 1995;16:322–353.

[27] Spinder T, Spijkstra JJ, van den Tweel JG, Burger CW, van Kessel H, Hompes PG, Gooren LJ.The effects of long term testosterone administration on pulsatile luteinizing

hormone secretion and on ovarian histology in eugonadal female to male transsexual subjects. *J. Clin. Endocrinol. Metab.* 1989 Jul;69(1):151-7.

[28] Dunaif A.Do androgens directly regulate gonadotropin secretion in the polycystic ovary syndrome? *J. Clin. Endocrinol. Metab.* 1986 Jul;63(1):215-21.

[29] Ehrmann DA, Rosenfield RL, Barnes RB, Brigell DF, Sheikh Z. Detection of functional ovarian hyperandrogenism in women with androgen excess. *N. Engl. J. Med.* 1992;327:157–162.

[30] Balen AH, Conway GS, Kaltas G, Techatrasak K, Manning PJ, West C, Jacobs HS. Polycystic ovary syndrome: the spectrum of the disorders in 1741 patients. *Human Reproduction* 1995; 10: 2107-11.

Ovarian Hypothesis

Ovarian dysfunction in PCOS is associated with an increased population of primordial follicles, suggesting that its origin may be in the fetal ovary [1]. The affected ovary may be genetically predisposed to secrete androgens excess, possibly in utero, probably in infancy and certainly at the onset of puberty [2,3]. The ovarian theory is originally based on the known stimulatory effect of LH on theca cell function and,on the increase, in classic PCOS, of serum LH levels at baseline and in response to GnRH . In fact, LH excess impairs hyperandrogenism through ovarian stimulus to androgenesis [4,5] Some clinical and experimental observations seem to deny the primary role of the LH increase in the pathogenesis of PCOS. In practice,the perplexity is based on these considerations: theca cells of polycystic ovaries secrete abnormal amounts of steroids in culture, whether before and after LH stimulation [6]

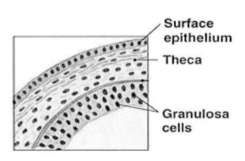

In the past, an alternative model of PCOS origin was also proposed , based on the hypothesis of a gonadotropin-dependent ovarian hyperandrogenism in which the central abnormality is an elevated intraovarian androgen concentration (6,7). It was suggested that women with PCOS have increased formation of 17α-hydroxy progesterone and androstenedione in response to LH because of abnormal enzymatic regulation of steroidogenesis (7,8,9).

Figure 5

Furthermore, when PCOS women receive LH analogue they exhibit hyperresponse of 17-hydroxyprogesterone and androstenedione that remain after normalization [9,10,11].Patients with androgen secreting ovarian neoplasms, as thecoma, have an high LH that returns to normal after tumour removal and, ovulation was often reported following ovarian wedge resection or ovarian cauterization [12,13,14]. Another consideration is based on the observation that the decrease in circulating androgens precede the fall in LH.Currently, several studies on pattern of ovarian steroid secretion,suggested that there is a generalized dysregulation, envoling the theca cell production, which is particularly prominent at the level of 17-hydroxylase and 17, 20-lyase activities [15].This is in contrast to normal women , who when given a single dose of a GnRH agonist, have a premature LH and follicle stimulating hormone increase that is of preovulatory measure and in whom plasma estradiol and estrone rise 3-fold within 24 hours [16]. It is important to remember that this process, in normal women is fairly efficient and there is relatively little elevation in the circulating estradiol precursors. Ovary is considered the main source of the hyperandrogenism in polycystic ovary syndrome. The former type of ovarian dysfunction typical of PCOS,has been found in more than half of hyperandrogenic patients, many of whom lack the classic criteria for the diagnosis of PCOS. An elevated plasma 17-hydroxyprogesterone response to GnRH agonist was found in 58% of hyperandrogenic patients.Interestingly, 96% of such responders had an abnormal dexamethasone androgen-suppression test, suggesting that it was also equally specific for PCOS.Impaired adrenal function is common in patients with PCOS; however, the androstenedione hyper response is less high than 17-hydroxyprogesterone hyper response [17]. Abnormal regulation of cytochrome P450 17 alpha is believed to cause the exaggerated 17-hydroxyprogesterone response to ACTH stimulation. However, in the study of Luboshitzky et al no differences statistically significant between PCOS and control groups were noted during the LDT (cortisol and 17 OH Progesterone levels before, and 30 and 60 minutes after the IV injection of 1 microg ACTH);while, the SDT (standard test: levels of cortisol and 17 OH Progesterone before, and 30 and 60 minutes after the IV injection of 250 microg ACTH) revealed exaggerated 17 OHP response to ACTH stimulation [18]. Therefore, the abnormal response is revealed by stimulation at a pharmacological dose (250 microg) but not by a physiological dose (1 microg). In any case, also this observation do not solve the question on whether the abnormal theca cell response is a consequence of residual thecal cell hyperplasia from antecedent LH stimulation,or not [19,20]. Adrenal glands may also be involved in the pathogenesis of PCOS. To investigate this possibility and to find out if buserelin test is able to distinguish PCOS patients from the patients with idiopathic hirsutism (IH), ACTH and buserelin tests were performed in 29 women with PCOS, 21 women with IH, and 20 control subjects (CS). Significantly higher basal and ACTH-stimulated levels of stimulated cortisol and DHEA-S in PCOS ,compared with controls and patients with IH, reflect that adrenal hyperactivity also plays a role in hyperandrogenemia seen in PCOS.

PCOS patients also possessed significantly higher basal and stimulated 17-hydroxyprogesterone levels, during buserelin testing , when compared with IH patients and CS. Because of the lack of the correlation between ACTH-stimulated and buserelin-stimulated 17-OH P levels, it is hard to say that adrenal hyperactivity seen in PCOS is the result of the dysregulation of cytochrome P450c17-alpha enzyme.These results suggest that buserelin test which is a GnRH analogue could distinguish at least some of the patients with PCOS from the other patients presenting with the common symptoms of hyperandrogenemia [21]. Today, many data are against such a primary role for LH excess in PCOS; mainly, it is known that ovarian hyperandrogenism can have the same frequency with or without the classic PCOS feature of LH excess;even though it could be supposed that these patients can secrete a LH molecule with enhanced bioactivity,or that gonadotropin levels inversely correlate with the adiposity of PCOS patients, and that the hyperinsulinemia of obesity amplifies the effect of normal gonadotropin levels [22,23,24,25]. LH as HCG,FSH and TSH (thyroid stimulating factor) is a α/ ß heterodimer with a common α subunit and a unique ß subunit. The ß subunit confers the hormonal specificity .In 1992, an immunological variant of LH (v-LH) was found in a healthy Finnish woman who was fertile and had normal levels of all other hormones measured. The gene encoding her LH ß was sequenced and two base changes in N-terminal region were identified. In practice, the first mutation in codon 8 changes tryptophan to arginine ,and the second in codon 15 changes isoleucine to threonine [26]. Following, it was showed that these mutations have a worldwide distribution [27, 28, 29]. V-LH showed in vitro an elevated bioactivity compared to that of normal LH [30].Besides, it seems that the LH action in carriers of the v-LH allele differ from that in non carriers. In addition, some studies supported the association of the v-LH mutations with high levels of serum E 2,T and SHBG in the follicular phase of the menstrual cycle, in obese PCOS women ,in menstrual disorders and in infertility [27,31,32, 33]. No differences were observed in LH pulsatility between normal control and women with homozygosis for the variant LH hormone; however, the altered bioactivity and in vivo kinetics of the variant might induce subtle changes in LH action [30]. Differences in circulatory kinetics of the two types of LH may explain the differences in LH function between women with ovulatory disorders and women with normal ovulatory cycles. In addition ,the maximal response of the variant LH to pituitary stimulation with GnRH seems to be greater than that of normal - type LH [34,35]. Within the last years, several other mutations of the LH ß subunit were discovered. Particularly ,in 1996 Roy reported seven novel mutations in LH beta-subunit gene identified by PCR-SSCP method. (Polymerase chain chain –SSCP) [36]. The increased LH secretion, as expressed by the LH/ FSH (follicle-stimulating hormone) ratio, is positively correlated with the increased free estradiol [19,37]. The LH/FSH ratio exhibit greater accuracy than total testosterone and average ovarian volume for evaluation of women with oligomenorrhea or anovulation. The LH/FSH ratio > 1 showed the best combination of sensitivity and specificity. A LH/FSH ratio of 2-3/ 1 is generally considered to indicate abnormal gonadotropin secretion. Body mass index(BMI) seems positively correlated with total testosterone in women with and without PCOS. However, BMI is negatively correlated with LH in PCOS but shows no correlation in non PCOS subjects.[38]. In any case, an increased LH-pulse frequency in PCOS , independent of BMI or adiposity, is well established. Obesity only seems to lower the LH pulse amplitude and the peak increment of LH in response to GnRH stimulation, but the LH pulse frequency in PCOS women is not influenced by BMI [27,39]. The downregulation response in normal women is because normal ovarian thecal cells respond to LH in a biphasic manner, increasing their steroid output in response to LH levels only to a point (at LH levels in the normal range for the early to midfollicular phase of the menstrual cycle), and ceasing to respond when LH levels exceed this The process of desensitization may in part involve downregulation of the number of LH receptor sites on thecal cells,and may be partly due to downregulation of thecal androgen biosynthesis by the local paracrine factors produced by the granulosa cells in response to LH.[40] .It seems that transforming growth factor-beta (TGF beta) could be produced by thecal - interstitial cells (TIC) ; consequently, TGF beta could be an autocrine regulator of TIC function. The study of Magoffin showed, in the rats, that the LH administration (50ng/ml) produced an important increase of androsterone level (100- fold at 2 days and 60-fold at 4 and 6 days).The concomitant treatment with TGF beta (10ng/ml) caused a 65% inhibition of aldosterone production at each time period. Furthermore, this experimental study reported a similar inhibition of androstenedione, while the progesterone resulted significantly increased. However, the progesterone increase was obtained only with the greatest doses of TGF beta($\geq$ 10 ng / ml). Particularly, TGF beta not interfered with the sensitivity of theca cells to LH. Besides, the synergistic stimulation of LH action by IGF-1 could be blocked by TGF beta. In addition seems that TGF beta alone or in combination with LH might increase the P450c17 without altering alpha protein content(17 alpha hydroxylase and 17,20 lyase)[40] .In PCOS, there is an escape from such desensitization and this implies that the ovarian dysfunction must be independent to LH excess. Normal theca cells are very sensitive to the downregulating effect of LH levels within the physiologic range [9,41] Normally, luteal progesterone (P) slows GnRH pulses favoring FSH synthesis and the later rise in FSH. While, hyperandrogenic women with PCO,exhibit exaggerated 17hydroxyprogesterone responses than those observed in normal women. Therefore, higher P level is required to suppress GnRH pulses indicating insensitivity to P feedback in hyperandrogenemia [8,42].Plasma 17-hydroxyprogesterone hyperresponsiveness to GnRH agonist testing is typical of polycystic ovary syndrome and other functional ovarian hyperandrogenism that does not meet criteria for the diagnosis of PCOS [8] .Anovulatory women with PCOS also have a higher luteinizing hormone (LH) and gonadotropin-releasing hormone (GnRH) pulse frequency and amplitude when compared to the normal midfollicular phase. This enhanced pulsatile secretion of GnRH was attributed to a reduction in hypothalamic opioid inhibition or to decreased sensitivity of the GnRH pulse generator to inhibition by ovarian steroids, particularly progesterone or to still unknown factors. Maximal stimulation of 17-hydroxyprogesterone and androstenedione in culture normally occurs at LH concentrations approximating the upper portion of the normal range for follicular phase serum LH levels, and a further increase in LH dosage leads to no further rise. Nevertheless, the possibility exists that the disproportionate 17-hydroxyprogesterone response to stimulation by gonadotropins in patients with PCOS and functional ovarian hyperandrogenism, might be explained by their LH levels on the LH-steroid dose-response curve being at a higher point where there could be incipient downregulation of 17,20-lyase at LH levels stimulatory to 17-hydroxylation.However, some researchers have shown that LH-steroid dose-response relationships during GnRH agonist tests are similarly abnormal in patients with or without elevated serum LH levels [8]. Following GnRH agonist administration, the responses of estradiol fall along the normal LH-steroid dose-response slope, but those of estradiol precursors do not. The apparent slope of the LH-steroid dose-response relationship is markedly abnormal for 17hydroxyprogesterone, above but parallel to normal for androstenedione, and slightly increased for testosterone. These data suggest that although 17,20-lyase efficiency is increased, it is increased less than that of 17-hydroxylation. These results also suggest that patients with functional ovarian hyperandrogenism, regardless of whether they have classic or nonclassic PCOS, have an LH-17-hydroxyprogesterone dose-response curve that is shifted upward and to the left. It was hypothesized that this earlier presentation of PCOS may relate to increased androgen sensitivity, indicated by androgen receptor gene CAG repeat length. Since the steroid responses do not fall along the normal LH-steroid dose-response curve, the defect in steroidogenesis must therefore be the result of escape from normal down- regulation of thecal cell secretion rather than over-stimulation by LH [43]. If we consider these results, then the fundamental defect underlying the androgen excess of PCOS is the ovarian hyper-responsiveness to gonadotropin action because of escape from downregulation and not a primary result of excess LH per se. The pattern of steroid secretion in polycystic ovary is thought to suggest a generalized dysregulation of ovarian androgen secretion, which is prominent at the level of 17 α-hydroxylase and 17,20 lyase activities. Furthermore, a primary dysregulation of ovarian P450c17 in the theca cell has been hypothesized.

References

[1] Webber LJ,Stubbs S,Stark J,Trew GH, Margara R,Hardy K,Franks S.Formation and early development of follicles in the polycystic ovary. *Lancet* 2003; 362(9389): 1017-21.

[2] Abbott DH, Dumesic DA, Franks S.Developmental origin of polycystic ovary syndrome - a hypothesis. *J. Endocrinol.* 2002 Jul;174(1):1-5. Review.

[3] Franks S,Mc Carthy MI,Hardy K.Development of polycystic ovarian syndrome:Involvement of genetic and environmental factors. *Int. J. Androl.* 2006;29:278-85.

[4] Blank SK, McCartney CR, Helm KD, Marshall JC.Neuroendocrine effects of androgens in adult polycystic ovary syndrome and female puberty. *Semin. Reprod. Med.* 2007 Sep;25(5):352-9. Review

[5] Blank SK, McCartney CR, Marshall JC.The origins and sequelae of abnormal neuroendocrine function in polycystic ovary syndrome. *Hum. Reprod. Update.* 2006 Jul-Aug;12(4):351-61. Review

[6] Gilling-Smith C, Story H, Rogers V, Franks S. Evidence for a primary abnormality of thecal cell steroidogenesis in the polycystic ovary syndrome. *Clin. Endocrinol. (Oxf)* 1997;47:93–99.

[7] Rosenfield RL. Hyperandrogenism in peripubertal girls. *Pediatr. Clin. North Am.* 1990 ;37(6):1333-58. Review.

[8] Rosenfield RL, Barnes RB, Ehrmann DA. Studies of the nature of 17-hydroxyprogesterone hyperresponsiveness to gonadotropin-releasing hormone agonist challenge in functional ovarian hyperandrogenism. *J. Clin. Endocrinol. Metab.* 1994;79:1686–1692.

[9] Barnes RB, Rosenfield RL, Burstein S, Ehrmann DA. Pituitary-ovarian responses to nafarelin testing in the polycystic ovary syndrome. *N. Engl. J. Med.* 1989; 320:559–565.

[10] Ibañez L, Hall JE, Potau N, Carrascosa A, Prat N, Taylor AE.. Ovarian 17-hydroxyprogesterone hyperresponsiveness to gonadotropin-releasing hormone (GnRH) agonist challenge in women with polycystic ovary syndrome is not mediated by luteinizing hormone hypersecretion: evidence from GnRH agonist and human chorionic gonadotropin stimulation testing. *J. Clin. Endocrinol. Metab.* 1996;81:4103–4107.

[11] Levrant SG, Barnes RB, Rosenfield RL. A pilot study of the human chorionic gonadotrophin test for ovarian hyperandrogenism. *Hum. Reprod.* 1997;12:1416–1420

[12] Dunaif A, Scully RE, Andersen RN, Chapin DS, Crowley WF Jr. The effects of continuous androgen secretion on the hypothalamic-pituitary axis in woman: evidence from a luteinized thecoma of the ovary. *J. Clin. Endocrinol. Metab.* 1984;59:389–393.

[13] Judd HL, Rigg LA, Anderson DC, Yen SS. The effects of ovarian wedge resection on circulating gonadotropin and ovarian steroid levels in patients with polycystic ovary syndrome. *J. Clin. Endocrinol. Metab.* 1976;43:347–355.

[14] Greenblatt E, Casper RF. Endocrine changes after laparoscopic ovarian cautery in polycystic ovarian syndrome. *Am. J. Obstet. Gynecol.* 1987;156:279–285.

[15] Wickenheisser JK, Nelson-DeGrave VL, McAllister JM.Human ovarian theca cells in culture. *Trends Endocrinol. Metab.* 2006 ;17(2):65-71.

[16] Ehrmann DA, Barnes RB, Rosenfield RL.Polycystic ovary syndrome as a form of functional ovarian hyperandrogenism due to dysregulation of androgen secretion. *Endocr. Rev.* 1995;16(3): 322-53

[17] Ehrmann DA, Rosenfield RL, Barnes RB, Brigell DF, Sheikh Z.Detection of functional ovarian hyperandrogenism in women with androgen excess.) *N. Engl. J. Med.* 1992 ;327(3):157-62.

[18] Luboshitzky R,Ishai A,Shen-Or Z,Herer P. Evaluation of the pituitary-adrenal axis in hyperandrogenemic women with polycystic ovary syndrome Neuro Endocrinol. *Lett.* 2003; 24(3-4):249-54.

[19] Rosenfield RL. Is polycystic ovary syndrome a neuroendocrine or an ovarian disorder? *Clin. Endocrinol. (Oxf)* 1997; 47:423–424.

[20] Sahin Y, Kelestimur F. 17-Hydroxyprogesterone response to buserelin testing in the polycystic ovary syndrome. *Clin. Endocrinol. (Oxf)* 1993;39:151–155.

[21] Kamel N, Tonyukuk V, Emral R, Corapçioğlu D, Baştemir M, Güllü SRole of ovary and adrenal glands in hyperandrogenemia in patients with polycystic ovary syndrome. *Exp. Clin. Endocrinol. Diabetes.* 2005 Feb;113(2):115-21.

[22] Fauser BC, Pache TD, Lamberts SW, Hop WC, de Jong FH, Dahl KD. Serum bioactive and immunoreactive luteinizing hormone and follicle-stimulating hormone levels in women with cycle abnormalities, with or without polycystic ovarian disease. *J. Clin. Endocrinol. Metab.* 1991;73:811–817.

[23] Imse V, Holzapfel G, Hinney B, Kuhn W, Wuttke W. Comparison of luteinizing hormone pulsatility in the serum of women suffering from polycystic ovarian disease using a bioassay and five different immunoassays. *J. Clin. Endocrinol. Metab.* 1992;74:1053–1061.

[24] Arroyo A, Laughlin GA, Morales AJ, Yen SS. Inappropriate gonadotropin secretion in polycystic ovary syndrome: influence of adiposity. *J. Clin. Endocrinol. Metab.* 1997;82:3728–3733.

[25] Taylor AE, McCourt B, Martin KA, Anderson EJ, Adams JM, Schoenfeld D, Hall JE. Determinants of abnormal gonadotropin secretion in clinically defined women with polycystic ovary syndrome. *J. Clin. Endocrinol. Metab*. 1997;82:2248–2256.

[26] Pettersson K, Ding YQ, Huhtaniemi I. An immunologically anomalous luteinizing hormone variant in a healthy woman. *J. Clin. Endocrinol. Metab*. 1992;74(1):164-71.

[27] Furui K,Suganuma S,Tsukahara S,Asada Y,Kikkawa F,Tanaka M, Ozawa T, Tomoda Y. Identification of two point mutations in the gene coding luteinizing hormone (LH) beta-subunut, associated with immunologically LH variants. *J. Clin. Endocrinol. Metab*. 1994;78(1): 107-13.

[28] Okuda K,Yamada T,Imoto H,Komatsubara H,Sugimoto O. Antigenic alteration of an anomalous human luteinizing hormone caused by two chorionic gonadotropin –type amino-acid substitutions. *Biochem. Biophys. Res. Commun*. 1994;200(1):584-90.

[29] Nilsson C,Pettersson K,Millar RP,Coerver KA , Matzuk MM,Huhtaniemi IT. Worldwide frequency of a common genetic variant of luteinizing hormone:an international collaborative research.International Collaborative Research Group. *Fertil. Steril*. 1997;67(6): 998-1004.

[30] Haavisto AM, Pettersson K,Bergendahl M,Virkamaki A., Huhtaniemi I. Occurrence and biological properties of a common genetic variant of luteinizing hormone. *J. Clin. Endocrinol. Metab*. 1995; 80(4): 1257-63.

[31] Rajkhowa M,Talbot JA,Jones PW,Pettersson K, Haavisto AM,Huhtaniemi I,Clayton RN. Prevalence of an immunological LH beta- subunit variant in a UK population of healthy women and women with polycystic ovary syndrome. *Clin. Endocrinol*. 1995: 43(3):297-303.

[32] Suganuma N,Furui K,Kikkawa F,Tomoda Y,Furuhashi M. Effects of the mutations (Tpr8 > Arg and Iie15> Thr) in huma luteinizing hormone(LH) beta-subunit on LH bioactivity in vitro and in vivo. *Endocrinology* 1996; 137(3):831-8.

[33] Takahashi K, Karino K, Kanasaki H, Miyazaki K. Altered kinetics of pituitary response to gonadotropin-releasing hormone with variant luteinizing hormone: correlation with ovulatory disorders. *Horm. Res*. 2004;61(1):27-32.

[34] Takahashi K,Kurioka H,Ozaki T,Kanasaki H,Miyazaki K,Karino K. Pituitary response to luteinizing hormone-releasing hormone in women with variant luteinizing hormone. *Eur. J. Endocrinol*. 2000;143(3):375-81.

[35] Roy AC, Liao WX, Chen Y, Arulkumaran S, Ratnam SS. Identification of seven novel mutations in LH beta-subunit gene by SSCP. Mol. *Cell. Biochem*. 1996;165(2):151-3

[36] Lobo RA, Granger L, Goehelsmann U, Mishell DR Jr. Elevations in unbound serum estradiol as a possible mechanism for inappropriate gonadotropin secretion in women with PCO. *J. Clin. Endocrinol. Metab*. 1981;52:156-8.

[37] Hsu MI, Liou TH, Liang SJ, Su HW,Wu CH, Hsu CS. Inappropriate gonadotropin secretion in polycystic ovary syndrome. *Fertil. Steril*. 2009;91(4): 1168-74.

[38] Morales AJ, Laughlin GA, Bützow T, Maheshwari H, Baumann G, Yen SSC 1996 Insulin, somatotropic, and luteinizing hormones axes in lean and obese women with polycystic ovary syndrome: common and distinct features. *J. Clin. Endocrinol. Metab*. 81:2854–2864.

[39] Rosenfield RL. Ovarian and adrenal function in polycystic ovary syndrome. *Endocrinol. Metab. Clin. North Am*. 1999;28:265–293.

[40] Magoffin DA,Gancedo B,Erickson GF. Transforming growth factor-beta promotes differentiation of ovarian thecal-interstitial cells but inhibits androgen production. *Endocrinology* 1989;125(4): 1951-8.

[41] Nobels F, Dewailly D. Puberty and polycystic ovarian syndrome: the insulin/insulin-like growth factor I hypothesis. *Fertil. Steril.* 1992;58:655–666.

[42] Burger CW, Korsen TJ, van Kessel H, van Dop PA, Caron FJ, Schoemaker J. Pulsatile luteinizing hormone patterns in the follicular phase of the menstrual cycle, polycystic ovarian disease (PCOD) and non-PCOD secondary amenorrhea. *J. Clin. Endocrinol. Metab.* 1985;61:1126-32.

[43] Rosenfield RL. Is polycystic ovary syndrome a neuroendocrine or an ovarian disorder? *Clin. Endocrinol.* (Oxf) 1997; 47:423–424.

Ovarian Steroid Biosynthesis

Although each cell type of the ovary possess the complete enzymatic complement required for steroid hormone synthesis,the predominant hormones formed differ among cell types. In the ovarian follicle, the Δ5-pathway is preferred for the formation of androgens and oestrogens, because theca cells of human ovary metabolize 17-OH Pregnenolone more efficiently than 17-OHP. The factors which determine what steroid is secreted by each cell type include the levels of gonodotrophin and gonodotrophin receptors, the expression of steroidogenic enzymes, and the availability of LDL cholesterol. A hallmark of PCOS is the excessive theca cell androgen secretion, which is directly linked to the symptoms of PCOS. It was also showed that increased androgen production is a stable steroidogenic phenotype of PCOS theca cells [1,2]. The theory that PCOS results from a primary abnormality of androgen biosynthesis was supported by Ehrmann *et al.*who affirmed that the dysregulation of the steroid biosynthesis and metabolism, prominently but not exclusively, involves P450c17 enzyme activities [3].These observations led to hypothesize that the hyperandrogenaemia associated with PCOS results from an intrinsic abnormality of ovarian theca cell steroidogenesis [4,5].

Steroid Secretion of Theca Cell

In an attempt to identify the biochemical basis for the increased testosterone production in PCOS theca cells, Nelson *et al.* examined 17β-hydroxysteroid dehydrogenase (17βHSD) isoform expression in long-term cultures of theca and granulosa cells isolated from normal and PCOS ovaries. 17βHSD-specific isoforms catalyze the final step in the conversion of androstenedione to testosterone.They reported that P450c17 and 3βHSD enzyme activities were increased by more than 500% and 1000%, respectively, in PCOS theca cells compared with controls, whereas 17βHSD enzyme activity was unaffected. They concluded that the increased synthesis of testosterone precursors could be the primary factor driving enhanced testosterone secretion in PCOS [5].Hence, although a number of researchers have proposed that

C17,20 lyase activity is disproportionately increased in PCOS, this new data suggests that both 17α-hydroxylase and C17, 20- lyase activities are coordinately increased in PCOS theca cells.Therefore,450c17 containing both 17 α-hydroxylase and 17,20-lyase activities ,seems to be the key factor in the formation of steroid hormones in the adrenals and in the gonads. These enzymatic activities are encoded by the gene CYP17 and their expression is strongly linked to levels of the LH in the ovary and of the ACTH in the adrenal cortex [6,7]. Furthermore, androgen secretion is also modulated by two other enzymes, not members of the P450gene: 3α-hydroxysteroid dehydrogenase type 2(3ß-HSD II),expressed in ovary and adrenal gland,and a proteic cholesterol carrier,from the outside to inside of the mitochondrial membrane (steroid acute regulatory protein). Although 17-OH progesterone response to ACTH is significantly higher in the patients with PCOS than in the control subjects, the lack of relationship between 17-OHprogesterone response to GnRH agonist buserelin and 17-OH progesterone response to ACTH stimulation suggest that the dysregulation of the cytochrome P450c 17alpha enzyme may not play a role in adrenal androgen excess seen in PCOS[8,9]. Thus, this dysregulation may be apparent as ovarian dysfunction alone, as adrenal dysfunction alone, or as both . Ovarian stimulation testing has suggested that ovarian hyperandrogenism is a result of dysregulation of the androgen-producing steroidogenic enzymes. On the other hand, ACTH stimulation testing is consistent with dysregulation of adrenal steroidogenic enzymes in about two-thirds of hyperandrogenic women [10].

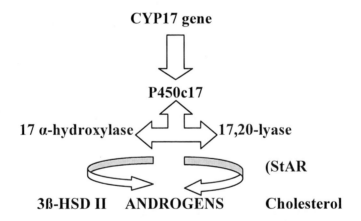

Figure 6

Although adrenal androgen concentrations may be elevated in women with PCOS, the weight of evidence suggests that in most cases, the ovary is the main contributor to excess androgen secretion. In 1993 Bain showed in the mouse that the four 3 ß HSD structural genes (Hsd3b) are closely linked within a segment of chromosome 3 that is conserved on human chromosome 1 [11,12].Several studies suggested that ovarian hyperandrogenemia is inherited as an autosomal dominant trait and that PCOS theca cells have a gene expression profile that is distinct from normal theca cells. Aldehyde dehydrogenase 6 and retinol dehydrogenase 2, which play a role in all-trans-retinoic acid biosynthesis and the transcription factor GATA, were included in the cohort of genes with increased mRNA abundance in PCOS theca cells. A recent study performed at Center for Research on Reproduction and Women's Health, University of Pennsylvania (Philadelphia) demonstrated that retinoic acid and GATA 6 increased the expression of 17alpha-hydroxylase, providing a functional link between altered gene expression and intrinsic abnormalities in PCOS theca cells [2].

Gonadotrophins and Growth Factors

Other evidence for a primary defect at the level of the ovary comes from the classic polycystic ovary morphology. The presence of many follicles with a high androgen to oestrogen ratio was first thought to represent a high rate of follicular atresia. Subsequently, the granulosa cells were shown to be viable and able to respond to FSH production [13]. The functional picture that emerges from arrested granulosa cells and very active theca cells is consistent with a blockage of FSH response, probably through various growth factors. As a consequence, the follicles are unable to successfully change their microenvironment from androgen dominance to oestrogen dominance, being the change essential for continued follicular growth and development. A number of peptides modulate gonadotrophin-dependent ovarian folliculogenesis and steroidogenesis acting by autocrine, paracrine and endocrine mechanisms

Hormonal interactions in early follicular phase.

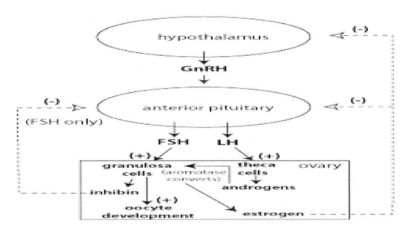

Table 5

Thus, LH stimulation of androgen synthesis appears to be augmented by factors such as inhibin and downregulated by factors such as activin, epidermal growth factor (EGF), transforming growth factor-α (TGF-α) and transforming growth factor-β1 (TGF-β1). It has long been known that inhibin augments LH-stimulated androstenedione production in cultured human theca cells, whereas activin has the opposite effect [14,15] As inhibin also has the ability to selectively inhibit FSH secretion, it was suggested that increased production of inhibin B from the multiple small viable follicles could also be a factor in suppressing FSH secretion [16]. Gonadotrophin-induced ovarian function is also known to be modulated by growth factors. In fact, IGFs and their receptors, binding proteins and proteases are important in normal ovarian follicle development. Overall, it is believed that IGFs stimulate ovarian cellular mitosis, inhibit apoptosis and increase steroidogenesis,mainly by enhancing P450scc enzyme activity and synergizing with LH to upregulate P450c17 production. It is interesting that the expression pattern of the components of the IGF system in the follicular fluid from polycystic ovaries was found to be the same as in atretic follicles, finding consistent with limitation of IGFs activity in PCOS [17,18]. GH itself may also be involved to the genesis and maintenance of hyperandrogenic chronic anovulation and polycystic ovarian morphology, at least in the subgroup of lean PCOS women in whom it is hypersecreted [19].GH actions on growth factors and their binding proteins are known to be similar to those of insulin [20]Recently, Gambineri et al reported that insulin-like factor 3(INSL3),a member of the relaxin-insulin family,could be related to a greater 17OH-progesterone response to buserelin , an index of ovarian hyperandrogenism. Besides,INSL3 levels seem positively related to ovarian follicle number[21].It was also suggested a role of leptin.Leptin, a product from the obesity gene, correlates positively with BMI but has also variation during the menstrual cycle where leptin levels peak in the luteal phase of the cycle,are in correlation with maximum progesterone levels [22].These changes suggest a direct physiological role for leptin in regulating ovarian function. Disruption of such an effect could play a role in menstrual irregularities generally observed in both obese and undernourished women and may offer a pathophysiological mechanism in women with PCOS [20,23].Most studies, however, report that leptin levels, in women with PCOS, do not differ significantly from normal controls, regardless of their bodyweight [24]. In addition there is no evidence for mutations of leptin or leptin receptor genes in women with polycystic ovary syndrome [25]. Nonetheless the different existing studies performed on intracellular signaling pathways, implicated in PCOS, steroidogenesis and androgen action, PCOS pathogenesis remains unclear . Is polycystic ovary syndrome a neuroendocrine or an ovarian disorder? [26].

References

[1] Strauss JF 3rd, Wood JR, Christenson LK, McAllister JM. Strategies to elucidate the mechanism of excessive theca cell androgen production in PCOS. Mol. *Cell. Endocrinol.* 2002;186:183–188.

[2] Wood JR, Nelson VL, Ho C, Jansen E, Wang CY, Urbanek M, McAllister JM, Mosselman S, Strauss JF 3rd.The molecular phenotype of polycystic ovary syndrome (PCOS) theca cells and new candidate PCOS genes defined by microarray analysis. *J. Biol. Chem.* 2003 ;278(29):26380-90.

[3] Ehrmann DA, Barnes RB, Rosenfield RL. Polycystic ovary syndrome as a form of functional ovarian hyperandrogenism due to dysregulation of androgen secretion. *Endocr. Rev.* 1995;16:322–353.

[4] Nelson VL, Legro RS, Strauss JF 3rd, McAllister JM. Augmented androgen production is a stable steroidogenic phenotype of propagated theca cells from polycystic ovaries. *Mol. Endocrinol.* 1999 Jun;13(6):946-57.

[5] Nelson VL, Qin KN, Rosenfield RL, Wood JR, Penning TM, Legro RS, Strauss JF 3rd,McAllister JM.The biochemical basis for increased testosterone production in theca cells propagated from patients with polycystic ovary syndrome. *J. Clin. Endocrinol. Metab.* 2001 Dec;86(12):5925-33.

[6] Magoffin DA,Gancedo B,Erickson GF. Transforming growth factor-beta promotes differentiation of ovarian thecal-interstitial cells but inhibits androgen production. *Endocrinology* 1989;125(4): 1951-8.

[7] John ME,Simpson ER,Waterman MR,Mason JI.Regulation of cholesterol side-chain cleavage cytochrome P-450 gene expression in adrenal cells in monolayer culture. *Mol. Cell. Endocrinol.* 1986; 45(2-3): 197-204.

[8] Sahin Y, Keleştimur F. 17-Hydroxyprogesterone responses to gonadotrophin-releasing hormone agonist buserelin and adrenocorticotrophin in polycystic ovary syndrome: investigation of adrenal and ovarian cytochrome P450c17alpha dysregulation. *Hum. Reprod.* 1997 May;12(5):910-3.

[9] Rosenfield RL, Barnes RB, Cara JF, Lucky AW. Dysregulation of cytochrome P450c 17 alpha as the cause of polycystic ovarian syndrome. *Fertil. Steril.* 1990 May;53(5):785-91. Review.

[10] Ehrmann DA, Rosenfield RL, Barnes RB, Brigell DF, Sheikh Z. Detection of functional ovarian hyperandrogenism in women with androgen excess. *N. Engl. J. Med.* 1992;327:157–162.

[11] Bain PA,Meisier MH, Taylor BA,Payne AH.The genes encoding gonadal and nongonadal forms of 3beta-hydroxysteroid dehydrogenase/delta 5-delta 4 isomerase are closely linked on mouse chromosome 3.*Genomics* 1993; 16(1):219-23.

[12] Rhéaume E,Sirois I,Latrie F,Simard J.Codon 367 polymorphism of the human type 3 beta-hydroxysteroid dehydrogenase/isomerase gene (HS5DB3) *Nucleic Acids Res.* 1991; 19(21): 6060.

[13] Almahbobi G, Anderiesz C, Hutchinson P, McFarlane JR, Wood C, Trounson AO. Effects of epidermal growth factor, transforming growth factor alpha and androstenedione on follicular growth and aromatization in culture. *Clin. Endocrinol.* (Oxf). 1996 ;44(5):571-80.

[14] Hsueh AJ, Dahl KD, Vaughan J, Tucker E, Rivier J, Bardin CW, Vale W. Heterodimers and homodimers of inhibin subunits have different paracrine action in the modulation of luteinizing hormone-stimulated androgen biosynthesis. *Proc. Natl. Acad. Sci. U S A.* 1987 Jul;84(14):5082-6.

[15] Hillier SG. Regulatory functions for inhibin and activin in human ovaries. *J. Endocrinol.* 1991 Nov;131(2):171-5. Review.

[16] Lockwood GM, Muttukrishna S, Groome NP, Matthews DR, Ledger WL.Mid-follicular phase pulses of inhibin B are absent in polycystic ovarian syndrome and are initiated by successful laparoscopic ovarian diathermy: a possible mechanism regulating emergence of the dominant follicle. *J. Clin. Endocrinol. Metab.* 1998 May;83(5):1730-5.

[17] Cataldo NA, Giudice LC.Insulin-like growth factor binding protein profiles in human ovarian follicular fluid correlate with follicular functional status. *J. Clin. Endocrinol. Metab.* 1992 ; 74(4): 821-9.

[18] San Roman GA, Magoffin DA Insulin-like growth factor binding proteins in ovarian follicles from women with polycystic ovarian disease: cellular source and levels in follicular fluid. *J. Clin. Endocrinol. Metab.* 1992 ;75(4):1010-6.

[19] Morales AJ, Laughlin GA, Bützow T, Maheshwari H, Baumann G, Yen SSC Insulin, somatotropic, and luteinizing hormones axes in lean and obese women with polycystic ovary syndrome: common and distinct features. *J. Clin. Endocrinol. Metab.* 1996 ; 81:2854–2864.

[20] Conway GS, Jacobs HS, Holly JM, Wass JA. Effects of luteinizing hormone, insulin, insulin-like growth factor-I and insulin-like growth factor small binding protein 1 in the polycystic ovary syndrome. *Clin. Endocrinol.* (Oxf). 1990 Nov;33(5):593-603.

[21] Gambineri A,Patton L,De Iasio R,Palladoro F,Pagotto U,Pasquali R.Insulin-like factor 3: a new circulating hormone related to luteinizing hormone-dependent ovarian hyperandrogenism in the polycystic ovary syndrome. J.Clin.Endocrinol.Metab.2007; 92(6): 2066-73.

[22] Hardie L, Trayhurn P, Abramovich D, Fowler P. Circulating leptin in women: a longitudinal study in the menstrual cycle and during pregnancy. *Clin. Endocrinol.* (Oxf). 1997 ;47(1):101-6.

[23] Jacobs HS, Conway GS.Leptin ,polycystic ovaries and polycystic ovary sindrome. *Hum. Reprod. Update* 1999; 5(2): 166-71. Review.

[24] Rouru J, Anttila L, Koskinen P, Penttilä TA, Irjala K, Huupponen R, Koulu M Serum leptin concentrations in women with polycystic ovary syndrome. *J. Clin. Endocrinol. Metab.* 1997 Jun;82(6):1697-700.

[25] Oksanen L, Tiitinen A, Kaprio J, Koistinen HA, Karonen S, Kontula K.No evidence for mutations of the leptin or leptin receptor genes in women with polycystic ovary syndrome. *Mol. Hum. Reprod.* 2000 Oct;6(10):873-6.

[26] Rosenfield RL. Is polycystic ovary syndrome a neuroendocrine or an ovarian disorder? *Clin. Endocrinol.* (Oxf) 1997; 47:423–424.

Insulin Resistance Hypothesis

The first recognition of an association between glucose intolerance and hyperandrogenism was made by Achard and Thiers (1921) and was called "the diabetes of bearded women" [1]. Several years after this first report, Burghen showed in PCOS women the association of hyperandrogenism with hyperinsulinemia. Burghen and colleagues reported that these women, had basal and glucose-stimulated hyperinsulinemia ,suggesting the presence of insulin resistance and the possibility that it might have etiological significance [2]. Attention was also focused on the association of hyperandrogenism and insulin resistance with acanthosis nigricans (AN) in 1976, when Kahn and colleagues described a distinct disorder affecting adolescent girls, which they designated as "type A syndrome".These girls were virilized showing increased muscle bulk, clitoromegaly, temporal balding, deepening of the voice and had extreme insulin resistance with diabetes mellitus as well as striking AN [3].Therefore, this study established the relationship between severity of hyperinsulinemia and degree of clinical expression of AN. After the recognition of Kahn, several researchers noted that acanthosis nigricans occurred frequently in obese hyperandrogenic women [4,5,6,7,8,9].These observations were also accompanied by extensive research on the relationship between insulin and gonadal function [10,11,12].The presence of hyperinsulinemia in PCOS women, independent of obesity, was confirmed worldwide through different studies [7,13,14,15,16] . The association between insulin resistance and PCOS is now well known, and currently PCOS is considered a syndrome characterized by a metabolic disorder in which hyperinsulinemia and insulin resistance play a key role.There are substantially three possible mechanisms contributing to the state of insulin resistance: peripheral target tissue resistance, decreased hepatic clearance, or increased pancreatic sensitivity. Studies with the euglycaemic clamp technique indicate that insulin resistance is a common feature of the syndrome, and both obese and nonobese women with the syndrome are more insulin-resistant and hyperinsulinaemic than age- and weight-matched normal women[15,17,18]. However, obese PCOS women had significantly decreased insulin sensitivity compared with nonobese PCOS women [19].For example, Morales *et al.* demonstrated reduced insulin sensitivity in lean PCOS compared with lean controls, a further decrease in obese controls and a twofold further reduction in obese PCOS, suggesting that obesity is additive to insulin resistance related to PCOS [20]. Consistent with the degree of insulin resistance, the manifestation of compensatory hyperinsulinaemia in lean PCOS women was incipient, being evident only in response to meals. Collectively, these observations indicate that insulin resistance is a common finding in women with PCOS independent of obesity and that insulin resistance in obese PCOS is composed of dual contributions, one unique to PCOS and the other obesity-specific.Not all studies, however,have shown insulin resistance in lean PCOS subjects.Reports using an intravenous glucose tolerance test, a continuous glucose infusion model or a hyperinsulinaemic euglycaemic clamp found normal insulin action in normal weight PCOS patients [21,22].There are several possible reasons for these discrepancies. The composition of study groups varies depending on local diagnostic criteria; there is no standard definition and assessment of insulin resistance; ethnic variations in central adiposity, insulin sensitivity and the prevalence of a positive family history of type 2 diabetes are rarely taken into account.In any case,decreased insulin sensitivity and pancreatic β-cell secretory dysfunction have been reported in PCOS [23,24]. The β-cell defect increased secretion of insulin under basal conditions and decreased secretion after meals resulting in insufficient insulin secretion to compensate for the degree of insulin resistance. The decreased postprandial secretory responses in these patients resembles the β-cell dysfunction of type 2 DM and are much more pronounced in PCOS women who have a first-degree relative with type 2 DM, suggesting an increased risk for developing glucose intolerance. Weight loss results in significantly improved insulin resistance, but the β-cell defect remains, suggesting that it may be the primary abnormality in PCOS [25].However, Rodin *et al.* have showed that polycystic ovaries unlike type 2 DM, were not associated with a defect in the secretion of insulin.[26].Finally, a reduction in the insulin clearance rate due to decreased hepatic insulin extraction has been reported by some investigators to be partially responsible for the elevations in insulin concentration by some investigators [27] . Several groups have focused their attention on the mechanisms of insulin signalling in order to define the pathogenesis of insulin resistance in PCOS. Insulin action is mediated through a protein tyrosine kinase receptor. Tyrosine autophosphorylation increases the insulin receptor's tyrosine kinase activity, whereas serine phosphorylation inhibits it. The tyrosine-phosphorylated insulin receptor phosphorylates intracellular substrates, such as IRS-1 and IRS-2 (insulin receptor substrate-1 and -2) inducing the signal transduction and the actions of insulin.A potential mechanism for insulin resistance in at least 50% of PCOS women appears to be related to excessive serine phosphorylation of insulin receptor. A factor extrinsic to the insulin receptor, presumably a serine-threonine kinase, causes serine phosphorylation of the insulin receptor, leading to inhibition of signalling [17,28] It is believed that the defect in insulin action is limited to glucose metabolism, whereas other biologic actions of insulin, including those involved in steroidogenesis, are not impaired. Interestingly, serine phosphorylation of IRS-1 appears to be the mechanism of TNF-α-mediated insulin resistance of obesity. Serine phosphorylation also appears to modulate the activity of the key regulatory enzyme of androgen biosynthesis, P450c17, present in both the adrenal and ovarian steroidogenic tissue. Thus, serine phosphorylation has been shown to increase enzyme activity and androgen synthesis [29]. It is therefore possible that a single defect as serine phosphorylation might produce both the insulin resistance and the hyperandrogenism in a subgroup of PCOS women.IGF-I is similar to the control value, suggesting that the metabolic signalling defect is in another pathway or downstream of this signalling step in PCOS fibroblasts.The hypothesis for the existence of a postreceptor defect in insulin action in PCOS is also consistent with reports of molecular studies showing no structural abnormality in the insulin receptor [30,31].

Hyperinsulinaemia and Hyperandrogenism.

Several studies have demonstrated a positive correlation between fasting insulin levels and androgen levels [[2,9,32]

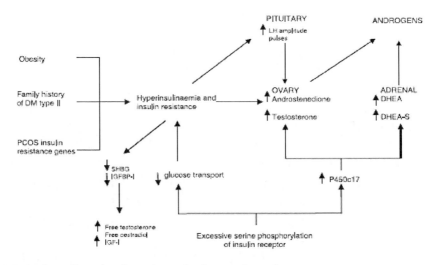

Table 6. Mechanism of hyperinsulinaemia causing hyperandrogenism

Furthermore, the severity of hyperinsulinaemia well correlates with the degree of clinical expression of the syndrome [4,5]. Whether hyperandrogenism results from the hyperinsulinaemia of insulin resistance, or vice versa, has been debated since this correlation was demonstrated. Most of the evidence supports hyperinsulinaemia as the primary factor. In fact, some experiments demonstrated that the decrease of hyperandrogenaemia by bilateral oophorectomy or administration of a GnRH-agonist has not induced changes in the hyperinsulinaemic state. Besides,it is well known that in PCOS antiandrogen therapy did not alter insulin sensitivity [33,34,35,36]. It is possible, however, that androgens may contribute in some extent to the associated insulin resistance of PCOS, as some investigators have found that insulin resistance was partially reversed during androgen suppression or antiandrogen treatment (37,38). In summary, these findings indicate that endogenous androgens do not play a central pathophysiologic role in sustaining insulin resistance in women with PCOS and that disordered insulin action precedes the increase in androgens. It is generally accepted that hyperinsulinaemia augments androgen production in PCOS. During puberty, insulin resistance develops probably because of the increase in sex steroids and growth hormone, resulting in secondary increase in insulin and IGF-1, which leads to a decrease in the sex hormone binding globulin (SHBG) and would allow to a greater sex steroid activity for pubertal development. Thus, PCOS can be considered as a state of exaggerated puberty or hyperpuberty. After puberty, the insulin and IGF-1 levels progressively decline in most patients, resulting in normalization of the clinical and morphological picture. In subjects with PCOS, the higher levels persist either because hyperinsulinemia persists or because,in the meantime, another pathogenic factor has taken over its role. In the latter instance, hyperinsulinemia probably only served as an inducing event. Despite evidence that insulin promotes ovarian androgen production in PCOS,the exact mechanism on cellular level remains unclear. Initially, insulin cross-reaction with the IGF-I receptor ,similar in structure to insulin receptor , was proposed as a possible mechanism of insulin mediated hyperandrogenism ,on the ovarian thecal cells.In view of the known actions of IGF-I in augmenting the thecal androgen response to LH , activation of IGF-I receptors by insulin would lead to increased androgen production in thecal cells [39,40].However, insulin has been shown to bind the IGF-I receptor with an affinity of 50-500 times lower than that of IGF-I. The cross-over effect of insulin with the type-I IGF receptor therefore is an important consideration at high insulin levels [41].The existence of hybrid and atypical insulin/IGF-I receptors which consist of a combination of α- and β-subunits of both receptors have also been described [42]. It is believed that these receptors can bind insulin and IGF-I with similar affinity. Also, it has been proposed that insulin has specific actions on steroidogenesis acting through its own receptor [43,44]. This pathway was supported by in vitro studies of both granulosa and thecal cells [45,46,47.48]. Interestingly,Willis et al using anti-insulin receptor and antitype-I IGF receptor antibodies, not only demonstrated that insulin effects on human granulosa cell steroidogenesis in vitro must be mediated via its own receptor, but also excluded both the insulin-type-I IGF hybrid receptor or the type-I IGF receptor as possible insulin action-mediated receptors [46]. Preliminary studies suggest that insulin enhances the amplitude of LH pulses but not their frequency in obese women with PCOS [48,49]. This is consistent with a previous report showing that there is a general concordance of the diurnal pattern of LH levels and of insulin levels in these women [50]. The insulin resistance in at least 50% of PCOS women appears to be related to excessive serine phosphorylation of the insulin receptor. A factor extrinsic to the insulin receptor, presumably a serine/threonine kinase, causes this abnormality and it is an example of an important new mechanism for human insulin resistance related to factors controlling insulin receptor signaling. Serine phosphorylation appears to modulate the activity of the key regulatory enzyme of androgen biosynthesis,the P450c17. It is thus possible that a single defect produces both the insulin resistance and the hyperandrogenism in some PCOS women. Studies in which insulin levels have been suppressed by insulin-lowering agents suggest that insulin might also contribute to changes in ovarian androgen secretion through effects at the pituitary level. An alternative possibility is that the reduced secretion of LH with these therapies could be secondary to high progesterone levels following ovulation. Insulin receptors have been identified in human pituitary tissue and insulin was found to stimulate gonadotropin release in vitro. Furthermore, insulin-mediated increase of ovarian cytochrome P450c17 activity, as an additional mechanism of insulin action in a subgroup of obese PCOS women has been showed. In fact, these studies reported a decrease in serum insulin concentrations with metformin,followed by a reduction of ovarian P450c17 activity,as demonstrated by a substantial reduction in the response of serum 17α-hydroprogesterone to the administration of leuprolide [49,51,52,53]. Another report revealed that hyperinsulinaemia may stimulate cytochrome P450c17 activity in the andrenal gland tissue of women with PCOS [45]. There are two other important actions of insulin which contribute to hyperandrogenism in PCOS: the inhibition of hepatic synthesis of serum sex hormone-binding globulin, which allows more free androgen and oestrogen to be bioavailable, and the inhibition of hepatic production of IGFBP-1, which allows an increase in circulating levels of IGF-I and greater local activity [54,55]. This is now known to be the mechanism for the frequently observed inverse correlation between peripheral insulin and SHBG levels. This relationship is so strong that SHBG concentrations are good markers for hyperinsulinaemic insulin resistance, and reduced SHBG concentration is a predictor for the development of type 2 DM [56,57].The clinical implication of these findings is that amelioration of hyperandrogenism in women with PCOS may be achieved by interventions that improve insulin sensitivity and reduce circulating insulin levels. Indeed, weight loss in women with PCOS improves the endocrine and ovarian dysfunction , while the pharmacological approach with agents that either decrease insulin secretion, like diazoxide or somatostatin , or that improve insulin sensitivity, like metformin or troglitazone have demonstrated conclusively that a reduction in serum insulin levels is associated with a reduction of ovarian androgen secretion in PCOS [48,58,59,60,61,62,63]. The improvement of serum androgen levels with different drug classes, with different mechanism of action, suggests an effect mediated by reduction in circulating insulin levels, although a direct ovarian effect especially of the insulin-sensitizing agents can not be excluded. These changes were independent of changes in body weight, although for metformin some controversy still exists . The insulin-sensitizing agents,metformin and troglitazone, not only reduce circulating insulin concentrations, but also reverse the metabolic and endocrine anomalies and more recently, restoring menstrual abnormalities and improving the reproductive outcome in anovulatory PCOS women [64,65,66,67]. In conclusion, recent knowledges lead to consider the insulin hypothesis more consistent than the others. Current knowledges strongly suggest that insulin is acting through its own receptors,rather than the IGF-I receptors, in PCOS in order to augment not only ovarian and adrenal steroidogenesis but also pituitary LH release. Indeed, the defect in insulin action appears to be selective and affecting glucose metabolism but not cell growth. Since PCOS usually has a menarchal age of onset, this makes it a particularly appropriate disorder in which to examine the ontogeny of defects in carbohydrate metabolism and for ascertaining large three-generation kindreds for positional cloning studies to identify NIDDM genes. Although the presence of lipid abnormalities, dysfibrinolysis, and insulin resistance would be predicted to place PCOS women at high risk for cardiovascular disease. Appropriate prospective studies are then necessary to directly assess this. However,if insulin resistance and hyperinsulinaemia have an important pathogenetic role in PCOS, why are not all patients with hyperinsulinaemia also hyperandrogenic; like many women with type 2 DM? Furthermore, why ovaries appear to be insulin-responsive in an insulin-resistant state? Indeed, does insulin activate a signalling system separate from glucose transport to stimulate steroidogenesis? It has been showed that although 82% of women with type 2 DM had polycystic ovaries in ultrasound, only 52% had clinical evidence of hyperandrogenism and/or menstrual disturbance, suggesting that hyperinsulinaemia alone is not sufficient for the expression of the syndrome [68].

References

[1] Achard C, Thiers J Le virilisme pilaire et son association a l'insuffisance glycolytique (diabete des femmes a barb). *Bull. Acad. Natl. Med.* 1921; 86:51–64.

[2] Burghen GA, Givens JR, Kitabchi AE. Correlation of hyperandrogenism with hyperinsulinism in polycystic ovarian disease. *J .Clin. Endocrinol. Metab.* 1980; 50:113–116.

[3] Kahn CR, Flier JS, Bar RS, Archer JA, Gorden P, Martin MM, Roth J. The syndromes of insulin resistance and acanthosis nigricans. N Engl J Med .1976; 294:739–745

[4] Conway GS,Jacobs HS.Hirsutism. *BMJ* 1990; 301(6753): 619-20.

[5] Robinson S, Kiddy D, Gelding SV, Willis D, Niththyananthan R, Bush A, Johnston DG, Franks S. The relationship of insulin insensitivity to menstrual pattern in women with hyperandrogenism and polycystic ovaries. *Clin. Endocrinol.* (Oxf)1993; 39:351–355.

[6] Flier JS, Eastman RC, Minaker KL, Matteson D, Rowe JW Acanthosis nigricans in obese women with hyperandrogenism. Characterization of an insulin-resistant state distinct from the Type A and B syndromes. *Diabetes* 1985; 34:101–107.

[7] Dunaif A, Barbieri RL, Ryan KJ Hyperandrogenism, insulin resistance, and acanthosis nigricans syndrome: a common endocrinopathy with distinct pathophysiologic features. *Am. J. Obstet. Gynecol.* 1983; 147:90.

[8] Dunaif A, Hoffman AR, Scully RE, Flier JS, Longcope C, Levy LJ, Crowley Jr WF The clinical, biochemical and ovarian morphologic features in women with acanthosis nigricans and masculinization. *Obstet. Gynecol* 1985;66:545–552.

[9] Stuart CA, Peters EJ, Prince MJ, Richards G, Cavallo A, Meyer WJ Insulin resistance with acanthosis nigricans: the roles of obesity and androgen excess. *Metabolism* 1986; 35:197–205.

[10] Peters EJ, Stuart CA, Prince MJ Acanthosis nigricans and obesity: acquired and intrinsic defects in insulin action. Metabolism 1986;35:807–813.

[11] Poretsky L, Kalin MF The gonadotropic function of insulin. *Endocr. Rev.* 1987; 8:132–141.

[12] Dunaif A, Hoffman AR Insulin resistance and hyperandrogenism: clinical syndromes and possible mechanisms. In: Pancheri P, Zichella L (eds) Biorhythms and Stress in the Physiopathology of Reproduction. Hemisphere Publishing Co, Washington, DC, 1988; pp 293–317.

[13] Taylor SI, Cama A, Accili D, Barbetti F, Quon J, Sierra MDLL, Suzuki Y, Koller E, Levy-Toledano R, Wertheimer E, Moncada VY, Kadowaki H, Kadowaki T Mutations in the insulin receptor gene. *Endocr. Rev.* 1992; 13:566–595.

[14] Shoupe D, Kumar DD, Lobo RA Insulin resistance in polycystic ovary syndrome. *Am. J. Obstet. Gynecol.* 1983; 147:588–592.

[15] Chang RJ, Nakamura RM, Judd HL, Kaplan SA Insulin resistance in nonobese patients with polycystic ovarian disease. *J. Clin. Endocrinol. Metab.* 1983;57:356–359.

[16] Barbieri RL, Ryan KJ Hyperandrogenism, insulin resistance, and acanthosis nigricans syndrome: a common endocrinopathy with distinct pathophysiologic features. *Am. J. Obstet. Gynecol.* 1983; 147:90.

[17] Dunaif A, Futterweit W, Segal KR, Dobrjansky A Profound peripheral insulin resistance, independent of obesity, in the polycystic ovary syndrome. *Diabetes* 1989; 38:1165–1174

[18] Dunaif A Polycystic ovary syndrome and obesity. In: Bjorntorp P, Brodoff BN (eds) Obesity. *J.B. Lippincott. Co. Philadelphia*, 1992; 594–605

[19] Dunaif A. Hyperandrogenic anovulation (PCOS): A unique disorder of insulin action associated with an increased risk of non-insulin dependent diabetes mellitus. *American Journal Medicine (Suppl* 1A) 1995; 98: 1A-33A.

[20] Morales AJ, Laughlin GA, Bützow T, Maheshwari H, Baumann G, Yen SSC 1996 Insulin, somatotropic, and luteinizing hormones axes in lean and obese women with polycystic ovary syndrome: common and distinct features. *J. Clin. Endocrinol. Metab.* 81:2854–2864

[21] Dale 1992 Dale PO, Tanbo T, Vaaler S, Abyholm T. Body weight, hyperinsulinemia, and gonadotropin levels in the polycystic ovarian syndrome: evidence of two distinct populations. *Fertil. Steril.* 1992;58:487–491

[22] Ovesen P, Moller J, Ingerslev HJ, Jorgensen JOL, Mengel A, Schmitz O, George K, Alberti MM, Moller N. Normal basal and insulin-stimulated fuel metabolism in lean women with the polycystic ovary syndrome. *J. Clin. Endocrinol. Metab.* 1993;7:1636–1640

[23] Ehrmann DA, Barnes RB, Rosenfield RL. Polycystic ovary syndrome as a form of functional ovarian hyperandrogenism due to dysregulation of androgen secretion. *Endocr. Rev.* 1995;16:322–353.

[24] Dunaif A, Finegood DT ß-Cell dysfunction independent of obesity and glucose intolerance in the polycystic ovary syndrome. *J. Clin. Endocrinol. Metab.* 1996; 81:942–947

[25] Holte J, Bergh T, Berne C, Wide L, Lithell H 1995 Restored insulin sensitivity but persistently increased early insulin secretion after weight loss in obese women with polycystic ovary syndrome. *J. Clin. Endocrinol. Metab.* 1995; 80:2586–2593

[26] Rodin DA, Bano G, Bland JM, Taylor K, Nussey SS. Polycystic ovaries and associated metabolic abnormalities in Asian women. *Clinical Endocrinology* 1998; 49: 91-99.

[27] O'Meara NM, Blackman JD, Ehrmann DA, Barnes RB, Jaspan JB, Rosenfield RL, et al . Defects in beta cell function in functional ovarian hyperandrogenism. *J. Clin. Endocrinol. Metab.* 1993;76:1241-7.

[28] Dunaif A. Insulin resistance and the polycystic ovary syndrome: mechanisms and implications for pathogenesis. *Endocrine. Reviews.*1997; 18: 774-800.

[29] Zhang L, Rodriguez H, Ohno S, Miller WL. Serine phosphorylation of human P450 C17 increases 17, zo-lyase activity: Implications for adrenarche and the PCOS. *Proc. Natl. Acad. Sci.* 1995;92:10619-23.

[30] Conway 1994 Conway GS, Avey C, Rumsby G. The tyrosine kinase domain of the insulin receptor gene is normal in women with hyperinsulinaemia and polycystic ovary syndrome. *Hum. Reprod.* 1994 Sep;9(9):1681-3.

[31] Sorbara 1994 Dunaif A, Sorbara L, Delson R, Green G Ethnicity and polycystic ovary syndrome are associated with independent and additive decreases in insulin action in Caribbean Hispanic women. *Diabetes* 1993; 42:1462–1468

[32] Lobo RA, Goebelsmann U, Horton R Evidence for the importance of peripheral tissue events in the development of hirsutism in polycystic ovary syndrome. *J. Clin. Endocrinol. Metab.* 1983; 57: 393 - 397

[33] Nagamani M, Dinh TV, Kelver ME Hyperinsulinemia in hyperthecosis of the ovaries. *Am. J. Obstet. Gynecol.* 1986; 154:384–389 40.

[34] Dunaif A, Green G, Futterweit W, Dobrjansky A.Suppression of hyperandrogenism does not improve peripheral or hepatic insulin resistance in the polycystic ovary syndrome.*J. Clin. Endocrinol. Metab.* 1990 Mar;70(3):699-704.

[35] Dunaif A,Green G,Phelps RG,Lebwohl M,Futterweit W,Lewy L.Acanthosis nogricans,insulin action and hyperandrogenism:Clinical ,histological and biochemical findings.*J. Clin. Endicrinol. Metab.*1991;73:590-5.

[36] Diamanti-Kandarakis E, Kouli C, Tsianateli T, et al. A survey of PCOS in Greek population. 79th Annual Meeting of the Endocrine Society, Minneapolis, MN, 1997.1995

[37] .Elkind-Hirsch K,Marrioneaux O,Bhushan M,Vernor D,Bhushan R.Comparison of single and combined treatment with exenatide and metformin on menstrual cyclicity in overweight women with polycystic ovary syndrome.*J.Clin.Endocrinol. Metab.* 2008; 93(7): 2670-2678.

[38] Moghetti P, Tosi F, Castello R, Magnani CM, Negri C, Brun E, Furlani L, Caputo M, Muggeo M. The insulin resistance in women with hyperandrogenism is partially reversed by antiandrogen treatment: evidence that androgens impair insulin action in women. *J. Clin. Endocrinol. Metab.* 1996 Mar;81(3):952-60.

[39] Bergh C, Carlsson B, Olsson JH, Selleskog U, Hillensjo T. Regulation of androgen production in cultured human thecal cells by insulin like growth factor-1 and insulin. *Fertil. Steril.* 1993;59:323-31

[40] Cara 1990 Caro JF, Dohm LG, Pories WJ, Sinha MK 1989 Cellular alterations in liver, skeletal muscle, and adipose tissue responsible for insulin resistance in obesity and Type II diabetes. *Diabetes. Metab. Rev.* 1989; 5:665–689

[41] Jacobs SL, Metzger DA, Dodson WC, Haney AF. Effect of age on response to human menopausal gonadotropin stimulation.*J. Clin. Endocrinol.Metab.* 1990 Dec;71(6):1525-30.

[42] Siddle K, Soos MA, Field CE, Navé BT.Hybrid and atypical insulin/insulin-like growth factor I receptors.*Horm. Res*. 1994;41 Suppl 2:56-64; discussion 65. Review.

[43] Poretsky L, Grigorescu F, Seibel M, Moses AC, Flier JS.Distribution and characterization of insulin and insulin-like growth factor I receptors in normal human ovary.*J. Clin. Endocrinol. Metab*. 1985 Oct;61(4):728-34.

[44] Poretsky L, Cataldo NA, Rosenwaks Z and Guidice L. The Insulin-related regulatory system in health and disease. *Endocrine. Reviews*. 1999; 20: 535-82.

[45] Franks S Polycystic ovary syndrome. *N. Engl. J. Med*. 1995; 333:853–861

[46] Willis D,Mason H,Gilling-Smith C,Franks S.Modulation by insulin of follicle-stimulation hormone and luteinizing hormone actions in human granulosa cells of normal and polycystic ovaries.*J.Clin.Endocrinol.Metab*. 1996; 81:302-9.

[47] Barbieri RL, Makris A, Ryan KJ.Insulin stimulates androgen accumulation in incubations of human ovarian stroma and theca.*Obstet. Gynecol*. 1984 Sep;64(3 Suppl): 73S-80S.

[48] Nestler JE. Insulin regulation of human ovarian androgens.*Hum. Reprod*.1997; 12:53-62 .

[49] Nestler JE, Jakubowicz DJ. Decreases in ovarian cytochrome P450c17 alpha activity and serum free testosterone after reduction of insulin secretion in polycystic ovary syndrome.*N. Engl. J. Med*. 1996 Aug 29;335(9):617-23.

[50] Yen SS, Apter D, Bützow T, Laughlin GA Gonadotrophin releasing hormone pulse generator activity before and during sexual maturation in girls: new insights.*Hum. Reprod*. 1993 Nov;8 Suppl 2:66-71.

[51] Unger RH, Diabetic hyperglycemia: link to impaired glucose transport in pancreatic beta cells.*Science*. 1991 Mar 8;251(4998):1200-5. Review.

[52] Adashi EY, Rock JA, Guzick D, Wentz AC, Jones GS, Jones HW Jr.Fertility following bilateral ovarian wedge resection: a critical analysis of 90 consecutive cases of the polycystic ovary syndrome.*Fertil. Steril*. 1981 Sep;36(3):320-5.

[53] Nestler JE, Jakubowicz DJ, Evans WS, Pasquali R Effects of metformin on spontaneous and clomiphene-induced ovulation in the polycystic ovary syndrome. *N. Engl. J. Med*. 1998; 338:1876 1880

[54] Bach LA.The insulin-like growth factor system: basic and clinical aspects.*Aust. N. Z. J. Med*. 1999 Jun;29(3):355-61. Review.

[55] LeRoith D, McGuinness M, Shemer J, Stannard B, Lanau F, Faria TN, Kato H, Werner H, Adamo M, Roberts CT Jr. Insulin-like growth factors.*Biol. Signals*. 1992 Jul-Aug;1(4):173-81. Review.

[56] Lindstedt G, Lundberg PA, Lapidus L, Lundgren H, Bengtsson C, Björntorp P.Low sex-hormone-binding globulin concentration as independent risk factor for development

Polycystic Ovarian Syndrome: Epidemiology, Aetiology and Pathogenesis 83

of NIDDM. 12-yr follow-up of population study of women in Gothenburg, Sweden.*Diabetes.* 1991 Jan;40(1):123-8.

[57] Nestler JE. Relation of adrenal androgen to insulin levels. *Ann. Intern. Med.* 1993 May 15;118(10):826.

[58] Kiddy DS, Hamilton-Fairley D, Bush A, Short F, Anyaoku V, Reed MJ, Franks S.Improvement in endocrine and ovarian function during dietary treatment of obese women with polycystic ovary syndrome.*Clin. Endocrinol. (Oxf).* 1992 Jan;36(1):105-11.

[59] Guzick D. PCOS: Symptomatology, pathophysiology and epidemiology. *Am. J. Obstet. Gynaecol.* 1998;179:S89-93.

[60] Nestler JC, Barlascini CO, Matt DW, Steingold KA, Plymate SR, Clore JN, et al . Suppression of serum insulin by diazoxide reduces serum testosterone levels in obese women with Polycystic Ovarian Syndrome. *J. Clin. Endocrinol. Metab.* 1989;68:1027-32.

[61] Prelevic GM, Wurzburger MI, Balint-Pesic L, Nesic JS. Inhibitory effect of somatostatin on secretion of luteinising hormone and ovarian steroids in PCOS. *Lancet* 1990;336:900-3.

[62] Velezquez EM, Mendoza S, Hamer T, Sosa F, Glueck CJ. Metformin therapy in polycystic ovary syndrome reduces hyperinsulinaemia, insulin resistance, hyperandrogenaemia, and systolic blood pressure, while facilitating normal menses and pregnancy. *Metabolism* 1994; 43: 647-54.

[63] Ehrmann DA, Schneider DJ, Sobel BE, Cavaghan MK, Imperial J, Rosenfield RL, Polonsky KS. Troglitazone improves defects in insulin action, insulin secretion, ovarian steroidogenesis, and fibrinolysis in women with polycystic ovary syndrome. *J. Clin. Endocrinol. Metab.* 1997; 82:2108–2116.62.

[64] Mitwally MF, Kuscu NK, Yalcinkaya TM. High ovulatory rates with use of troglitazone in clomiphene-resistant women with polycystic ovary syndrome.*Hum. Reprod.* 1999;14(11):2700-3.

[65] Pirwany IR, Yates RW, Cameron IT, Fleming R. Effects of the insulin sensitizing drug metformin on ovarian function, follicular growth and ovulation rate in obese women with oligomenorrhoea.*Hum. Reprod.* 1999 ;14(12):2963-8.

[66] Moghetti P, Castello R, Negri C, Tosi F, Perrone F, Caputo M, Zanolin E, Muggeo M. Metformin effects on clinical features, endocrine and metabolic profiles, and insulin sensitivity in polycystic ovary syndrome: a randomized, double-blind, placebo-controlled 6-month trial, followed by open, long-term clinical evaluation. *Endocrinol. Metab.* 2000 ;85(1):139-46.

[67] Vandermolen DT, Ratts VS, Evans WS, Stovall DW, Kauma SW, Nestler JE.Metformin increases the ovulatory rate and pregnancy rate from clomiphene citrate in patients with polycystic ovary syndrome who are resistant to clomiphene citrate alone.*Fertil. Steril.* 2001 ;75(2):310-5.

[68] Conn JJ, Jacobs HS, Conway GS.The prevalence of polycystic ovaries in women with type 2 diabetes mellitus.*Clin. Endocrinol. (Oxf).* 2000 ;52(1):81-6.

Altered Cortisol Metabolism Hypothesis

The presence of defects in ovarian and adrenal steroidogenesis of women with infertility has been reported in several laboratory and clinical studies [1,2,3]. Besides,elevated androgens as well as abnormal regulation of the hypothalamic-pituitary-adrenal (HPA) axis and elevated cortisol clearance rates are well known features in obese women [4]. However, changes in cortisol metabolism mainly due to extra-adrenal factors have been observed in lean as well as in obese women with infertility. Several isolated or combined enzyme deficiencies were reported in a third of women with irregular cycles with a substantial number of subjects exhibiting a diminished 11-hydroxylase activity [5]. An important study analysed the calculated 11-deoxy cortisol/cortisol ratios, indicative for 11-hydroxylase activity, in women with normogonadotrophic ,normoestrogenic oligomenorrhoea and clomiphene citrate-resistant infertility,compared with lean and obese ovulatory controls. Infertility was commonly observed in obese women who frequently showed clinical features of pseudo-hypercortisolism, even though their morning serum cortisol concentrations were normal or even low, but their 24 h free urinary cortisol excretion usually was normal or even high, meaning that although cortisol production in adipose tissue is high the clearance rate was also increased [6]. Obese individuals, displaying features of the metabolic syndrome, have evidence of an altered peripheral handling of glucocorticoids through a reinforcement of peripheral 11-HSD, Type 1. This enzyme system enhances the local production of cortisol, particularly in visceral adipose tissues [7,8].

The imbalance between cortisol and its precursor steroid,11-deoxycortisol, as observed in infertile women, mirrors an insufficient cortisol production in relation with its high clearance rate.

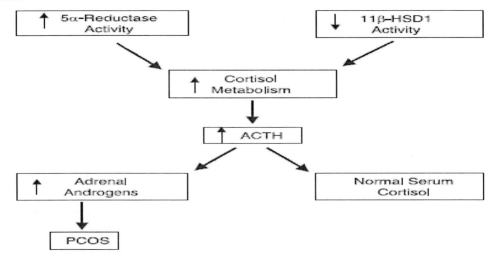

Table 7

Local cortisol production in peripheral tissues (11-HSD, Type 1 in visceral fat) may compensate this minute systemic low cortisol status..In conclusion, abnormal baseline 11-deoxycortisol/cortisol conversions were found in 88% of women with clomiphene citrate-resistant normo-gonadotrophic normo-estrogenic oligomenorrhoea. This

Polycystic Ovarian Syndrome: Epidemiology, Aetiology and Pathogenesis   85

abnormality disappears almost completely after ACTH administration, thus excluding overt CAH and suggesting an alternative operational pathway in non-adrenal tissues.Androgen excess in women with polycystic ovary syndrome may be ovarian and/or adrenal in origin, and an increased adrenal production was found in almost 25% of PCOS women likely as a result of a genetic trait or secondary to ovarian hormonal secretion [9,10,11]. In peripheral tissues, corticosteroid hormone action is modulated,in part, by the activity of 11 ß hydroxysteroid dehydrogenases . 11 ß HSD 2 inactivates cortisol and inactive cortisone in the kidney ,while 11 ß HSD 1 performs the reverse reaction activating active cortisol from inactive cortisone in the liver and adipose tissue. It is important to remember that loss of 11 HSD 2 activity in the kidney may lead to cortisol-induced mineralcorticoid excess ,while loss of hepatic 11 ß HSD 1 activity improves insulin sensitivity through a reduction in cortisol induced gluconeogenesis and hepatic glucose output. Conversely , increased activity of 11 ß HSD 1 in omental adipose tissue can stimulates glucocoticoid-induced adipocyte differentiation which may lead to central obesity. Stewart *et al.* first documented increased total cortisol metabolite excretion in the urine of PCOS women using gas chromatography and mass spectrometry,compared to controls. In particular, they found that the ratio of 5α to 5β cortisol metabolites were higher in PCOS subjects than in controls, indicating enhanced 5α-R activity [12]. This steroidogenic enzyme is responsible for both 5α-reduction of testosterone to 5α-dihydrotestosterone in the skin and of cortisol to 5α-dihydrocortisol in the liver.Therefore, it was suggested that increased activity of 5α-R mediates both hirsutism and enhanced hepatic cortisol metabolism. Rodin *et al* found evidence for dysregulation of 11βHSD enzyme activity in PCOS women. In particular, they found that the levels of 11-hydroxy to 11-oxo cortisol metabolites were lower in PCOS women than in controls, indicating impaired activity of 11βHSD1 (13). Hence, two isoenzymes of 11βHSD catalyse the interconversion of active cortisol to inactive cortisone and vice versa. 11βHSD1 is an oxoreductase mainly expressed in human liver and adipose tissue, responsible for cortisone to cortisol conversion. Impaired activity of this enzyme is compatible with increased metabolic clearance of cortisol, resetting of ACTH secretion, and with generalized adrenocortical overactivity. Because liver and adipose tissue are also targets of insulin action, they speculated that the dysregulation of this enzyme might be the result of hyperinsulinaemia. Alternatively, they suggested that 11βHSD dysregulation could be due to hyperandrogenaemia itself. Increased peripheral metabolism of cortisol may occur through two ways:

- enhanced irreversible inactivation of cortisol by 5α-reductase in liver
- impaired reversible interconversion of cortisone by 11ß-hydroxysteroid dehydrogenase type 1(11ß HSD1)in liver and adipose tissue.

Increased peripheral cortisol metabolism either by increased 5 α-reductase activity and increased inactivation of cortisol or by impaired 11 ß-HSD type 1 activity and impaired regeneration of cortisol results in compensatory increase of ACTH secretion via a decrease in the negative feedback signal, maintaining normal plasma cortisol concentrations at the expense of adrenal androgen excess [12,13,14]. A positive correlation between 5α-reductase and BMI has been found as well as a positive correlation was also found between 5α-reductase and the homeostasis model insulin resistance index (HOMA-R). While, no correlation was found between 11 ß-HSD 1 activity and insulin insensivity or BMI (15).The mechanism of the 5α-R and/or 11βHSD1 activity in women with PCOS remain still uncertain. Although, more than half of women with PCOS may be overweight, and obesity may cause abnormalities of cortisol metabolism; however,this mechanism cannot fully account for abnormalities of 5α-R and 11βHSD1 activities in PCOS. Stewart et al. have found increased 5α-R activity in PCOS subjects, compared with controls of similar weights [12]. Similarly, the altered 11βHSD1 activity in PCOS reported by Rodin et al. was also confirmed in lean PCOS subjects [13,14]. Recently, Walker et al.have also excluded the increased production of endogenous inhibitors of 11βHSD1, measured in urine, as a mechanism of abnormal cortisol metabolism in PCOS (16). Another proposed mechanism is that high oestrogen levels in PCOS, especially in the form of oestrone, could downregulate 11βHSD1 activity in liver. However, recent evidence suggests that oestrogen does not have a potent effect on 11βHSD1 activity in humans [17]. Finally, the association between the activities of these enzymes with insulin resistance and hyperinsulinaemia in women with PCOS, needs to be clarified and might explain the altered cortisol metabolism in these women. Non-obese individuals with hypertension may have subtle adrenal 11-hydroxylase or peripheral 11-HSD Type 2 deficiencies, resulting in mild mineralocorticoid excess. Obese individuals, displaying features of 'the metabolic syndrome', have evidence of an altered peripheral handling of glucocorticoids through a reinforcement of peripheral 11-HSD, Type 1. This enzyme system enhances the local production of cortisol, particularly in visceral adipose tissues [7, 8].Therefore, in obesity, reactivation of cortisone to cortisol by 11ß-HSD1 in liver is impaired, so that plasma cortisol levels tend to fall, and there may be a compensatory effect. These changes, observed in cortisol metabolism, are mainly due to extra-adrenal factors in lean as well as obese women with infertility. Abnormal baseline 11-deoxycortisol/ cortisol conversions were found in 88% of women normogonadotrophic, normoestrogenic with oligomenorrhoea and associated clomiphene citrate-resistance [17]. This abnormality disappeared almost completely after ACTH administration, thus excluding overt CAH and suggesting an alternative operational pathway in non-adrenal tissues. Further studies are needed to compare the effects of interventions such as dietary programmes or insulin-sensitizing agents, to investigate cortisol metabolism, and ultimately to improve ovulation and pregnancy rates for these women [18,19].

References

[1] Gilling-Smith, C., Story, H., Rogers, V. and Franks, S. Evidence for a primary abnormality of thecal cell steroidogenesis in the polycystic ovary syndrome *Clin. Endocrinol* (Oxf.1997; 47: 93–99.

[2] Gonzalez, F.Adrenal involvement in polycystic ovary syndrome. *Semin. Reprod. Endocrinol.* 1997;15: 137–157.

[3] Rosenfield, R.L.Ovarian and adrenal function in polycystic ovary syndrome. *Endocrinol. Metab. Clin. North. Am.* 1999; 28: 265–29

[4] Strain G.W, Zumoff B, Strain J.J., Levin J,Fukushima, D.K. Cortisol production in obesity. *Metabolism* 1980; 293(29): 980–985.

[5] Eldar-Geva T., Hurwitz A., Vecsei P., Palti Z., Milwidsky A,Rosler F. Secondary biosynthetic defects in women with late-onset congenital adrenal hyperplasia. *N. Engl. J. Med.* 1990., 323, 855–863.

[6] Prelevic, G.M., Wurzburger, M.I. and Balint-Peric, L. 24-Hour serum cortisol profiles in women with polycystic ovary syndrome. *Gynecol. Endocrinol.* 1993; 7, 179–184.

[7] Rask, E., Olsson T., Soderberg S., Andrew R., Livingstone D.E., Johnson O, Walker, B.R. Tissue-specific dysregulation of cortisol metabolism in human obesity. *J. Clin. Endocrinol. Metab.* 2001; 86, 1418–1421.

[8] Rask, E., Walker, B.R., Soderberg, S., Livingstone, D.E., Eliasson, M., Johnson, O., Andrew, R. and Olsson, T. Tissue-specific changes in peripheral cortisol metabolism in obese women: increased adipose 11beta-hydroxysteroid dehydrogenase type 1 activity. *J. Clin. Endocrinol. Metab.* 2002; 87, 3330–3336.

[9] Ehrmann DA, Rosenfield RL, Barnes RB, Brigell DF, Sheikh Z.Detection of functional ovarian hyperandrogenism in women with androgen excess. *N. Engl. J. Med.* 1992; Jul 16;327(3):157-62.

[10] Turner EI, Watson MJ, Perry LA, White MC.Investigation of adrenal function in women with oligomenorrhoea and hirsutism (clinical PCOS) from the north-east of England using an adrenal stimulation test. *Clin. Endocrinol.* (Oxf). 1992; Apr;36(4):389-97.

[11] Moran C, Azziz R.The role of the adrenal cortex in polycystic ovary syndrome. *Obstet. Gynecol. Clin. North Am.* 2001; Mar;28(1):63-75. Review.

[12] Stewart PM, Shackleton CH, Beastall GH, Edwards CR.5 alpha-reductase activity in polycystic ovary syndrome. *Lancet.* 1990; Feb 24;335(8687):431-3.

[13] Rodin A, Thakkar H, Taylor N, Clayton R.Hyperandrogenism in polycystic ovary syndrome. Evidence of dysregulation of 11 beta-hydroxysteroid dehydrogenase. *N. Engl. J. Med.* 1994 ;Feb 17;330(7):460-5.

[14] Chin D, Shackleton C, Prasad VK, Kohn B, David R, Imperato-McGinley J, Cohen H, McMahon DJ, Oberfield SE. Increased 5alpha-reductase and normal 11beta-hydroxysteroid dehydrogenase metabolism of C19 and C21 steroids in a young population with polycystic ovarian syndrome. *J. Pediatr. Endocrinol. Metab.* 2000; Mar;13(3):253-9.

[15] Tsilchorozidou T,Honour JW,Conway GS.Alterated cortisol metabolism in polycystic ovary syndrome:insulin enhances 5 α-reduction but not the elevated adrenal steroid production rates. *J. Clin. Endocrinol. Matab.* 2003;88(12):5907-13.

[16] Walker BR, Rodin A, Taylor NF, Clayton RN.Endogenous inhibitors of 11beta-hydroxysteroid dehydrogenase type 1 do not explain abnormal cortisol metabolism in polycystic ovary syndrome. *Clin. Endocrinol.* (Oxf). 2000; Jan;52(1):77-80.

[17] Finken MJ,Andrews RC,Andrew R,Walker BR.Cortisol metabolism in healthy young adults: sexual dimorphism in activities of A-ring reductases,but not 11beta-hydroxysteroid dehydrogenases . *J. Clin. Endocrinol. Metab.*1999 Sep;84(9):3316-21. .

[18] Kirchengast, S. and Huber, J. Body composition characteristics and body fat distribution in lean women with polycystic ovary syndrome. *Hum. Reprod.* 2001; 16: 1255–1260.

[19] Dolfing JG., Tucker K.E.,Lem.C.M, Uittenbogaart J,.Verzijland JC, Schweitzer D.H Low 11-deoxycortisol to cortisol conversion reflects extra-adrenal factors in the majority of women with normo-gonadotrophic normo-estrogenic infertility. *Hum. Reprod.* 2003;Vol. 18, No. 2, 333-337.

Genetics Aspects of PCOS

Polycystic ovary syndrome has been for many years one of the most controversial entities in gynecological endocrinology. The exact cause of PCOS is not known. but familial aggregation of this syndrome is now well established. The familial clustering of PCOS cases and the growing evidence that the interaction between multiple genetic and environmental factors may lead to the development of this syndrome, have stimulated many genetic investigations [1,2]. There is an inheritable component of PCOS which means women with this condition frequently have a mother or sister with PCOS.There is a fifty percent chance of getting PCOS if the mother has this condition. Effectively, the high incidence of PCOS in first degree relatives of the affected and the different existing studies suggest a dominant inheritance [3,4,5]. There are also ethnic and racial variations in the prevalence of PCOS [6] . Several observations reported so far have been made on families of white European descent, with none from those of south Asian descent [7,4]. The only large study in twins revealed an incidence of 50% for PCO in monozygotic and dizygotic twins, but with strong discordance. These data suggest a complex inheritance pattern, perhaps polygenic, which seems to be linked to insulin resistance [8]. A study evaluated data from 1325 monozygotic twins, 1191 dizygotic twins (711 women from same sex-twin pairs and 480 women from opposite-sex twin pairs),745 sisters of twins,and 218 spouses of male twins.The conclusion showed that the prevalence of PCOS is not different in women from opposite-sex and same sex twin pairs, sisters, or spouses. Therefore, the possible androgen exposure of the female fetus, caused by a shared intrauterine environment with a male fetus,does not result in PCOS-like trait.[9]. On average,the probability about the occurrence of hirsutism and oligomenorrhoea among sisters of the proband is about 50%, of PCO 73%, of hyperandrogenaemia 87% and of hyperinsulinaemia 66% , to which hyperinsulinaemia was later included [3,5,6,10] A recent report of a large number of sisters of affected women showed that 22% of sisters had well characterised PCOS,and another 24% had hyperandrogenaemia with regular cycles [7]. Several phenotypes of PCOS are reported to occur within a given family, which supports a heterogeneous genetic basis with variable expression of a monogenic trait or an oligogenic trait [7,11]. Several genes have been considered in the pathogenesis of the syndrome or of some symptoms.

Familial Studies

Studies of first-degree relatives of women with PCOS reveal familial clustering of the disease, particularly hyperandrogenemia. A prospective evaluation found that 46% of the sisters of PCOS patients were hyperandrogenemic suggesting a dominantly inherited trait controlling androgen levels [12]. Another investigation evaluating 367 families of predominantly European origin, with at least one PCOS woman,showed the linkage between PCOS and 19 STRs. Particularly, the strongest evidence was observed with D19S884. In conclusion,this study revealed a PCOS suscptibility locus map very close to D19S884.[13]. Some studies considered the metabolic phenotype in the brothers of women with PCOS.The results showed that the brothers have dyslipidemia as well as evidence for insulin resistance similar to that of their systers with PCOS. Cholesterol, LDL cholesterol , and triglyceride levels were significantly higher in brothers compared with control men,whereas HDL cholesterol levels were similar in the two groups. Moreover, fasting insulin , proinsulin levels and the homeostatic index of insulin resistance (HOMA-IR) were significantly higher whereas, fasting proinsulin/ insulin ratios did not differ in brothers compared with control men.These findings support the hypothesis that some features of PCOS are heritable and are not sex specific [4,14,15,16]. Going et al studied 1st degree relatives of 29 women affected by PCOS and 10 asymptomatic control volunteers of reproductive age. Sibling of the PCOS probands were affected for a segregation ratio of 55%, which is considered as autosomal dominant inheritance with nearly complete penetrance ,in comparison to the control families with segregation ratio of 25% [17]. Increased prevalence of frontal baldness in male relatives was first reported in 1979 [18].

References

[1]   Givens JR. Familial polycystic ovarian disease. *Endocrinology and Metabolism Clinics of North America* 1988; 17: 771-781. 27.

[2]   Carey AH, Chan KL, Short F et al. Evidence for a single gene effect causing polycystic ovaries and male pattern baldness. *Clinical Endocrinology* 1993; 38: 653-8.

[3]   Cooper DN, Clayton JF. DNA polymorphism and the study of disease associations. *Human Genetics* 1988; 78: 299-312.

[4]   Norman RJ, Masters S, Hague W. Hyperinsulinaemia is common if family members of women with polycystic ovary syndrome. *Fertility Sterility* 1996; 66: 942-7.

[5]   Legro RS,Spielman R,Urbanek M,Driscolll D,Strauss JF 3rd, Dunaif A. Phenotype and genotype in polycystic ovary syndrome. *Recent Prog. Horm. Res.* 1998;53:217-56.

[6]   Jakubowski L.Genetic aspects of polycystic ovary syndrome. *Endokrynol .Pol.* 2005; 56(3): 285- 93.

[7]   Hague WM, Adams J, Reedres ST et al. Familial polycystic ovaries: a genetic disease? *Clinical Endocrinology* 1988; 29: 593-605).

[8] Jahanfar S, Eden JA, Warren P et al. A twin study of polycystic ovary syndrome. *Fertility and Sterility* 1995; 63: 478-86.

[9] Kuijper EA,Vink JM,Lambalk CB,Boomsma DI. Prevalence of polycystic ovary syndrome in women from opposite -sex twin pairs. *J. Clin. Endocrinol.Metab.* 2009; 94(6): 1987-90.

[10] Lunde O, Magnus, P, Sandvik L et al. Familial clustering in the polycystic ovarian disease. *Gynaecology and Obstetrics* 1989; 28: 23-30.

[11] Franks S, Gharani N, Waterworth D, Batty S, White D, Williamson R, McCarthy M. The genetic basis of polycystic ovary syndrome. *Human Reproduction* 1997; 12: 2641-48.

[12] Strauss JF,3rd.Some new thoughts on the pathophysiology and genetica of polycystic ovary syndrome. *Ann. NY Acad. Sci.* 2003: 997:42-8.

[13] Ubbanek M,Woodroffe A,Ewens KG,Diamanti-Kandarakis E,Legro RS,Strauss JF 3rd, Dunaif A,Spielman RS.Candidate gene region for polycystic ovary syndrome on chromosome 19 p13.2. *J. Clin. Endocrinol. Metab.* 2005; 90(12): 6623-9.

[14] Sam S,Coviello AD, Sung Yeon-Ah, Legro RS,Dunaif A. Metabolic Phenotype in the brothers of women with Polycystic Ovary Syndrome. *Diabetes Care* 2008;31(6):1237-41.

[15] Colilla S,Cox NJ,Ehrmann DA,Heritability of insulin secretion and insulin action in women with polycystic ovary syndrome and their first degree relatives. *J. Clin. Endocrinol. Metab.* 2001;86: 2027-2031.18.

[16] Sam S,Sung Y,Legro RS,Dunaif A.Evidence for pancreatic ß-cell dysfunction in brothers of women with PCOS. *Metabolism* 2007;57: 84-89.

[17] Going JJ, Gusterson BA. Molecular pathology and future developments. *Eur. J. Cancer.* 1999 35:1895-1904.

[18] Ferriman D, Purdie AW.The inheritance of polycystic ovarian disease and a possible relo premature balding. *Clinical Endocrinology* 1979; 11: 291-300.

Genes mainly involved in the pathogenesis of PCOS

- steroid hormone biosynthesis and metabolism(

StAR,CYP11,CYP17,CYP19,HSD17B1-3, HSD3B1-2),

- gonadotropin and gonadal hormones action (ACTR1,ACTR2A-

B,FS,INHA,INHBA-B, INHC,SHBG,LHCGR,FSHR,MADH4 ,AR),

- insulin secretion and action (IGF-1, IGF1R, IGFBPl1-3,INS VNTR,IR,INSL,

IRS1-2, PPARG) .

- obesity and energy regulation (MC4R,OB,OBR,POMC,UCP2-3),

Molecular Genetic Studies in PCOS

Genetic association studies are used to investigate genes or genetic markers that might be associated with a particular disease phenotype or trait. These studies rely on the identification and characterization of natural variants or polymorphisms in the DNA sequence among individuals. If an association is present, a particular variant will be seen more often than expected by chance in an individual carrying the trait. Variants fall into several categories, depending on where they occur relative to a gene. First, variants can occur within or outside a gene. Those that occur within a gene may occur within an exon, an intron or regulatory regions. Regulatory regions control gene transcription and include the promoter region upstream of the gene and the 3'-untranslated region downstream of the protein-coding region. Variants within a gene can be functional or silent. Functional variation within a gene can be the direct cause of a phenotype abnormality or may increase susceptibility to a disease. Because PCOS is characterized by endocrinological abnormalities, polymorphisms in genes encoding sex hormones or regulators of their activity have been investigated. Several genes have been considered in the pathogenesis of the syndrome or of some symptoms.

Genes involved in ovarian and adrenal steroid hormones biosynthesis and metabolism

CYP11a gene which converts cholesterol to pregnenolone, is a rate-limiting step in androgen biosynthesis. This conversion is catalyzed by the P 450 cytochrome side chain cleavage enzyme, encoded by CYP11,a gene located at 15q24 [1]. Different studies showed the association between hyperandrogenism and a microsatellite polymorphism of the CYP11 in PCOS patients [1,2,3,4]. However,subsequent large scale analysis did not confirm the role of CYP11a polymorphism in the hyperandrogenism [5].Mutations of CYP21 gene were also investigated .The conversion of 17-hydroxyprogesterone into 11-deoxycortisol is catalyzed by the 21-hydroxylase enzyme encoded by CYP21[6].It was showed that children with premature pubarche and adolescent girls with functional hyperandrogenism could be heterozygous for mutations in CYP21. In fact ,women with functional hyperandrogenism show a well known increased 17-hydroxyprogesterone response to ACTH stimulation [7]. It was hypothesized that this earlier presentation of PCOS could be related to increased androgen sensitivity and indicated by androgen receptor gene CAG repeat length. This polymorphism was genotyped in 181 Barcelona girls (age, 10.9 yr; range, 4-19 yr) who had presented with PP, and in 124 Barcelona control girls. PP girls had shorter mean CAG number than Barcelona controls (PP vs. controls: P = 0.003) and greater proportion of short alleles 20 repeats or less (37.0% vs.24.6%, P = 0.002). Among post-menarcheal PP girls (n = 69),shorter CAG number was associated with higher 17-hydroxyprogesterone levels post-leuprolide (P = 0.009), indicative of ovarian hyperandrogenism, higher testosterone levels,acne and hirsutism scores, and more menstrual cycle irregularities.This study suggested that ovarian hyperandrogenism risk may be related to both low birth weight and shorter mean CAG number. In summary, shorter androgen receptor gene CAG number, indicative of increased androgen sensitivity, increases risks for PP and subsequent ovarian hyperandrogenism [8]. The response to ACTH appears to be closely related to altered factors regulating glucose-mediated glucose disposal,increased peripheral metabolism of cortisol, and to a less extent to the effects of extra-adrenal androgens,insulin resistance,hyperinsulinemia or obesity. Furthermore, DHEAS levels and response of adrenal androgens to ACTH seem relatively constant over time and are closely correlated between PCOS patients and their siblings suggesting that this abnormality is an inherited trait in PCOS [6]. Although ovaries are the main source of increased androgens in the syndrome, between 20 and 30% of women with PCOS have adrenal androgen excess, primarily detectable by elevated dehydroepiandrosterone sulfate (DHEAS) levels. Patients with PCOS show a generalized hypersecretion. The bulk of evidence points to the ovary being their source. Theca interna cells in PCO atretic follicles are the main site of excess androgen production. It seems that the theca interna cells and the granulosa cells from PCOS show abnormal steroidogenetic function,while the localization of P-450(17alpha,lyase) and P-450arom (aromatase cytochrome) in PCOS is essentially identical to that in the normal ovary [9].It was hypotesized that PCOS ovaries could have decreased levels of c-fos transcription factor. This factor could inhibit 17 alpha-hydroxylase 17,20 lyase activity in the human ovary, and its decreased expression seen in PCOS may lead to elevated transcription,resulting in increased production of androgens [10]. Another study focused on the role of an activating single/nucleotide polymorphism (SNP) at position/71 of the promoter of 17 beta/ hydroxysteroid dehydrogenase type 5 gene (71A/G HSD 17B5 SNP)in polycystic ovarian syndrome.The results showed that this variant can contribute to the severity of hyperandrogenemia in women with PCOS but this is not a major component of the molecular pathogenetic mechanism of PCOS [11]. In any case, androgen excess in PCOS seems to be, even in part ,a heritable trait. Studies on polymorphisms in the genes of two isoforms of 5 alpha-reductase (SRD5A1 and SRD5A2) suggest an important role of both isoforms. The Leu allele of the Val89Leu variant in SRD5A2 seems associated with protection against PCOS modestly reducing 5alpha-reductase activity. Haplotypes in SRD5A1 but non SRD5A2 were also associated with the degree of hirsutism in affected women. While, haplotypes with both genes were associated with PCOS risk. Only the SRD5A1 haplotypes seem important because of their influence on hair follicle and hirsutism [12]. An interesting study performed at Sinai Medical Center of Los Angeles showed this genetic evidence, suggesting a potential role of DHEA sulfotransferase (SULT2 A1),but non steroid sulfatase (STS) in the inherited androgens excess of PCOS.[13].

References

[1]   Franks S,Gilling-Smith C,Gharani N,McCarthy M.Pathogenesis of polycystic ovary syndrome:evidence for a genetically determined disorder of ovarian androgen production. *Hum. Fertil.* 2000;3:77-79.

[2] Gharani N, Waterworth DM, Batty S et al. Association of the steroid synthesis gene CYP11 a with polycystic ovary syndrome and hyperandrogenism. *Human Molecular Genetics* 1997; 6: 397-402.

[3] Diamanti-Kandarakis E,Bartzis MI,Bergiele AT,Tsianateli TC,Kouli CR.Microsatellite polymorphism (tttta)n at-528 base pairs of gene CYP11a influences hyperandrogenemia in patients with polycystic ovary syndrome. *Fertil. Steril.*2000; 4:735-741.

[4] Wang Y,Wu XK,Cao YX et al. Microsatellite polymorphism of (tttta)n in the promoter of CYP11a gene in Chinese women with polycystic ovary syndrome. *Zhonghua Yi Xue Za Zhi* 2005;85: 3396-400.

[5] Tan L,Zhu G.Relationship between the microsatellite polymorphism of CYP11a gene and the pathogenesis of hyperandrogenism of polycystic ovary syndrome in Chinese. *Chin. J. Med.Gen.* 2005; 22:216-218.

[6] Azziz R,Bradley ELJr, Potter HD,Boots LR. Adrenal androgen excess in women lack of a role for 17-hydroxylase and 17,20lyase dysregulation. *J. Clin. Endocrinol. Metab.* 1995; 80.400-405.

[7] Ibanez L, de Zegher F, Poteau N. Premature pubarche, ovarian hyperandrogenism and the polycystic ovary syndrome: from a complex constellation to a simple sequence of prenatal onset. *J. Endocrinol. Invest.* 1998; 21(9): 558-66.

[8] Ibanez L,Ong KK,Mongan N,Jaaskelamen J, Marcos MV, Hughes IA,De Zegher F. Dunger DB. Androgen receptor gene CAG repeat polymorphism in the development of ovarian hyperandrogenism. *J. Clin. Endocrinol. Metab.* 2003; 88(7): 3333.

[9] Tamura T,Kitawaki J,Yamamoto T,Osawa Y, Kominami S,Takemori S,Okada H.Immunohistochemical localization of 17 alpha-hydroxylase /C17-20 lyase and aromatase cytocrome P-450 in polycystic human ovaries. *J. Endocrinol.* 1993; 139 (3):503-9.

[10] Beshay VE,Havelock JC, Sirianni R, Ye P,Suzuki T,Rainey WE, Carr BR. The mechanism for protein kinase C inhibition of androgen production and 17 alpha-hydroxylase expression in a theca cell tumour model. *J. Clin. Endocrinol. Metab.* 2007; 92(12):4802-9.

[11] Marioli DJ,Saltamavros AD,Vervita V,Koika V,Adonakis G,Decavalas G,Markou KB,Georgopoulos NA. Association of the 17/hydroxysteroid dehydrogenase type 5 gene polymorphism (/71A/G HSD17B5 SNP) with hyperandrogenemia in polycystic ovary syndrome (PCOS). *Fertil.Steril.* 2009; 92(2): 648/52). 1.

[12] Goodarzi MO,Shah NA,Antoine HJ,Pall M,Guo X,Azziz R. Variants in the 5 alpha-reductase type 1 and type 2 genes are associated with polycystic ovary syndrome and the severity of hirsutism in affected women. *J. Clin. Endocrinol. Metab.* 2006; 91(10):4085-91.

[13] Goodarzi MO,Antoine HJ,Azziz R. Genes for enzymes regulating dehydroepiandrosterone sulfonation are associated with levels of dehydroepiandrosterone sulfate in polycystic ovary syndrome. *J. Clin. Endocrinol. Metab.* 2007; 92(7): 2659/64.

Genes involved in gonadotropin and gonadal hormones action

LH as HCG,FSH and TSH (thyroid stimulating factor) is a α/ ß heterodimer with a common α subunit and a unique ß subunit. The ß subunit confers the hormonal specificity. In 1992, an immunological variant of LH (V-LH) was found in a healthy Finnish woman who was fertile and had normal levels of all other hormones measured. The gene encoding her LH ß was sequenced and two base changes in N-terminal region were identified. In practice, the first mutation in codon 8 changes tryptophan to arginine and the second in codon 15 changes isoleucine to threonine [1] Later, it was showed that these mutations have a worldwide distribution [2,3,4] V-LH showed in vitro an elevated bioactivity compared to that of normal LH [5].Besides, it seems that the LH action in carriers of the V-LH allele might differ from that in non carriers. In addition, some studies supported the association of the V-LH mutations with high levels of serum E 2,T and SHBG in the follicular phase of the menstrual cycle in obese PCOS women ,in menstrual disorders and in infertility [6,7.8] No differences were observed in LH pulsatility between normal control and women with homozygosis for the variant LH hormone; however, the altered bioactivity and in vivo kinetics of the variant might induce subtle changes in LH action [5]. Differences in circulatory kinetics of the two types of LH may explain the differences in LH function between women with ovulatory disorders and women with normal ovulatory cycles. In addition ,the maximal response of the variant LH to pituitary stimulation with GnRH seems to be greater than that of normal -type LH [9,10]. Particularly,in 1996 Roy reported seven novel mutations in LH beta-subunit gene identified by PCR-SSCP method. (Polymerase chain –SSCP) [10,11]. Although some studies reported that obese PCOS patients had a higher frequency of the heterozygous V-LH compared with obese controls,other studies failed to find any association with PCOS [12].Thus,the functional role of the V-LH remains until now evasive but it seems not to be crucial in the pathogenesis of PCOS. Polymorphisms in the follicle stimulating hormone beta subunit (FSH) were mainly found in South East Asian populations [13].The FSH receptor (FSHR) is localized on chromosome 2p21.The portion of chromosome 2 including the gene codifying the receptor of FSH can display point mutations that cause variations in the aminoacid sequence. Consequently, the functional properties may be enhanced or impaired. Therefore, FSHR inactivating mutations may cause primary or secondary amenorrhea, infertility and premature ovarian failure..On the contrary,activating mutations may predispose to ovarian hyperstimulation syndrome, secondary to exogenous FSH administration or spontaneous [14].A single natural loss of function mutation of the FSHR has been reported ; however when many European women were examined for FSHR mutations the results were negative. Later, Beau et al found the partial loss of function mutation of the FSHR in a patient with secondary amenorrhea and very high plasna gonadotropin concentrations,especially FSH, contrasting with normal sized ovaries and antral follicles up to 5mm at ultrasonography [15].Several Finnish families were identified displaying an inherited pattern of ovarian dysgenesis leading to underdeveloped ovaries and primary amenorrhea. Genetic studies revealed a mutation Ala189Val/ homozigous in all affected women evaluated The Ala189Val mutation of the FSHR gene results in a complete block of FSH action in vivo. The failure of hCG to increase both ovarian estradiol and testosterone secretion emphasizes the possible contribution of FSH in regulating ovarian androgen synthesis,and supports the theory that both gonadotropins are necessary for appropriate ovarian steroidogenesis in humans .Another identified mutation as heterozigous is the Asp567Gly. [16,17]. In 2003,Meduri et al reported a new inactivating mutation of the FSH receptor in a patient showing a homozygous Pro (519)Thr.This mutation totally impaired adenylate cyclase stimulation in vitro.; a complete block in the follicular maturation after the first stage was also observed. The woman showed complete FSH resistance and infertility associated with the persistence of a high number of small follicles[18]. In the meantime, polymorphisms of the FSH receptor gene do not appear to have pathophysiological significance with regard to ovarian function [19]. Nevertheless,a recent study suggested that the polymorphisms of the FSH receptor gene might play a role in genetic susceptibility to PCOS (20). Increased levels of oestradiol result from peripheral aromatisation of excess androgens, and from follicle stimulating hormone induced ovarian follicular secretion. Plasma inhibin-B is elevated in women with PCOS. Inhibin stimulating androgen production and androgens in turn stimulating inhibin secretion, establishing a vicious circle within the ovary that inhibits ovulation..Some researches found that inhibin A concentrations increase with increasing follicle size resulting in higher follicular fluid concentrations in dominant follicles from normal women compared with PCOS follicles. So, the inhibin A deficiency may play a role in the follicular arrest associated with PCOS [21,22,23].Although ovarian follicle recruitment and growth remain unaffected, the selection of a dominant preovulatory follicle does not occur in PCOS [11]. The physiological role of intraovarian activin (beta-beta)and inhibin (alpha/beta)dimers in human is unclear. However,recent studies have provided a mechanism of inhibin action that is consistent with its role in reproduction and may expand inhibin function to tissues outside the reproductive axis [24]. The identification of follistatin as a beta-subunit-specific high affinity binding protein has added complexities for the interpretation of the precise role of these ovarian peptides.Although,the study of Roberts et al could clarify several aspects of the inhibin/activin/follistatin system action. Granulosa cells of the small antral follicle have the potential to form all dimers of inhibin and activin.and their autocrine and paracrine actions may be modulated by follistatin in both granulosa cells and thecal cell layers. With the growth of the dominant follicle, beta-beta subunit mRNA is no longer detectable in any cell type ,and beta-A subunit expression emerges in the thecal cell along with continued abundant expression of beta A-subunit in the granulosa cell. In the corpus luteum the inhibin-activin-follistatin system appear to function in an autocrine fashion.[25]. Follistatin is an activin-binding protein that neutralizes the biological activity of activin in vivo and in vitro and is expressed in multiple tissues, including the ovary, pituitary, adrenal cortex, and pancreas [26]. Activin, a member of the transforming growth factor-ß superfamily, modulates the production of androgens by ovarian thecal cells, the development of ovarian follicles, and the secretion of FSH by the pituitary and insulin by pancreatic ß-cells [27,28]. Because follistatin inhibits the activity of activin, altered follistatin activity would be expected to affect follicular development, ovarian androgen production, pituitary FSH secretion, and insulin release. All these processes have been shown to be perturbed in PCOS Female transgenic mice that overexpress follistatin, display reduced serum levels of FSH and arrested folliculogenesis (23,25,29). In 1999,Urbanek et al carried out a multicenter study using the same diagnostic criteria for PCOS and tested 37 candidate genes for PCOS from 150 families with at least one affected member.They found that follistatin gene with the strongest evidence remained significant even after correction for multiple testing [30].Follistatin is a glycosylated polypeptide homologous to epidermal growth factor which binds to activin thereby reducing serum follicle stimulating hormone levels and increasing ovarian androgen production. Furthermore,follistatin levels have recently considered as a marker for inflammation [30]. Extensive sequencing of the follistatin gene identified variants at 17 sites, but none of these seem to be likely etiological agents in PCOS. No common variants were detected in the coding regions of follistatin [31,32].The one potential exception is a locus on chromosome 19p13.2, which is now thought to be in the region of the fibrillin 3 (FBNN3) gene. Fibrillins are modulators of TGFβ proteins, but their potential role in PCOS remains to be determined [33].Recent studies draw also attention to role of anti-Mullerian hormone in polycystic ovaries. Anti-Müllerian hormone(AMH) is a dimeric glycoprotein, a member of the transforming growth factor (TGF) superfamily. It is produced exclusively in the gonads and is involved in the regulation of follicular growth and development. In the ovary AMH is produced by the granulosa cells of early developing follicles and seems to be able to inhibit the initiation of primordial follicle growth and FSH-induced follicle growth. Hence, AMH is largely expressed throughout folliculogenesis. From the primary follicular stage towards the antral stage,serum levels of AMH may represent both the quantity and quality of the ovarian follicle pool. In women with PCOS, the AMH levels, after metformin therapy, are 2 to 3-fold higher than in healthy women. Furthermore,the levels correlate positively with those of serum androstenedione and testosterone and with follicle count and negatively with age. AMH levels, the number of antral follicles and ovarian volume decreased significantly during metformin treatment. Considering these correlations, AMH measurement could be used to assess ovarian ageing, to diagnose polycystic ovaries-PCOS and to evaluate treatment efficacy [34] The reduction of AMH in follicles greater than 9 mm from normal ovaries appears to be an important requirement for the selection of the dominant follicle. AMH production per granulosa cells was 75 times higher in anovulatory PCOS, compared with normal ovaries. The increase in AMH may contribute to failure of follicle growth and ovulation seen in polycystic ovary syndrome [35] An interesting study showed that serum concentrations of AMH are increased in prepubertal daughters of PCOS mothers, suggesting that these girls appear to show evidence of an altered follicular development during infancy and childhood [36].The commonest characteristic of PCOS is a disturbance in the selection of the dominant follicle resulting in anovulation. It was showed that genotype and allele frequencies for the AMH Ile (49)Ser (rs10407022) and AMH type II receptor-482 A>G polymorphisms are similar in PCOS women and controls. Nevertheless, PCOS carriers of the AMH (49)Ser allele less often have polycystic ovaries , lower follicle numbers and lower androgen levels, compared with non carriers. Furthermore, it was showed "in vitro" that the bioactivity of the AMH (49) Ser protein is diminished, compared with the AMH (49) Ile protein. In conclusion, genetic variants in the AMH and AMH type II receptor gene do not influence PCOS susceptibility. However, the data might suggest that the AMH Ile (49) polymorphism contribute to the severity of the PCOS phenotype [37]. A clearer understanding of its role in ovarian physiology might help clinicians to find a key role for AMH measurement in the field of reproductive medicine [38]. The post GnRH agonist rise in FSH and LH levels did not influence AMH values..Poor response in IVF, indicative of a diminished ovarian reserve, is associated with reduced baseline serum AMH concentrations. In line with recent observations it appears that AMH may reflect ovarian follicular status better than the usual hormone markers and can be used as a marker for ovarian ageing [39,40].An interesting laboratory-based study considering the theory of an intrinsic abnormality of early follicle development in PCOS, evaluated the proportion of primordial and primary follicles in normal and PCOS women with regular menses or with anovulation . The aim of this study was to establish whether the accelerated transition of follicles from primordial to primary stages in PCO women is due to increased granulosa cell (GCs) division. This parameter was measured by the expression of minichromosome maintenance protein2(MCM2) The results showed that granulosa cell proliferation was increased in anovulatory PCO compared with both normal and ovulatory PCO ,with an increased proportion of preantral follicles with MCM2-positive granulosa cells.The number of GCs differed significantly among the three types of ovary at the transitional and primary stages. This was accompanied by an altered relationship between oocyte growth and GC division/ cuboidalization. The data of this research could explain the increased proportion of primary follicles in PCOS [41]. A Chinese study found that the number of hypodiploidy cells associated with apoptosis in granuòosa cells of PCOS was significantly higher than that in normal ovary. PDCD5(a apoptosis protein) –positive cells were mainly observed in cytoplasm. Consequently,these researchers postulated that PDCD5 is an important apoptosis regulating factor in granulosa cells of PCOS and normal ovary,which might be involved in the pathogenesis of PCOS [42]. Excessive granulosa cell activity may be implicated in the abnormal follicular dynamic of the syndrome [43]. In women with PCOS, Xita et al found subnormal levels of SHBG, and a microsatellite repeat in the promoter of the SHBG gene linked to PCOS susceptibility [44]. Although in other studies, evaluating different populations,the p.D327N polymorphism in this gene was not found to influence PCOS susceptibility [45,46].

References

[1]   Pettersson K, Ding YQ, Huhtaniemi I. An immunologically anomalous luteinizing hormone variant in a healthy woman. *J. Clin. Endocrinol. Metab*. 1992;74(1):164-71.

[2]   Furui K,Suganuma S,Tsukahara S,Asada Y,Kikkawa F,Tanaka M, Ozawa T, Tomoda Y. Identification of two point mutations in the gene coding luteinizing hormone (LH)

beta-subunut, associated with immunologically LH variants. *J. Clin. Endocrinol. Metab.* 1994;78(1): 107-13.

[3] Okuda K,Yamada T,Imoto H,Komatsubara H,Sugimoto O. Antigenic alteration of an anomalous human luteinizing hormone caused by two chorionic gonadotropin –type amino-acid substitutions. *Biochem. Biophys. Res. Commun.* 1994;200(1):584-90.

[4] Nilsson C,Pettersson K,Millar RP,Coerver KA , Matzuk MM,Huhtaniemi IT. Worldwide frequency of a common genetic variant of luteinizing hormone:an international collaborative research. International Collaborative Research Group. *Fertil. Steril.* 1997;67(6): 998-1004.

[5] Haavisto AM, Pettersson K,Bergendahl M,Virkamaki A., Huhtaniemi I. Occurrence and biological properties of a common genetic variant of luteinizing hormone. *J. Clin. Endocrinol. Metab.* 1995; 80(4): 1257-63.

[6] Rajkhowa M,Talbot JA,Jones PW,Pettersson K, Haavisto AM,Huhtaniemi I,Clayton RN. Prevalence of an immunological LH beta- subunit variant in a UK population of healthy women and women with polycystic ovary syndrome. *Clin. Endocrinol.* 1995: 43(3):297-303.

[7] Suganuma N,Furui K,Kikkawa F,Tomoda Y,Furuhashi M. Effects of the mutations (Tpr8 > Arg and Iie15> Thr) in human luteinizing hormone(LH) beta-subunit on LH bioactivity in vitro and in vivo. *Endocrinology* 1996; 137(3):831.

[8] Takahashi K, Karino K, Kanasaki H, Miyazaki K. Altered kinetics of pituitary response to gonadotropin-releasing hormone with variant luteinizing hormone: correlation with ovulatory disorders. *Horm. Res.* 2004;61(1):27-32.

[9] Takahashi K,Kurioka H,Ozaki T,Kanasaki H,Miyazaki K,Karino K. Pituitary response to luteinizing hormone-releasing hormone in women with variant luteinizing hormone. *Eur. J. Endocrinol.* 2000;143(3):375-81.

[10] Roy AC, Liao WX, Chen Y, Arulkumaran S, Ratnam SS. Identification of seven novel mutations in LH beta-subunit gene by SSCP. Mol. *Cell. Biochem.* 1996;165(2):151-3.

[11] Lobo RA, Granger L, Goehelsmann U, Mishell DR Jr. Elevations in unbound serum estradiol as a possible mechanism for inappropriate gonadotropin secretion in women with PCO. *J. Clin. Endocrinol. Metab.* 1981;52:156-8.

[12] Elter K,Erel CT,Cine N,Ozbek U,Hacihanefioglu B,Ertungealp E.Role of the mutations Trp8-Arg and Ile15-Thr of the human luteinizing hormone ß subunit in women with polycystic ovary syndrome. *Fertil. Steril.* 1999;71:425-430.

[13] Liao WX,Tong Y,Roy AC,Ng SC. New Accl polymprphisms in the follicle stimulating hormone beta subunit gene and its prevalence in three South East Asian populations. *Human Heredity* 1999;49:181-2.

[14] Lussiana C,Guani B,Mari C,Restagno G,Massobrio M,Revelli A.Mutations and polymorphisms of the FSH receptor (FSHR) gene:clinical implications in female fecundity and molecular biology of FSHR protein and gene. *Obstet. Gynecol. Surv.* 2008;63(12):785-95.

[15] Beau I, Touraine P, Meduri G,Gougeon A, Desroches A,Matuchansky C,Milgrom E,Kuttenn F,Misrahi M. A novel phenotype related to partial loss of function mutations of the follicle stimulating hormone receptor. *J. Clin. Invest.* 1998;102(7):1352-9.

[16] Vaskivuo TE,AittomakiK,AnttonenM,Ruokonen A, Herva R,Osawa Y,Heikinheimo M , Huhtaniemi I,Tapanainen JS.Effects of follicle –stimulating hormone(FSH) and

human chorionic gonadotropin in individuals with an inactivating mutation of the FSH receptor. *Fetil. Steril.* 2002; 78(1):108-13.

[17] Gromoll J,Simoni M,Nordhoff V,Behre HM,De Geyter C,Nieschlag E.Functional and clinical sequences of mutations in the FSH receptor. *Mol. Cell Endocrinol.* 1996; 125(1-2):177-82.

[18] .Meduri G,Touraine P,Beau I,Lahuna O,Desroches A,Vacher-Lavenu MC,Kuttenn F,Misrahi M.Delayed puberty and primary amenorrhea associated with a novel mutation of the human follicle-stimulating hormone receptor:clinical,histological,and molecular studies. *J. Clin. Endocrinol. Metab.* 2003;88(8):3491-8.

[19] Conway GS,Conway E,Walker C,Hoppner W,Gromoll J,Simoni M.Mutation screening and isoform prevalence of the follicle stimulating hormone receptor gene in women with premature ovarian failure,resistant ovary syndrome and polycystic ovary syndrome. *Clin. Endocrinol.* (Oxf) 1999;51(1):97-99.

[20] Du J,Zhang W,Guo L,Zhang Z,Shi H,Wang J,Zhang H,Gao L,He L.Two FSHR variants, haplotypes and meta-analysis in Chinese women with premature ovarian failure and polycystic ovary syndrome . *Mol. Genet. Metab.* 2010;Epub ahead of print

[21] Knight PG,Glister C.Potential local regulatory functions of inhibins,activins and follistatin in the ovary. *Reprod.* 2001;121:503-512.

[22] Welt CK. Regulation and function of inhibins in the normal menstrual cycle. *Semin. Reprod. Med.* 2004 Aug;22(3):187-93.

[23] Fujiwara T,Sidis Y,Welt C,Lambert-Messerlian G,Fox J,Taylor A,Schneyer A.Dynamics of inhibin subunit and follistatin mRNA during development of normal and polycystic ovary syndrome follicle. *J. Clin. Endocrinol. Metab.* 2001; 86(9):4206-15.

[24] Cook RW, Thompson TB,Jardetzky TS, Woodruff TK.Molecular biology of inhibin action. *Semin. Reprod. Med.* 2004; 22(3):269-76.

[25] Roberts VJ,Barth S,el-Roely A,Yen SS.Expression of inhibin/ activin subunits and follistatin messenger ribonucleic acids and proteins in ovarian follicles and the corpus luteum during the human menstrual cycle. *J. Clin. Endocrinol. Metab.* 1993<77(5): 1402-10.

[26] Legro RS, Spielman R, Urbanek M, Driscoll D, Strauss JF, Dunaif A. 1998 Phenotype and genotype in polycystic ovary syndrome. *Recent Prog. Horm. Res.* 53:217–256.

[27] Shibata H, Kanzaki M, Takeuchi T, Miyazaki J, Kojima I. 1996 Two distinct signaling pathways activated by activin A in glucose responsive pancreatic beta-cells lines. *J. Mol. Endocrinol.* 16:249–258.

[28] Mather JP, Moore A, Li RH. 1997 Activins, inhibins, and follistatins; further thoughts on a growing family of regulators. *Proc. Soc. Exp. Biol. Med.* 215:209–222.

[29] Guo Q, Kuma TR, Woodruff T, Hadsell LA, DeMayo FJ, Matzuk MM. 1998 Overexpression of mouse follistatin causes reproductive defects in transgenic mice. *Mol. Endocrinol.* 12:96–106. 28.

[30] Chen MJ, Yang WS, Chen HF, Kuo JJ,Ho HN,Yang ys, Chen SU. Increased follistatin levels after oral contraceptive treatment in obese and non-obese women with polycystic ovary syndrome. *Hum. Reprod.* 2010;25(3):779-85.

[31] Urbanek M, Legro RS, Driscoll DA, Azziz R, Ehrmann DA, Norman RJ, Strauss JF 3rd, Spielman RS, Dunaif A. Thirty-seven candidate genes for polycystic ovary

syndrome: strongest evidence for linkage is with follistatin. *Proc. Natl. Acad. Sci. U S A.* 1999 ;96(15):8573-8.

[32] Urbanek M,Wu X,Vickery KR et al.Allelic variants of the follistatin gene in polycystic ovary syndrome. *J. Clin. Endocrinol. Metab.* 2000;85: 4455-4461.

[33] Stewart DR, Dombroski BA,Urbanek M, Ankener W,Ewens KG,Wood JR,Legro R. S,Strauss J. F, Dunaif III A.,Spielman RS. Fine Mapping of Genetic Susceptibility to Polycystic Ovary Syndrome on Chromosome 19p13.2 and Tests for Regulatory Activity. *J. Clin. Endocrinol. Metab.* 2006;Vol. 91, No. 10 4112-4117.

[34] Piltonen T, Morin-Papunen L, Koivunen R, Perheentupa A, Ruokonen A, Tapanainen JS.Serum anti-Müllerian hormone levels remain high until late reproductive age and decrease during metformin therapy in women with polycystic ovary syndrome. *Hum. Reprod.* 2005 Jul;20(7):1820-6.

[35] Pellatt 2007 Pellatt L, Hanna L, Brincat M, Galea R, Brain H, Whitehead S, Mason H. Granulosa cell production of anti-Müllerian hormone is increased in polycystic ovaries. *J. Clin. Endocrinol. Metab.* 2007 Jan;92(1):240-5.

[36] Sir-Patermann T,Codner E,Maliqueo M, Echiburu B,Hitschfeld C,Crisosto N,Perez-Bravo F, Recabarren SE,Cassoria F. Increased anti-Mullerian hormone serum concentrations in prepubertal daughters of women with polycystic ovary syndrome. *J. Clin. Endocrinol. Metab.* 2006;91(8): 3105-9.

[37] Kevenaar ME,Laven JS, Fong SL, Uitterlinden AG, de Jong FH, Themmen AP, Visser JA. A functional anti-mullerian hormone gene polymorphism is associated with follicle number and androgen levels in polycystic ovary syndrome patients. *J. Clin. Endocrinol. Metab.* 2008;93(4):1310-6.

[38] La Marca A, Volpe A. Anti-Müllerian hormone (AMH) in female reproduction: is measurement of circulating AMH a useful tool? *Clin. Endocrinol.*(Oxf)2006; 64(6): 603-10.

[39] Fanchin R,Schonauer LM, Righini C,Guibourdenche J,Frydman R,Taieb J.Serum anti-Mullerian hormone is more strongly related to ovarian follicular status than serum inhibin B,estradiol,FSH and LH on day 3. *Hum. Reprod.* 2003; 18(2): 323-7.

[40] van Rooij IA, Broekmans FJ, te Velde ER,Fauser BC,Bancsi LF,de Jong FH, Themmen AP. Serum anti-Mullerian hormone levels : a novel measure of ovarian reserve. *Hum. Reprod.* 2002; 17(12): 3065-71.

[41] Stubbs SA,Stark J,Dilworth SM, Franks S,Hardy K. Abnormal preantral folliculogenesis in polycystic ovaries is associated with increased granulosa cell division. *J. Clin. Endocrinol. Metab.* 2007; 92(11):4418-26.).

[42] Sun CL,Qiao J,Hu ZX,Zhuang T, Chen YY. Expression of novel apoptosis-related protein PDCD5 in granulosa cells of polycystic ovary syndrome. *Beijing Da Xue Xue Bao* 2005;37(5):476-9.

[43] Nardo LG,Yates AP,Roberts SA,Pemberton P,Laing I. The relationship between AMH, androgens,insulin resistance and basal ovarian follicular status in non-obese subfertile women with and without polycystic ovary syndrome. *Hum. Reprod.* 2009: 24(11): 2917-2923.

[44] Xita N, Tsatsoulis A, Chatzikyriakidou A, Georgiou I. Association of the (TAAAA)n repeat polymorphism in the sex hormone-binding globulin (SHBG) gene with polycystic ovary syndrome and relation to SHBG serum levels. *J. Clin. Endocrinol. Metab.* 2003; 88:5976–5980.

[45] Ferk P, Teran N, Gersak K. The (TAAAA)n microsatellite polymorphism in the SHBG gene influences serum SHBG levels in women with polycystic ovary syndrome. *Hum. Reprod.* 2007; 22:1031–1036.

[46] Bendlova B, Zavadilova J, Vankova M, Vejrazkova D, Lukasova P, Vcelak J, Hill M, Cibula D, Vondra K, Starka L, et al. Role of D327N sex hormone-binding globulin gene polymorphism in the pathogenesis of polycystic ovary syndrome. *J. Steroid. Biochem. Mol. Biol.* 2007; 104:68–74.

Genes involved in insulin secretion and metabolism

The increased risk of type 2 diabetes and cardiovascular disease in women with PCOS has led to numerous association studies in genes related to these diseases. The insulin gene (INS) is located between the genes for tyrosine hydroxylase and for IGF-II at 11p15.5 and include variable tandem repeats (VNTR) embedded at the 5regulatory region of INS [1]. Insulin gene (INS) variable number of tandem repeats (VNTR) polymorphism, particularly in class I and III alleles, is linked to an increased susceptibility to type 2 diabetes and high birth weight. The transcriptional activity of the longer polymorphic region of the class III, containing approxymately 157 repeats, is greater than that of the classes II and I which comprise the shorter polymorphisms [2].Waterworth et al found that class III alleles were frequent in PCOS women and particularly in those with anovulation [3].It seems that class III alleles are transmitted more commonly from fathers than from mothers to affected daugther [4,5].The study of Huxtable et al may suggest that the microsatellite polymorphism 5 of the INS gene is associated with several phenotypes,including type I diabetes, PCOS and birth weight. They found that there was no significant association between diabetes and the INS-VNTR genotype but they supported that the variation within the TH-INS-IGF2 could influence type 2 diabetes susceptibility. In addition,it has been shown that class III alleles and paternal class alleles transmission were significantly related to increased number of PCOS features and to reduced insulin sensitivity among women with PCOS [5]. A microsatellite polymorphism, located outside the insulin receptor(INSR) gene, could influence INSR gene expression in the ovary [6].Insulin acts on the normal ovary by a receptor mediated stimulation of steroidogenesis. Ovarian effects of increased insulin are described in women with diabetes mellitus, obesity, syndrome of extreme insulin resistance and PCOS [7]. The efficacy of insulin sensitising agents such as metformin in the treatment of PCOS supports this hypothesis [8].Metformin, an insulin-sensitizing drug often used in women with PCOS to induce ovulation, is believed to act via phosphorylation of IRS proteins:IRS-1 and IRS-2. The insulin receptor substrates IRS-1 and IRS-2 are proteins that participate in the insulin signal transduction pathway. Extensive investigations on a possible association between the p.G972R polymorphism in the IRS-1 gene and PCOS have been carried out, with both positive and negative results[9,10,11,12,13]. The polymorphism was associated with symptoms of PCOS across four different studies [9,14,15,16].The activation of the insulin receptor after insulin binding requires the autophosphorylation of the ß subunit of the insulin receptor.When, IRS-1 is dysfunctional, IRS-2 can act on intracellular transmission of the insulin signal but it requires higher insulin concentration for activation than in normal condition [17,18]. Investigations into the pG1057D polymorphism in the IRS-2 gene have failed to show an association with susceptibility to PCOS but have linked this polymorphism with blood glucose levels in women with PCOS [12,13,14,15].It seems that the Gly972Arg IRS-1 could be more prevalent in insulin resistant PCOS patients than in non-insulin resistant patients and control[15]. In addition,Gly972Arg carriers are more obese,more insulin resistant and have higher fasting insulin levels than the other PCOS women and controls [10].

Calpains

Calpain-10 is a cysteine protease that could play a role in insulin secretion and action [19]. Its gene (CAPN10) is associated with type 2 diabetes, and potential associations between five different polymorphisms and PCOS have been investigated. No associations were found between the UCSNP43, UCSNP19, UCSNP63 polymorphisms and PCOS, although there were some links with the symptoms of PCOS [20,21,22]. In particular,it was reported as a single nucleotide polymorphism of the calpan-10 gene could influence hirsutism [22]. In the CAPN10 gene, two different Spanish studies found an association between either the SNP UCSNP44 or UCSNP45 and PCOS susceptibility [21,22].These associations were not observed in a German study [13]. Some studies found that variation in the gene CAPN10 encoding calpain 10 is associated with type 2 diabetes [23].Ehrmann et al reported the association between the 121/121 haplotype of this gene and higher insulin levels in African-American women and an increased risk of PCOS in both African American and white women [20]. Nonetheless, other investigations have had coonflicting results about the relation of these polymorphisms with PCOS [24].

Insulin-Like Growth Factors

The variant ApaI RFLP in the insulin-like growth factor-2 (IGF-2) gene has been linked to PCOS susceptibility in Caucasian women, whereas polymorphisms in genes encoding IGF-1, IGF-1 receptor and IGF-2 receptor seem not be associated. Of three variants investigated in the paraoxonase gene (PON1),the 108C/T variant was linked to PCOS susceptibility in Caucasian women [25]. The p.L55M polymorphisms was not associated with PCOS, but was linked with a higher BMI and greater insulin resistance in women who were homozygotic for the 55M polymorphism compared with carriers of the common 55L allele.This polymorphism is believed to contribute to impaired insulin function by increasing levels of oxidative stress in women with PCOS. The remaining investigated polymorphism (p.Q192R) was associated with neither susceptibility nor phenotype, although insulin resistance does not affect the ovary, thus enabling the excess insulin to cause ovarian androgen hypersecretion [26,27]. Obese women with PCOS are more insulin resistant than non-obese controls, suggesting that obesity and PCOS exert independent effects on insulin resistance. But weight loss restores insulin sensitivity only in some, and insulin resistance is described also in non-obese PCOS subjects . Insulin resistance in PCOS is more prominent in anovulatory women than equally hyperandrogenaemic women with regular menses [26]. It is now clear that PCOS is often associated with profound insulin resistance as well as with defects in insulin secretion. These abnormalities, together with obesity, explain the substantially increased prevalence of glucose intolerance in PCOS. Moreover,since PCOS is an extremely common disorder, PCOS-related insulin resistance is an important cause of NIDDM in women . The insulin resistance in at least 50% of PCOS women appears to be related to excessive serine phosphorylation of the insulin receptor. A factor extrinsic to the insulin receptor, presumably a serine/threonine kinase, causes this abnormality and is an example of an important new mechanism for human insulin resistance related to factors controlling insulin receptor signaling. Serine phosphorylation appears to modulate the activity of the key regulatory enzyme of androgen biosynthesis, P450c17. It is thus possible that a single defect produces both the insulin resistance and the hyperandrogenism in some PCOS women . Recent studies strongly suggest that insulin is acting through its own receptor ,rather than the IGF-I receptor, in PCOS to augment not only ovarian and adrenal steroidogenesis but also pituitary LH release [28].Indeed, the defect in insulin action appears to be selective, affecting glucose metabolism but not cell growth. Since PCOS usually has a menarchal age of onset, this makes it a particularly appropriate disorder in which to examine the ontogeny of defects in carbohydrate metabolism. Although the presence of lipid abnormalities, dysfibrinolysis, and insulin resistance would be predicted to place PCOS women at high risk for cardiovascular disease, appropriate prospective studies are necessary to directly assess this. Hence, it seems that the VNTR polymorphism might affect the presence of hyperinsulinemia and insulin resistance in some PCOS phenotypes [29]. Nevertheless this evidence, in other investigations the association between insulin gene, PCOS and hyperandrogenism were not found.[30]. However,these evaluations were often based on exclusivive ultrasonographic criteria and this hamper definitive conclusions.The insulin receptor is encoded by the insulin receptor gene (INSR) located at the chromosome 19 [31].The activation of the insulin receptor after insulin binding requires the autophosphorylation of the ß subunit of the insulin receptor. A number of variants of other genes involved in insulin resistance, type 2 diabetes and/or obesity have been investigated but failed to show an association with PCOS: apolipoprotein E (APOE), C2 (FOXC2), glycogen synthetase 1 (GYS1),and protein tyrosine phosphatase 1B (PTPN1)[13,25,32,33].

References

[1]   Jiunien C.VanHeyningen V.Report of the committee on the genetic constitution of chromosome 11.Cytogenet. *Cell Genet.* 1990;55:153-169.

[2] Bell GI,Selby MJ,Rutter WJ.The highly polymorphic region near the human insulin gene is composed of simple tandemly repeating sequences. *Nature* 1982;295:31-35.

[3] Waterworth DM, Bennett ST, Gharani N, McCarthy MI, Hague S, Batty S, et al. Linkage and association of insulin gene VNTR regulatory polymorphism with polycystic ovary syndrome. *Lancet* 1997; 349: 986-90.

[4] Bennett ST,Told JA, Waterworth DM. Association of insulin gene VNTR polymorphism with polycystic ovary syndrome(letter). *Lancet* 1997; 349:1771-1772.

[5] Huxtable SJ, Saker PJ, Haddad L, Walker M, Frayling TM, Levy JC, Hitman GA, O'Rahilly S, Hattersley AT, McCarthy MI. Analysis of parent-offspring trios provides evidence for linkage and association between the insulin gene and type 2 diabetes mediated exclusively through paternally transmitted class III variable number tandem repeat alleles. *Diabetes*. 2000 Jan;49(1):126-30.

[6] Tucci S, Futterweit W, Concepcion Es, Greenberg DA, Villanueva R. et al. Evidence for association of polycystic ovary syndrome in Caucasian women with a marker at the Insulin Receptor Gene Locus. *Journal of Clinical Endocrinology and Metabolism* 2001, 86: 446-9.

[7] Poretsky L, Cataldo NA, Rosenwaks Z and Guidice L. The Insulin-related regulatory system in health and disease. *Endocrine Reviews* 1999; 20: 535-82.

[8] Velezquez EM, Mendoza S, Hamer T, Sosa F, Glueck CJ. Metformin therapy in polycystic ovary syndrome reduces hyperinsulinaemia, insulin resistance, hyperandrogenaemia, and systolic blood pressure facilitating normal menses and pregnancy. *Metabolism* 1994; 43: 647-54.

[9] Sir-Petermann T, Angel B, Maliqueo M, Santos JL, Riesco MV, Toloza H, Perez-Bravo F. Insulin secretion in women who have polycystic ovary syndrome and carry the Gly972Arg variant of insulin receptor substrate-1 in response to a high-glycemic or low-glycemic carbohydrate load. *Nutrition* 2004; 20:905–91.

[10] Dilek S, Ertunc D, Tok EC, Erdal EM, Aktas A. Association of Gly972Arg variant of insulin receptor substrate-1 with metabolic features in women with polycystic ovary syndrome. *Fertil. Steril.* 2005; 84:407–412.

[11] Baba T, Endo T, Sata F, Honnma H, Kitajima Y, Hayashi T, Manase K, Kanaya M, Yamada H, Minakami H, et al. Polycystic ovary syndrome is associated with genetic polymorphism in the insulin signaling gene IRS-1 but not ENPP1 in a Japanese population. *Life Sci.* 2007; 81:850–854.

[12] Ehrmann DA, Tang X, Yoshiuchi I, Cox NJ, Bell GI. Relationship of insulin receptor substrate-1 and -2 genotypes to phenotypic features of polycystic ovary syndrome. *J. Clin. Endocrinol. Metab.* 2002; b87:4297–4300.

[13] Haap M, Machicao F, Stefan N, Thamer C, Tschritter O, Schnuck F, Wallwiener D, Stumvoll M, Haring HU, Fritsche A. Genetic determinants of insulin action in polycystic ovary syndrome. *Exp. Clin. Endocrinol. Diabetes* 2005; 113:275–281.

[14] Villuendas G, Botella-Carretero JI, Roldan B, Sancho J, Escobar-Morreale HF, San Millan JL. Polymorphisms in the insulin receptor substrate-1 (IRS-1) gene and the insulin receptor substrate-2 (IRS-2) gene influence glucose homeostasis and body mass index in women with polycystic ovary syndrome and non-hyperandrogenic controls. *Hum. Reprod.* 2005; 20:3184–3191.

[15] El Mkadem SA, Lautier C, Macari F, Molinari N, Lefebvre P, Renard E, Gris JC, Cros G, Daures JP, Bringer J, et al. Role of allelic variants Gly972Arg of IRS-1 and

Gly1057Asp of IRS-2 in moderate-to-severe insulin resistance of women with polycystic ovary syndrome. *Diabetes* 2001; 50:2164–2168.

[16] Witchel SF, Kahsar-Miller M, Aston CE, White C, Azziz R.Prevalence of CYP21 mutations and IRS1 variant among women with polycystic ovary syndrome and adrenal androgen excess. *Fertil. Steril.* 2005 Feb;83(2):371-5.

[17] Burks DJ,White MF.IRS proteins and beta-cell function. *Diabetes* 2001; 50(Suppl.1): 140-145.

[18] White MF.IRS proteins and the common path to diabetes. *Am. J. Physiol. Endocrinol. Metab.* 2002; 283: 413-22.

[19] Sreenan SK,Zhou YP,Otani K et al. Calpains play a role in insulin secretion and action. *Diabetes* 2001;50:2013-2020.

[20] Ehrmann DA,Schwarz PEH,Hara M et al.Relationship of calpain-10 genotype to phenotypic features of polycystic ovary syndrome. *J. Clin. Endocrinol. Metab.* 2002; 87:1669-1673.

[21] Gonzalez A, Abril E, Roca A, Aragon MJ, Figueroa MJ, Velarde P, Ruiz R, Fayez O, Galan JJ, Herreros JA, et al. Specific CAPN10 gene haplotypes influence the clinical profile of polycystic ovary patients. *J. Clin. Endocrinol. Metab.* (2003) 88:5529–5536.

[22] Escobar-Morreale HF, Peral B, Villuendas G, Calvo RM, Sancho J, San Millan JL. Common single nucleotide polymorphisms in intron 3 of the calpain-10 gene influence hirsutism. *Fertil. Steril.* (2002) 77:581–587.

[23] Horikawa Y,Oda N,Cox NJ et al.Genetic variation in the gene encoding calpain-10 is associated with type 2-diabetes mellitus. *Nat. Genet.* 2000;26:163-75.

[24] Haddad L,Evans JC,Gharani N et al.Variation within the type 2 diabetes susceptibility gene calpain-10 and polycystic ovary syndrome. *J. Clin. Endocrinol. Metab.* 2002; 87:2606-2610

[25] San Millan JL,Corton M,Villuendas G,Sancho J,Peral B,EscobarMorreale HF.Association of the polycystic ovary syndrome with genomic variants related to insulin resistance,type 2 diabetes mellitus,and obesity. *J. Clin. Endocrinol. Metab.* 2004;89:2640-2646.

[26] Dunaif A. Insulin resistance and the polycystic ovary syndrome: mechanisms and implications for pathogenesis. *Endocrine Reviews* 1997; 18: 774-800. 15.

[27] Franks S, Gilling-Smith C, Willis D. Insulin action in the normal and polycystic ovary Endocrinology and Metabolism Clinics of North America 1999; 28: 361-378.

[28] Diamanti-Kandarakis E,Argyrakopoulou G,Economou F,Kandaraki E,Koutsilieris M.Defects in insulin signaling pathways in ovarian steroidogenesis and other tissues in polycystic ovary syndrome. *J. Steroid Biochem. Mol. Biol.* 2008;109(3-5):242-6.

[29] Michelmore K, Ong K,Mason S et al.Clinical features in women with polycystic ovaries: relationships to insulin sensitivity,insulin gene VNTR and birth weight. *Clin. Endocrinol.* 2001;55: 439-446.

[30] Calvo RM,Telleria J,Sancho J,San Millan JL,Escobar-Morreale HF.Insulin gene variable number of tandem repeats regulatory polymorphism is not associated with hyperandrogenism in Spanish women. *Fertil. Steril.* 2002;77:666-668.

[31] Goldfine OD.The insulin receptor :molecular biology and transmembrane signalling. *Endocrine Rev.*1987;8:235-255.

[32] Heinonen S, Korhonen S, Hippeläinen M, Hiltunen M, Mannermaa A, Saarikoski S. Apolipoprotein E alleles in women with polycystic ovary syndrome. *Fertil. Steril.* 2001; M;75(5): 878-80.

[33] Rajkhowa M. , Neary R. H., Kumpatla P,Game F. L, Jones PW, Obhrai M S,Clayton R. N. Altered Composition of High Density Lipoproteins in Women with the Polycystic Ovary Syndrome. *J. Clin. Endocrinol. Metab*. 2009; 82(10):3389-94.

Genes involved in obesity and energy modulation

During the last decade,the high prevalence of overweight or obesity in women with PCOS and the recent knowledge on endocrine function of adipose tissue have led to consider the eventual role of adipocytokines in the pathogenesis of PCOS. The studies of Hu et al and Menzaghi et al focused on two variants of adiponectin gene:T45G in exon 2 and G276T in intron 2 that might be associated with obesity,insulin resistance,and the risk of developing type 2-diabetes.[1,2].While, the results of subsequent studies are conflicting. In particular ,Xita et al showed that the distributions of genotypes and alleles of both polymorphisms were no different in women with PCOS and controls, indicating that the individual polymorphisms are not associated with increased risk for PCOS. However, carriers of the T45GG genotype had greater hyperinsulinemia, as estimated by the AUC insulin during the OGTT, than those with the G276T genotype , and this was independent of age and BMI. In addition, women with PCOS carriers of the genotype at position 276 had a higher BMI (P = 0.01) and greater AUC insulin (P = 0.01) than the others.The latter genotype was found less frequently among overweight/obese women with PCOS than in normal-weight individuals (P = 0.002). It is also showed that carriers of the G allele had a tendency for lower serum adiponectin than the other genotype [3].The results of this and other studies seems to deny the causative role of these polymorphisms of the adiponectin gene in the pathogenesis of PCOS.Although the presence of these variants could influence the phenotype of PCOS, its severity and the metabolic disturbances [4]. Recently,Tan et al examined the influence of genetic variants inducing susceptibility to obesity and/or type 2 diabetes mellitus (T2DM) on metabolic and PCOS specific traits in 386 women.They found a risk allele effect of FTO iintron 1 SNP on BMI of the affected PCOS women more significant than in general population [5].

References

[1] Hu FB,Doria A,Li T et al. Genetic variation at the adiponectin locus at risk of type 2 diabetes in women. *Diabetes* 2004;53:209-13.

[2] Menzaghi C,Ercolino T,Di Paola R et al. A haplotype at the adiponectin locus is associated with obesity and other features of the insulin resiatance syndrome. *Diabetes* 2002;51:2306-2312.

[3]   Xita N,Georgiou I,Chatzikyriakidou A et al.Effect of adiponectin gene polymorphisms on circulating adiponectin and insulin resistance indexes in women with polycystic ovary syndrome. *Clin. Chem.* 2005;51:416-23.

[4]   Escobar-Morreale HF,Villuendas G,Botella-Carretero JI et al.Adiponectin and resistin in PCOS:a clinical,biochemical and molecular study. *Hum. Reprod.* 2006;21:2257-226.

[5]   Tan S,Scherag A,Janssen OE,Hahn S,Lahner H,Dietz T,Scherag S,Grallrt H. et al.Large effects on body mass index and insulin resistance of fat mass and obesity associated gene(FTO) variants in patients with polycystic ovary syndrome (PCOS). *BMC Med. Genet.* 2010; 11-12.

Genes involved in low-grade inflammation

Women with PCOS may have chronic low-level inflammation; although polycystic ovary syndrome per se is not associated with increased chronic inflammation [1]. The actions of TNF are mainly mediated by type 1 or type 2 TNF receptors. Of the five polymorphisms in the TNF receptor 2 gene (TNFRSF1B), investigated in relation to PCOS, only p.M196R was found to be associated with PCOS susceptibility and hyperandrogenism [2].Furthermore TNF,a cytokine secreted by adipose tissue, seems to play a role in insulin resistance [3].It was suggested that the mutation 308 is associated with hyperandrogenism and 17-hydroxyprogesterone before and after GnRH stimulation [4]. In spite of this,it was also affirmed no association between the 308 polymorphism in the tumour necrosis factor alpha - promoter region and polycystic ovaries [5]. Other genes as type 2 TNF receptor gene, 597 G and 174 G polymorphisms in the promoter of the IL-6, and other variants of the IL-6 receptor have been associated with hyperandrogenism [6].In particular, it has been shown that the interleukin-6 -597G/A polymorphism is associated with PCOS susceptibility ; while, the 572G/C polymorphism seems not associated, and the 174G/C seems associated with susceptibility and not associated with but related to the PCOS phenotype [1,7,8].With respect to reproductive biology, IL1 has highly inflammatory features and is believed to affect the processes of fertilization and implantation [9]. While human granulosa and cumulus cells synthesize IL1RA, expression of paracrine-acting IL1 in the ovary, which could be involved in multiple steps leading to ovulation and, probably, influencing ovarian physiology [10]. Regarding this aspect of IL1, a study showed as PCOS patients suffering from anovulation show a clear tendency to have an IL1A polymorphism which may be responsible for the abnormal ovulation process of these patients [11]. Interleukin -6 , one of the cytokines of the glycoprotein 130 (gp130) family, may exert a short term insulin-sensitizing effect;whereas, in a long-term period it may induce insulin resistance. Serum sgp 130 seems inversely and independently associated with insulin sensitivity in women with PCOS [12].In conclusion,association of polymorphisms in the interleukin-6 receptor complex seem associated with obesity and hyperandrogenism [6,7]. In spite of these and other reports,. until now the link between polymorphisms of the TNF and IL-6 and PCOS remains controversial. In any case,one of the most prominent mediators of inflammation is the interleukin-1(IL1) family that consists of three different cytokines, the proinflammatory cytokines IL1α, IL1β and the physiological antagonist IL1 receptor antagonist (IL1RA)(13,14). IL1α and IL1β are produced by monocytes, macrophages, neutrophils and epithelial cells, affecting nearly every cell type [10,15]. The human genes encoding IL1α (IL1A) and IL1β (IL1B) are located within a 430 kb region on chromosome 2q14.2 [16,17]. A recent study showed that the 889C/T polymorphism in the IL1A gene is associated with PCOS, which was not the case for the 511C/T and 3953G/A polymorphisms in the IL1B gene. However,a rare allele combination of the IL1 gene was associated with high IL-1 beta plasma levels in healthy individuals [18,19]. Hence, interleukin-1 alpha but not interleukin-1 beta gene polymorphism could be associated with polycystic ovary syndrome [20]. In conclusion, the etiology of PCOS is still discussed controversially, but there is evidence that genetic factors play an important role [21,22].

References

[1] Mohlig M, Spranger J, Osterhoff M, Ristow M, Pfeiffer AF, Schill T, Schlosser HW, Brabant G, Schofl C. The polycystic ovary syndrome per se is not associated with increased chronic inflammation. *Eur. J. Endocrinol.* (2004) 150:525–532.

[2] Peral B, San Millan JL, Castello R, Moghetti P, Escobar-Morreale HF. Comment: the methionine 196 arginine polymorphism in exon 6 of the TNF receptor 2 gene (TNFRSF1B) is associated with the polycystic ovary syndrome and hyperandrogenism. *J. Clin. Endocrinol. Metab.* (2002) 87:3977–3983.

[3] Hotamisligil GS,Peraldi P, Budavari A,Ellis R,White MF,Spiegelman BM. IRS-1 mediated inhibition of insulin receptor tyrosine kinase activity in TNF-α and obesity may induced insulin resistance. *Sci.* 1996;271:665-668.

[4] Escobar-Morreale HF, Calvo RM,Sancho J,San Millan JL,TNF-α and hyperandrogenism : a clinical ,biochemical ,and molecular genetic study. *J. Clin. Endocrinol. Metab.* 2001;86: 3761-3767 3.

[5] Milner CR, Craig JE, Hussey ND, Norman RJ. No association between the -308 polymorphism in the tumour necrosis factor alpha (TNFalpha) promoter region and polycystic ovaries. *Mol. Hum. Reprod.* 1999; 5:5–9.

[6] Escobar-Morreale HF, Calvo RM, Villuendas G, Sancho J, San Millan JL. Association of polymorphisms in the interleukin 6 receptor complex with obesity and hyperandrogenism. *Obes. Res.* 2003; 11:987–996.

[7] Villuendas G, San Millan JL, Sancho J, Escobar-Morreale HF. The 597G and 174G-C polymorphisms in the promoter of the IL-6 gene are associated with hyperandrogenism. J. Clin. Endocrinol. Metab. 2002; 87:1134-1141.

[8] Walch K, Grimm C, Zeillinger R, Huber JC, Nagele F, Hefler LA. A common interleukin-6 gene promoter polymorphism influences the clinical characteristics of women with polycystic ovary syndrome. Fertil. Steril. (2004) 81:1638–1641.

[9] Sukhikh GT,Vanko L.V, Interrelationships between immune and reproductive systems in human, Russ. J. Immunol. 1999 ; 4:. 312–314.

[10] Gerard N, Caillaud M., A. Martoriati A, Goudet G, A.C. Lalmanach A.C The interleukin-1 system and female reproduction, *J. Endocrinol.* 2004; 180: 203-12

[11] Wang B,Zhou S, Wang J,Liu, F, Ni F, Liu C,Yan Y J, Cao Y, Ma X. Lack of association between interleukin-1a gene (IL-1a) C (-889) T variant and polycysticovarysyndrome in chinese women. *Endocrine* 2009;35(2): 198 203.

[12] Nikolajuk A,Kowalska I,Karczewska-Kupczewska M,Adamska A,Otziomek E, Wolczynski S,Kinalska I,Gorska M,Straczkowski M.Serum soluble glycoprotein 130 concentrations is inversely related to insulin sensitivity in women with polycystic ovary syndrome. *Diabetes* 2010; 59(4): 1026-9.

[13] Dinarello CA, Biology of interleukin 1, *FASEB J.* 1988;2:108–115.

[14] de los Santos M.J,Anderson D.J,Racowsky C., Simon C, Hill JA. Expression of interleukin-1 system genes in human gametes, *Biol. Reprod.* 1998; 59: 1419–1424.

[15] Dinarello C.A, Interleukin-1, interleukin-1 receptors and interleukin-1 receptor antagonist, *Int. Rev. Immunol.* 1998; 16:457–499.

[16] Nicklin M.J, Weith A and Duff G.W, A physical map of the region encompassing the human interleukin-1 alpha, interleukin-1 beta, and interleukin-1 receptor antagonist genes, *Genomics* 1994;19: 382–384.

[17] Pociot F, Molvig J., Wogensen L, Worsaae H , Nerup J, A TaqI polymorphism in the human interleukin-1 beta (IL-1 beta) gene correlates with IL-1 beta secretion in vitro, *Eur. J. Clin. Invest.* 1992; 22: 396–402.

[18] Licastro J. Hulkkonen, P. Laippala and M. Hurme, A rare allele combination of the interleukin-1 gene complex is associated with high interleukin-1 beta plasma levels in healthy individuals, *Eur. Cytokine Netw.* 2000; 11: 251–255.

[19] di Giovine FS, Takhsh E., Blakemore A.I.,Duff G.W. Single base polymorphism at −511in the human interleukin-1 beta gene (IL1 beta), Hum.Mol.Genet.1992;1: 45 20.

[20] Kolbus A, Walch K, Nagele F, Wenzl R, Unfried G, Huber JC. Interleukin-1 alpha but not interleukin-1 beta gene polymorphism is associated with polycystic ovary syndrome. *J. Reprod. Immunol.* 2007; 73:188–193.

[21] Franks S, Gharani N, Waterworth D, S. Batty S, D. White D, R. Williamson R,McCarthy M.The genetic basis of polycystic ovary syndrome, *Hum. Reprod.* 1997; 12: 2641–2648.

[22] Legro RS., The genetics of polycystic ovary syndrome, *Am. J. Med.* 1995;98:.9S–16S.

In:Polycystic Ovarian Syndrome: An Enigmatic...
Editor: Rosa Sabatini

ISBN: 978-1-61761-853-6
©2011 Nova Science Publishers, Inc.

Chapter III

Polycystic Ovarian Syndrome: Symptoms and Clinical Manifestations

Rosa Sabatini

Expert Family Planning Service. Department of Obstetrics and Gynecology
Policlinico-University of Bari . Piazza Giulio Cesare 11.70124. Bari. Italy

Polycystic ovary syndrome is a common and perplexing endocrine disorder of women in their reproductive years, with a prevalence of up to 10%. Clinical expression of the syndrome varies but commonly infrequent or prolonged menstrual periods, excess hair growth, acne and obesity can all occur in women with polycystic ovary syndrome (PCOS) .Menstrual abnormality may signal the condition in adolescence, or PCOS may become apparent later following weight gain or difficulty becoming pregnant. Recently, the European Society for Human Reproduction and Embryology and the American Society for Reproductive Medicine (ESHRE/ASRM) have achieved a new consensus regarding the definition of PCOS. This is now defined as the presence of any two of the following three criteria: polycystic ovaries; oligo-/anovulation; and/or clinical or biochemical evidence of hyperandrogenism (1). Polycystic ovarian syndrome affects approximately 5 million women in the United States and is the leading cause of female infertility. Fortunately,it is also one of the most treatable forms of infertility;however, patients often suffer from it too long because it is mistreated or unrecognized. Many patients are surprised to find that there are effective treatments available for virtually every symptom associated with their condition. The presentations of PCOS are heterogeneous and may change throughout the lifespan, starting from adolescence to post-menopausal age, and may have health impact later in life.

Initial symptoms

Clinical Features of PCOS	Incidence
Irregular menses	85%
Hirsutism	70%
Obesity	40%
Acne	35%
Skin pigmentation	3%

Polycystic Ovarian Syndrome first signs may be irregular and heavy periods, occasional amenorrhea, obesity, hirsutism and sometimes infertility. These symptoms are due to imbalance of various hormones. PCOS occurs in all races and communities and, it is rare above the age of 40 years but more common in the reproductive age and some cases are also seen in young teenagers [2]. Hyperandrogenism must be considered in any girl with premature pubarche, unusual acne, hirsutism, or androgenetic alopecia. An association with menstrual irregularity or obesity should raise the index of suspicion. The most common causes of hyperandrogenism present in a teenage girl are functional ovarian hyperandrogenism, and functional adrenal hyperandrogenism, which usually seem to be due to an exaggeration of adrenarche. The plasma-free testosterone is a more sensitive indicator of hyperandrogenism than is the total testosterone concentration. The pattern of response of plasma free testosterone, DHEAS, and cortisol to dex-suppression testing can be diagnostic of the source of androgen excess. The syndrome is a result of a functional hormonal disorder that disrupts normal ovarian function. Normally, the pituitary gland releases follicle stimulating hormone (FSH) which travels through the blood stream to the ovaries telling them to mature an egg. The follicle initially less than 2-6 mm in diameter matures until it reaches over 20 mm in diameter. This takes approximately 14 days. Once mature, the follicle sends back a signal to the brain indicating it is ready for ovulation.The pituitary gland then sends out a pulse of luteinizing hormone (LH), telling the ovary to release or ovulate the egg. The follicle rupture releases the egg to the surface of the ovary where the fallopian tube should pick it up. PCOS occurs when the hormonal signals are not carried through. Thus,follicles do not grow and release the egg, instead stay small, 2 to 6 mm in diameter each month. Over time, these small follicles build up resulting in an ovary packed with multiple small cysts.The reason why the ovary fails to respond to the FSH is not well understood. It is believed that there are elevated resistance factors that inhibit the ovaries' ability to function normally Some of these resistance factors are the androgens and the insulin-like growth factors. The ovary stays in a steady-state of no ovulation which is the hallmark of PCOS. These resistance factors are manifested in other areas of the body. Androgens in the skin cause hirsutism or male-type distribution of hair growth on the face, chest and abdomen. Increased activity in the oil gland of the hair follicle may also result in oily skin and acne. Nearly 70% of patients with PCOS have some degree of insulin resistance. Insulin is a hormone released into the blood stream by the pancreas. It works to drive blood glucose into cells . Insulin resistance means that more insulin is needed to achieve the same result as a person without PCOS. Patients with type II diabetes have the same condition. Indeed, PCOS patients are at a higher risk of developing type II diabetes.The reason for this insulin resistance is an intense area of research. Currently, it is believed to be related to an inherent defect within the cells signaling a mechanism to allow glucose to come into the cell. Due to the cellular resistance, PCOS patients have elevated levels of insulin and/or insulin-like growth factors which can then adversely affect the ovary. In addition, insulin promotes growth or body mass and weight retention. Because of this, PCOS patients have a very difficult time loosing weight regardless of how much they exercise and diet.The fundamental clinical features of PCOS include hirsutism and menstrual irregularities from the time of menarche. Obesity is present in approximately 50% of these patients, some of whom also carry a diagnosis of NIDDM . The biochemical abnormalities associated with the clinical picture include LH hypersecretion, hyperandrogenism, acyclic estrogen production, subnormal SHBG levels, and hyperinsulinemia. Hirsutism usually progresses slowly in patients with PCOS; however, in some cases the clinical presentation can resemble virilizing tumors, late-onset CAH, or Cushing syndrome. Virilization or rapidly progressive hirsutism requires immediate investigation to rule out a virilizing tumor. Goals of therapy for teenage patients include decreasing levels of bioavailable androgens, blockade of androgen action at target tissues, stabilization of the endometrium, and reduction of insulin resistance. Consideration of insulin-sensitizing agents,antiandrogens, topical treatments for acne and facial hair excess, and hair removal is dependent on the patient's symptoms and concerns. A healthy approach to eating, in some cases weight loss, and exercise are encouraged to reduce the risk of cardiovascular disease and type 2 diabetes mellitus. Management of the adolescent with PCOS is challenging and often requires a supportive, multidisciplinary team approach for optimal results [3].Although the original description of PCOS by Stein and Leventhal was published in 1935, the cause of PCOS remains unknown.This reason, coupled with the fact that PCOS-related insulin resistance, an important cause of NIDDM in women, is still an object of active investigation.

Chief complaints and/or clinical manifestations

Reproductive
Menstrual cycle disturbances
Overweight or Obesity and difficulty losing weight
Infertility
Miscarriage
Problems in pregnant PCOS women
Acne, androgenic alopecia, hirsutism, acanthosis nigricans

Depression

Metabolic
Impaired glucose tolerance
Type 2 diabetes mellitus
Dyslipidemia
Gestational diabetes
Sleep apnea
Cardiovascular disease
Nonalcoholic fatty liver disease
Chronic kidney disease
Cancer risk

Menstrual Disturbances

Irregular menses are the hallmark for an individual who does not ovulate regularly. Since the lack of ovulation is a central feature of the syndrome, many patients will suffer from infertility. Many of these women reported early menarche, often younger than 12 and have irregular periods which may persist longer than the normal first 1-2 years after puberty. It is reported that oligomenorrhea affects 50% and amenorrhea almost 39% of PCOS women. A study found that none of the biochemical findings of hyperandrogenaemia correlates consistently with the specific type of menstrual disorder [4]. Some studies reported that menstrual disorders are present in 62% of the adolescents not using hormonal contraception, 59% of which fulfilled the criteria for polycystic ovary syndrome [5]. Premenstrual syndrome may be more common and more severe. Estrogen dominance, high levels of estrogen compared to progesterone, causing more fat deposition around thighs and butt, still worse, PMS and sometimes premenstrual headache. After the age of 35 it increases the risk of fibroids with very heavy periods, often causing iron deficiency.

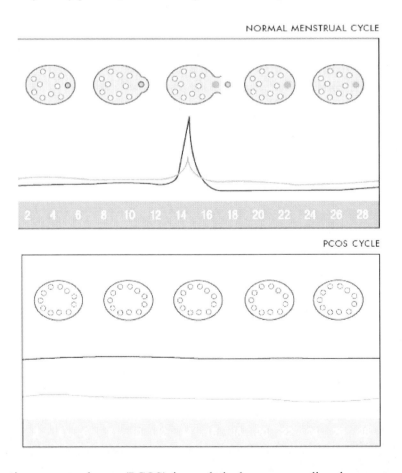

Polycystic ovary syndrome (PCOS) is a relatively common disorder among adolescent girls. The typical clinical features including menstrual irregularities and hirsutism are usually not apparent until middle to late adolescence. However, several studies suggest that PCOS may begin in early puberty. Young women with premature pubarche, a family history of

PCOS, Caribbean Hispanic and African American ancestry, and/or obesity are more likely to develop PCOS. Adolescents with PCOS may have elevated total or free testosterone, androstenedione, and luteinizing hormone levels, insulin resistance,and hyperinsulinemia. The laboratory evaluation and management of the adolescent with suspected PCOS should be individualized on the basis of the clinical features and symptoms. The cornerstone of most treatment strategies includes either a combination of oral contraceptive or progestin to decrease testosterone levels and regulate the menstrual cycle. Obesity is present in approximately 50% of these patients, some of whom also carry a diagnosis of NIDDM. The biochemical abnormalities associated with the clinical picture include LH hypersecretion, hyperandrogenism, acyclic estrogen production, subnormal SHBG levels, and hyperinsulinemia[6]. Goals of therapy for teenage patients include decreasing levels of bioavailable androgen, blockade of androgen action at target tissues, stabilization of the endometrium, and reduction of insulin resistance. A recent study evaluated the presence of insulin resistance as well as the incidence of polycystic ovary syndrome in adolescents with menstrual disorders.The patients were divided into two groups: group I (22 patients with menstrual irregularity), and group II (12 patients with regular menstrual cycles). BMI and Ferriman-Gallway index were calculated for all patients who also received a pelvic ultrasound. DHEAS, 17 OH-P , testosterone, TSH, LH, FSH and prolactin were measured. In addition, the glucose tolerance test was conducted with 75 mg dextrose and measurement of glucose and insulin. The results showed that ovary volume was larger in group I than in group II as DHEAS and testosterone levels were higher in patients with menstrual irregularity. In group I the Authors found two patients with diabetes mellitus and one patient with glucose intolerance. Sixteen patients in this group had clinical or hormonal characteristics of PCOS. The mean values of the area under the insulin curve (AUIC) were higher in patients with menstrual irregularities than in controls (P< 0.05). The presence of PCOS was detected in 95% of the adolescents with menstrual irregularity (7). Therefore, menstrual irregularity may be an early clinical sign of PCOS in adolescence. This hypothesis has been supported by several studies. A Brazilian investigation determined the hormonal, metabolic and ultrasonographic patterns of adolescents with menstrual irregularity since menarche, but without clinical signs of hyperandrogenism .These adolescents were divided in two groups: 13 adolescents with irregular cycles (IC) within the first 3 postmenarchal years (IC $\leq$ 3) and 15 adolescents having persistent irregular cycles for more than three postmenarchal years(IC > 3).These adolescents were compared with 15 adolescents with PCOS and 18 normal adolescents. The values of free testosterone, free androgen index, luteinizing hormone (LH) and LH/follicle-stimulating hormone (FSH) ratio were similar in IC $\leq$ 3, IC > 3 and PCOS, and higher than in the normal group (p < 0.005). The total testosterone and androstenedione levels were higher and sex hormone-binding globulin (SHBG) lower in PCOS only when compared with the normal group (p < 0.05). The ovarian volume was similar in IC $\leq$ 3 , IC > 3 and PCOS, and higher than in the normal group (p < 0.005). A higher incidence of polycystic structure was found in IC $\leq$ 3, IC > 3 and PCOS, whereas normal structure was more common in normal adolescents (p < 0.0005). There were no significant differences in glucose and insulin parameters between the groups. These results indicate that menstrual irregularity within the first postmenarchal years can be an early clinical sign of PCOS[8]. The amenorrhea and oligomenorrhoea symptoms seem to have a significant correlation with insulin resistance and these can be also associated to obesity, acanthosis and polycystic ovaries [9].Another study reported that two per cent of adolescents (aged 15-18) with regular menstrual cycles developed oligomenorrhoea, and 12 per cent of these with irregular menstrual cycles. Fifty-one per cent of the oligomenorrhoeic adolescents remained oligomenorrhoeic. Increased BMI, concentration of LH, androstenedione or testosterone, and polycystic ovaries were associated with persistence of oligomenorrhoea. Glucose/ insulin ratio as a marker for insulin resistance was not associated with an increased risk for oligomenorrhoea.Therefore, oligomenorrhoea at age 18 years is better predicted by menstrual cycle pattern at age 15 years than by LH or androgen concentrations or PCO at this age. Not only obese, but also normal weight oligomenorrhoeic adolescents have a high risk of remaining oligomenorrhoeic[10].Furthermore,it seems that in adolescents having oligomenorrhea with associated eating disorders, oligomenorrhea could be more persistent than in adolescents having secondary amenorrhea associated with eating disorders [4].

References

[1] Hart R.,Hickey M,Franks S. Definitions, prevalence and symptoms of polycystic ovaries and polycystic ovary syndrome. *Best Pract. Res. Clin. Obstet. Gynaecol*. 2004; 18(5):671-83. Review.

[2] Olutunmbi Y,Paley K,English JC3rd.Adolescent female acne : etiology and management. *J. Pediatr. Adolesc. Gynecol*. 2008;21(4):171-6.

[3] Driscoll DA. Polycystic ovary syndrome in adolescence. *Semin. Reprod. Med.* 2003; 21(3):301-7.

[4] Cupisti S,Dittrich R,Binder H,Beckmann MW,Mueller A. Evaluation of biochemical hyperandrogenemia and body mass index in women presenting with amenorrhea. *Exp. Clin. Endocrinol. Diabetes* 2007;115(5):298-302.

[5] Wiksten-Almstromer M, Hirschberg AL,Hagenfeldt K. Prospecive follow-up of menstrual disorders in adolescence and prognostic factors. *Acta Obstet. Gynecol. Scand.* 2008; 87(11): 1162-8.

[6] Gordon CM. Menstrual disorders in adolescents. Excess androgens and the polycystic ovary syndrome. *Pediatr. Clin. North Am*. 1999;46(3):519-43.

[7] Fernandes AR,de Sa Rosa e Silva AC,Romao GS, Pata MC,dos Reis RM.Insulin resistance in adolescents with menstrual irregularities. *J. Pediatr. Adolesc. Gynecol*. 2005;18(4): 269-74.

[8] Avvad CK,Holeuwerger R,Silva VC,Bordallo MA,Breitenbach MM. Menstrual irregularity in the first postmenarchal years: an early clinical sign of polycystic ovary syndrome in adolescence. *Gynecol. Endocrinol*. 2001;15(3):170-7.

[9] Gonzales Centeno A,Nahum Hernandez P,Mendoza R,Avala AR. Correlation between menstruation disorders and insulin resistance. *Ginecol. Obstet. Mex*. 2003;71:312-7

[10] van Hooff MH,Voorhorst FJ,Kaptein MB,Koppenaal C,Schoemaker J.Predictive value of menstrual cycle pattern, body mass index, hormone levels and polycystic ovaries at age 15 years for oligo-amenorrhoea at age 18 years. *Hum. Reprod*. 2004;19(2): 383-92.

Obesity

Obesity, ranging from 30-75% of cases, is strongly associated with PCOS. Increased body weight in PCOS is often due to increased visceral fat which is particularly associated with increased risk of cardiovascular disease, type 2 diabetes and hypertension. Therefore, Polycystic ovary syndrome is not only a reproductive endocrinopathy but also a metabolic disorder. In fact, it is associated with hyperinsulinemia, glucose intolerance, obesity and altered lipid profile.[1,2]. Insulin resistance is thought to be the uniting pathogenic factor in the associations between hypertension, glucose intolerance, obesity, lipid abnormalities and coronary artery disease, which together constitutes the metabolic syndrome [3].

Both hyperinsulinemia and dyslipidemia are risk factors for cardiovascular disease (CVD). Evidence of subclinical CVD has been reported in overweight PCOS women. [4]. It was also noted that women with PCOS may have dyslipidemia, increased blood pressure, plasminogen activator inhibitor and coronary artery calcification. Interesting observations pointed out the abnormal lipid profile difference between PCOS cases and controls which is mainly seen in women aged less than 45 years, while carotid artery changes are seen in PCOS women after 45 years

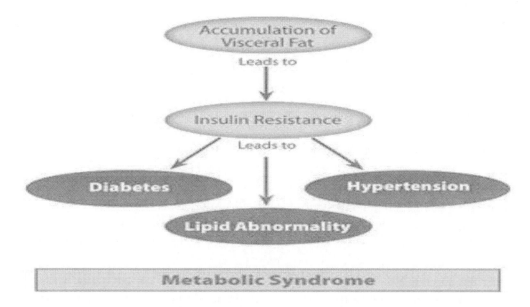

Interesting observations pointed out the abnormal lipid profile difference between PCOS cases and controls which is mainly seen in women aged less than 45 years, while carotid artery changes are seen in PCOS women after 45 years. Both hyperinsulinemia and dyslipidemia are risk factors for cardiovascular disease (CVD). Evidence of subclinical CVD has been reported in overweight PCOS women. [4]. It was also noted that women with PCOS may have dyslipidemia, increased blood pressure, plasminogen activator inhibitor and coronary artery calcification. Interesting observations pointed out the abnormal lipid profile difference between PCOS cases and controls which is mainly seen in women aged less than 45 years, while carotid artery changes are seen in PCOS women after 45 years. This indicates that dyslipidemia occurring at a younger age translates into atherosclerosis and cardiovascular disease later in life. Although obesity is often associated with metabolic disorders, lean women with PCOS also have been found to have hyperinsulinemia and dyslipidemia [5].Obesity induces, through the path of insulin resistance, high levels of insulin-related growth factors; these will stimulate theca cells to produce supranormal amounts of androgens and reduce SHBG synthesis by liver cells, thereby raising the proportion of free circulating testosterone. The resulting androgen excess is considered to contribute to the presence of an increased number of follicles in all stages as well as arrested maturation of FSH sensitive follicles. It is important to remember that obesity is considered a condition of SHBG imbalance.In fact, the levels of SHBG tend to decrease with increasing body fat and this induces an increased fraction of free androgens delivered to target sensitive tissues.The net balance,with the dominant role of insulin, which inhibits SHBG synthesis in the liver, may be responsible for the decrease of SHBG concentrations observed in obesity.Leptin is considered as one of the major peripheral signals that affects food intake and energy balance. The discovery of the adipocyte-produced hormone leptin has greatly changed the field of obesity research and our understanding of energy homeostasis. It is now accepted that leptin is the afferent loop informing the hypothalamus about the state of fat stores, with hypothalamic efferents regulating appetite and energy expenditure. Indeed, leptin has a role as a metabolic adaptator in overweight and fasting states. In adult life, there is experimental evidence that leptin is a permissive factor for the ovarian cycle, with a regulatory role exerted at the hypothalamic, pituitary, and gonadal levels, and with, in part, unexplained changes in pregnancy and postpartum [6] More recently, leptin has been shown to play a role in other target reproductive organs, such as the endometrium, placenta, and mammary gland, with corresponding influences on important physiological processes such as menstruation, pregnancy, and lactation. As a marker of whether nutritional stores are adequate, leptin may act in concert with gonadotropins and the growth hormone axis to initiate the complex process of puberty. Conditions in which nutritional status is suboptimal, such as eating disorders, exercise-induced amenorrhea, and functional hypothalamic amenorrhea, are associated with low serum leptin levels. Conditions with excess energy stores or metabolic disturbances,such as obesity and polycystic ovarian syndrome, often have elevated serum or follicular fluid leptin levels, raising the possibility that relative leptin deficiency or resistance may be at least partly responsible for the reproductive abnormalities that occur with these conditions. In conclusion, obesity is a classic condition of circulating leptin excess.The discrepancy between increased leptin blood levels and its central effects represents the leptin resistance [7]. There is evidence that leptin acts directly on the ovaries through functional receptors . Leptin influences the functioning of the ovary and the endometrium and interacts with the release and activity of gonadotrophins and with the hormones that control their synthesis [8] . Rapid weight gain and change in body type from lean to heavy coincide with pre-puberty central obesity. Obesity is a major health problem throughout the world. It, independent of polycystic ovary syndrome, is associated with anovulation ,and minimal weight loss alone should be considered to be an effective therapy for induction of ovulation in both obese and obese PCOS women. Women with a

BMI in excess of 35 kg/ m² should lose weight prior to conception and not prior to receiving infertility treatment.

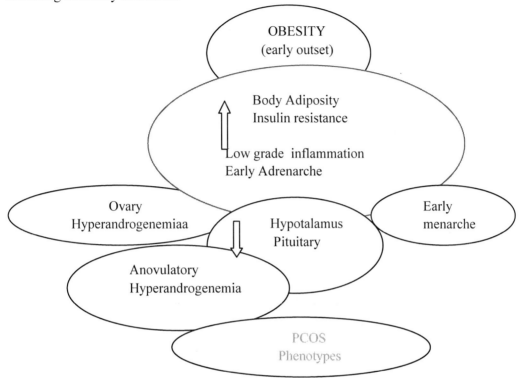

Intrinsic in this program is the use of contraception and high-dose folic acid during that period of preconceptual weight reduction [9]. Obesity affects approximately half of the general population and is thus a common problem among the fertile population. Obese women have a higher prevalence of infertility compared with their lean counterparts. Maternal morbility, mortality and fetal anomalies increase with obesity, and the success of assisted reproductive technology (ART) treatments is significantly reduced for obese women. The mainstay for treatment is weight loss, which improves both natural fertility and conception rates with ART. Assisted reproduction in obese women is preferable in those with a BMI of 30 kg/ m² or less [10]. Approximately half of all women with polycystic ovary syndrome are overweight or obese, and studies have reported endocrine and metabolic differences between lean and obese women with PCOS. Obesity contributes to anovulation, menstrual irregularities, and reduced conception rate. A study of Columbia University (New York) investigated early endocrine and metabolic alterations in adolescents with PCOS. An ethnically heterogeneous group of 48 adolescents was studied : 11 nonobese with PCOS [age 16.1 ± 1.9 yr; body mass index (BMI), 22.5 ± 1.5 kg/m²], 22 obese with PCOS (age 15.5 ± 1.4 yr; BMI, 35.9 ± 6.2 kg/m²), and 15 obese controls (age 14.4 ± 1.5 yr; BMI, 35.8 ± 7.1 kg/m²). The nonobese adolescents with PCOS demonstrated higher levels of LH, SHBG, Delta4-A, DHEAS, free IGF-I, dihydrotestosterone, and high-density lipoprotein, and lower low-density lipoprotein, compared with the obese PCOS group. Fasting levels of insulin and proinsulin were higher, and the fasting glucose to insulin ratio, quantitative insulin sensitivity check index, and composite insulin sensitivity index were lower in the obese compared with the nonobese PCOS subjects. Greater levels of LH and androgens, including total and free testosterone, Delta4-A, and DHEAS, and lower SHBG levels were found in the obese PCOS group compared with the obese controls.Adolescents with PCOS manifest clinical, metabolic, and endocrine features similar to those of adult women, and differences between non obese and obese women with PCOS may be detected in adolescence. These findings indicate a more pronounced alteration in the hypothalamo-pituitary-adrenal axis in non obese adolescents with PCOS and a more marked dysregulation of insulin levels and impairment of insulin sensitivity in their obese counterparts. The data also suggest differences in the IGF system between non obese and obese adolescents with PCOS [11]. The FTO gene has recently been shown to influence a person's predisposition to obesity, and is the first gene to be associated convincingly with susceptibility to PCOS. The FTO gene is known to influence weight. There are two versions of this gene, one of which is associated with increased weight gain and susceptibility to development of obesity..This gene shows genetic evidence to corroborate the well established link between PCOS and obesity. PCOS is a common condition affecting up to 1 in 10 women of childbearing age and is a leading cause of infertility. PCOS affects the ovaries and is characterized by irregular periods and excessive hair growth . The syndrome is strongly associated with obesity,and it is thought that the prevalence of PCOS will increase with rising levels of obesity [12]. Low adiponectin and ghrelin levels in PCOS patients could be caused by insulin resistance as well as high testosterone levels. A recent study performed in 51 obese hirsute women and 63 weight-matched female controls evaluated adiponectin and ghrelin levels in PCOS. Relationships between adiponectin, ghrelin, leptin, body composition, testosterone and insulin were examined. Measurements of body composition included waist-hip-ratio (WHR), BMI and whole body dual-energy X-ray absorptiometry scan measures of body fat mass. Measurements of fasting levels of adiponectin , ghrelin, leptin, androgen status, oestradiol, lipid variables and insulin during follicular phase were also performed. The results of this research showed that obese hirsute PCOS patients demonstrated significantly lower adiponectin levels than weight-matched controls, suggesting a very high risk for the metabolic syndrome. Furthermore, ghrelin levels decreased in hirsute PCOS patients and showed a significant, negative correlation with testosterone, independent of body composition [13]. In conclusion,obesity, particularly the abdominal phenotype, may be partly responsible for insulin resistance and associated hyperinsulinemia in women with PCOS. Therefore, obesity-related hyperinsulinemia may play a key role in favoring hyperandrogenism in these women. Other factors such as increased estrogen production rate, increased activity of the opioid system and of the hypothalamic-pituitary-adrenal axis, decreased sex hormone binding globulin synthesis and, possibly, high dietary lipid intake, may be additional mechanisms by which obesity favors the development of hyperandrogenism in PCOS.

References

[1] Legro RS, Finegood D, Dunaif A. A fasting glucose to insulin ratio is a useful measure of insulin sensitivity in women with polycystic ovary syndrome. *J. Clin. Endocrinol. Metab.* 1998; 83: 2694-8.

Polycystic Ovarian Syndrome: Symptoms and Clinical Manifestations 121

[2] Dokras A, Bochner M, Hollinrake E, Markham S, Vanvoorhis B, Jagasia DH. Screening women with polycystic ovarian syndrome for metabolic syndrome. *Obstet. Gynecol.* 2005;106:131-7.

[3] Apridonidze T, Essah PA, Iuorno MJ, Nestler JE. Prevalence and characteristics of the metabolic syndrome in women with polycystic ovary syndrome. *J. Clin. Endocrinol. Metab.* 2005;90:1929-35.

[4] Meyer C, McGrath BP, Teede HJ. Overweight women with PCOS have evidence of subclinical cardiovascular disease. *J. Clin. Endocrinol. Metab.* 2005;90:5711-6.

[5] Talbott EO, Zborowski JV, Sutton-Tyrell K, McHugh-Pemu KP, Guzick DS. Cardiovascular risk in women with polycystic ovary syndrome. *Obstet. Gynecol. Clin. North Am.* 2001;28:111-33.

[6] Casanueva FF,Diequez C.Neuroendocrine regulation and actions of leptin. *Neuroendocrinol.* 1999; 20(4): 317-63.

[7] Moschos S,Chan JL,Mantzoros CS. Leptin and reproduction:a review. *Fertil. Steril.* 2002; 77(3) : 433-44.

[8] Mitchell M, Amstrong DT,Robker RL,Norman RJ. Adipokines :implications for female fertility and obesity. *Reproduction* 2005;130(5): 583-97.

[9] Nelson SM,Fleming RF. The preconceptual contraception paradigm:obesity and infertility. *Hum. Reprod.* 2007;22 (4): 912-5.

[10] Wilkes S, Murdoch A. Obesity and female fertility : a primary care perspective. *J. Fam. Plann. Repro . Health Care* 2009;35(3): 181-185.

[11] Silfen ME,Denburg MR, Manibo AM,Lobo RA,Jaffe R,Ferin M, Levine LS,Oberfield SE.Early endocrine, metabolic, and sonographic characteristics of polycystic ovary syndrome (PCOS): comparison between nonobese and obese adolescents. *Clin. Endocrinol. Metab.* 2003; 88(10):4682-8.

[12] Frayling TM, Timpson NJ, Weedon MN et al. (2007) A common variant in the FTO gene is associated with body mass index and predisposes to childhood and adult obesity. *Science* 316: 889-894.

[13] Glintborg D,Andersen M,Hagen C,Frystyk J,Hulstrom V,Flyvbjerg A,Hermann AP. Evaluation of metabolic risk markers in polycystic ovary syndrome (PCOS). Adiponectin, ghrelin, leptin and body composition in hirsute PCOS patients and controls. *Eur. J. Endocrinol.* 2006 ;155(2):337-39.

Infertility and PCOS

Polycystic ovary syndrome is the most common cause of anovulatory infertility, affecting 5-10% of the women in childbearing age and 20% of those presenting with subfertility. Furthermore,almost 50% of PCOS women suffer from insulin resistance and obesity and reproductive function is strongly dependent on body weight and metabolic status. In fact, a high blood insulin level, as a consequence of insulin resistance, is one of the major reasons for ovulation failure. In addition, several studies highlighted the link between obesity and infertility. Obesity contributes to anovulation, menstrual irregularities, and reduced conception rate .Furthermore, maternal morbility and mortality as well as fetal anomalies and perinatal complication are increased with obesity. It is well known as a low-calorie diet may lead to weight loss and enhance fertility, in women with PCOS [1]. Several studies have shown that weight loss can decrease male hormone levels, induce the return of menstrual periods, and enhance fertility in women with PCOS. However, an ideal weight-loss diet has not been established for the condition. Obesity is a major health problem across the world. Recent studies suggest that obese patients should be denied for treatment of any kind aiming to improve ovulation rates and achieve pregnancy until they have reduced their BMI.It was suggested that this approach is not a resolution of the problem, but, indeed, may amplify the maternal and perinatal complications attributed to fertility centers. Obesity independent of polycystic ovary syndrome is associated with anovulation and a minimal weight loss alone is an effective therapy for induction of ovulation in both obese women and obese PCOS women. Consequently, lifestyle programmes encouraging weight loss should be considered to be an ovulation induction therapy and a due consideration for a potential pregnancy in an obese woman given. It was proposed that women with a BMI in excess of 35 kg m^2 should lose weight prior to conception and not prior to receiving infertility treatment.Therefore, clinicians undertaking the management of infertility in obese women should adopt measures to reduce their body mass prior to exposing them to the risks of pregnancy. It was advocate that this approach should be aggressively managed including pharmacological strategies; intrinsic in this programme is the use of contraception and an high-dose folic acid administration during that period of preconceptual weight reduction [2].Furthermore, it seems that women who are obese by 18 years old are more likely to report PCOS and infertility and less likely to get pregnancy, compared with women who became obese later in life [3].To investigate the relationship between body mass index and intercourse compliance six hundred twenty-six infertile women with PCOS (mean age of 28.1 ± 4 years and mean BMI 35.2 ± 8.7 kg/m^2) were evaluated . Overall, body mass index was not associated with increased intercourse compliance.However, patients with BMI ≥ 35 were less likely to ovulate than patients with BMI <35,and they tend to be more compliant with intercourse frequency in ovulatory cycles than patients with BMI <35. Therefore,an elevated BMI in infertile women with PCOS is not associated with poor intercourse compliance [4].The regulation of reproduction is obtained by a complex hypothalamus/pituitary/ovary hormonal system. There are a lot of ovarian peptides, playing an essential role in the regulation of this system. However, the mechanisms of their action are not exactly known.Inhibins are glycoproteins mainly produced in the ovaries and taking part in the regulation of menstrual cycle. They consist of glycosylated alpha subunit and one of two beta subunits, inhibin A and inhibin B. There are many studies about possible use of inhibins in reproductive medicine. Recent data indicate the role of inhibin A in obstetrics. The measurement of inhibin B can provide useful information about ovarian reserve, and plays an important role in assisted reproductive techniques. Inhibin B can be also regarded as potential marker of premature ovarian failure and ovarian recovery in hypothalamic disturbances [5]. Important marker of ovarian reserve is also the Anti-Mullerian Hormone (AMH). Generally , AMH levels decrease with age and in patients with ovarian failure is undetectable or greatly reduced depending from the number of antral follicles in the ovaries. In PCOS patients, the AMH levels are increased [6]

Polycystic ovary syndrome , one of the most frequent endocrine diseases, affects approximately 5%-10% of women in childbearing age and constitutes the most common cause of female sterility; regardless of the need or not for treatment, a change in lifestyle is essential for the treatment and ovulation to be restored. Obesity is the principal reason for modifying lifestyle since its reduction improves ovulation and the capacity for pregnancy lowering the risk of miscarriage and later complications that may occur during pregnancy (gestational diabetes, pre-eclampsia, etc).When lifestyle modification is not sufficient, the first step in ovulation induction is clomiphene citrate. The second-step recommendation is either exogenous gonadotrophins or laparoscopic ovarian surgery. Recommended third-line treatment is in vitro fertilization. Metformin use in PCOS should be restricted to women with glucose intolerance [7]. A retrospective study evaluated sex ratio and pregnancy complications in PCOS patients More than half (54%) of the singleton pregnancies were conceived spontaneously. More complications were seen in pregnancies achieved while using metformin than without .Compared to spontaneous conception, more boys than girls were born in singleton pregnancies after in vitro fertilization/ intracytoplasmatic sperm injection treatment (p = 0.004).Therefore,it seems that in women with PCOS the mode of conception may influence both the rate of pregnancy complications and the offspring sex ratio [8]. The Cochrane Database Syst Rev.2009 reported that clinical pregnancy rates are improved for metformin versus placebo (OR = 3.86) and for metformin and clomiphene versus clomiphene alone (OR =1.48). In the studies that compared metformin and clomiphene alone, there was no evidence of an improved live birth rate but the OR resulted in improved clinical pregnancy rate in the clomiphene group (OR = 0.63); although, there was significant heterogeneity.There was also evidence that ovulation rates in PCOS women are improved with metformin versus placebo(OR 2.12) and with metformin and clomiphene versus clomiphene alone (OR = 3.46).Metformin was also associated with a significantly higher incidence of gastrointestinal disturbance, but no serious adverse effects were reported.Therefore,it seems that metformin may be still of benefit in improving clinical pregnancy and ovulation rates. However, there is no evidence that metformin improves live birth rates whether it is used alone or in combination with clomiphene, or when compared with clomiphene. Therefore, the use of metformin in improving reproductive outcomes in women with PCOS appears to be limited [9].Frequently, low ovulatory and pregnancy rates were reported with clomiphene citrate (CC) in anovulatory PCOS patients.The metformin and clomiphene combination resulted in a significantly higher rate of ovulation. The pregnancy rate was 8% with CC and 24% with metformin and CC. The CC group also ovulated at a similar rate as that of the control group. The ovulatory rate and the pregnancy rate with the metformin-CC combination was found to be higher when compared with CC alone. Metformin increased the ovulatory rate in CC failures, also implying increased sensitivity to CC [10]. Miscarriage, multiple pregnancy rates and adverse events were poorly reported. Clomiphene was effective in increasing pregnancy rate compared to placebo (OR 5.8) like clomiphene plus dexamethasone treatment compared to clomiphene alone.(OR 9.46) No evidence of a difference in effect was found between clomiphene versus tamoxifen or clomiphene in conjunction with human chorionic gonadotrophin (hCG) versus clomiphene alone. No evidence of a difference in effect on pregnancy rate was found with any of the other comparisons This review shows evidence supporting the effectiveness of clomiphene citrate and clomiphene in combination with dexamethasone for pregnancy rate only. There is limited evidence on the effects of these drugs on outcomes such as miscarriage. Evidence in favor of these interventions is flawed due to the lack of evidence on live births [11]. On the other hand, women who received metformin showed a significantly higher number of good quality embryos and implantation rate when compared with the placebo controls. Despite the transfer of a similar number of embryos, an insignificant increased in the pregnancy rate along with significant reduction in the abortion rate was observed in the metformin-treated group as compared with the placebo controls. No fetal abnormalities were encountered in the babies born in the metformin-treated group. It is concluded that metformin affects positively the quality of both oocytes and embryos without a significant increase in the pregnancy rate. It decreases significantly the rates of abortion and ovarian hyperstimulation syndrome [12].The N, N' dimethyl-biguanide(Metformin) is an antidiabetic drug that increases glucose utilization in insulin-sensitive tissues. As Polycystic Ovary Syndrome and diabetes share some altered parameters such as abnormal glucose- insulin ratio, altered lipidic metabolism and insulin-resistance syndrome , the use of metformin has become increasingly accepted and widespread in the treatment of PCOS.Currently, metformin is used to induce ovulation and during early pregnancy in PCOS patients, however, a complete knowledge of the metformin action has not been achieved yet [13]. Treatment of normogonadotropic anovulatory infertility (World Health Organization class 2, or WHO2) is performed by induction of ovulation using clomiphene citrate (CC), followed by follicle-stimulating hormone (FSH) in cases of treatment failure.Not all patients will become ovulatory or will conceive with this treatment.Others,exhibiting multifollicular instead of monofollicular development,may encounter complications such as ovarian hyperstimulation and multiple pregnancy. Recently,introduced alternative treatment interventions such as insulin-sensitizing drugs, aromatase inhibitors, or laparoscopic electrocautery of the ovaries may offer the possibility to improve the efficacy of the classical ovulation induction algorithm. Based on initial patient characteristics, it may be possible to identify specific patient subgroups with altered chances of success or complications while using one of these interventions. Regarding CC and FSH ovulation induction, this has been performed using multivariate prediction models. This approach may enable us to improve safety, cost-effectiveness, and patient convenience in ovulation induction [14]. A systematic review and meta-analysis of pregnancy outcome after metformin use for polycystic ovary syndrome (PCOS)was conducted.All pertinent studies from 1966 to September 2004.were considered. After adjustment for publication bias, metformin treatment in the first trimester was associated with a statistically significant (57%) protective effect. The malformation rate in the disease-matched control group was approximately 7.2%, statistically significantly higher than the rate found in the metformin group (1.7%). On the basis of the data available today, there is no evidence of an increased risk for major malformations when metformin is taken during the first trimester of pregnancy[15]. Another study performed at the Cholesterol Center, Jewish Hospital of Cincinnati (USA) investigated on the capacity of metformin (2.55 g/day). to facilitate conception in 72 oligoamenorrhoeic women with polycystic ovary syndrome (PCOS), and to safely reduce the rate of first trimester spontaneous abortion (SA), together with an increase of the number of live births without teratogenicity.Outcome measures included number of first trimester SA, live births, normal ongoing pregnancies ≥ 13 weeks, gestational diabetes (GD), congenital defects (CD), birthweight and height, as well as weight, height, and motor and social development during the first 6 months of life. Metformin therapy during pregnancy in women with PCOS was safely associated with reduction in spontaneous abortions and in gestational diabetes, was not teratogenic, and did not adversely affect birthweight or height,or motor and social development at 3 and 6 months of life [16].Ultimately, a review evaluated the evidence in using of aromatase inhibitors for ovulation induction and pregnancy in patients with polycystic ovary syndrome .Trials using intrauterine insemination methods for pregnancy were excluded.The resulting articles were divided into 2 groups:aromatase inhibitor use in clomiphene-resistant patients and their use in treatment-naïve patients. Accepted pharmacologic treatments for women with PCOS and infertility include clomiphene citrate, gonadotropins, and gonadotropin-releasing hormone (GnRH) analogs. Each medication has variable efficacy rates and adverse effects. Therefore, other treatments are needed for a subset of women with PCOS and infertility. Evidence suggests that nonsteroidal aromatase inhibitors, specifically letrozole and anastrozole, may have ovulation-inducing effects by inhibiting androgen-to-estrogen conversion. Further trials with aromatase inhibitors have demonstrated efficacy for increased endometrium thickness, ovulation rates, and pregnancy rates when used in clomiphene citrate-resistant or treatment-naïve patients. Hence, aromatase inhibitors might be a good tool in selected cases but some researchers suggest further trials, comparing aromatase inhibitors with clomiphene citrate, before that this treatment can be recommend routinely for ovulation induction in women with PCOS and infertility. However, aromatase inhibitors may be considered in a subset of this population, specifically women who are clomiphene citrate resistant or those who, after discussion of risks and benefits, are not candidates for clomiphene citrate, gonadotropins, or GnRH analogs [17]. A study evaluating the effects of letrozole versus clomiphene citrate reported that the levels of serum estradiol and progesterone were significantly higher in the CC group . However, ovulation occurred in 67.5% of the cycles in letrozole group and 70.9% in clomiphene group. While, the pregnancy rate per cycle was 15.1% in the letrozole and 17.9% in the clomiphene group [18]. Another study reported ovulation occurring in 185/285 cycles (64.9%) in the letrozole group versus 207/297 cycles (69.6%) in the combined metformin-CC group, without statistically significant difference. The total number of follicles was significantly more in the combined metformin-CC group . A nonsignificant increase in endometrial thickness on the day of hCG administration was observed in the letrozole group . No statistically significant difference regarding the pregnancy rate (PR) was observed between both groups(14.7% vs. 14.4%). Letrozole and combined metformin-CC are equally effective for inducing ovulation and achieving pregnancy in patients CC-resistant PCOS [19]. A clinical trial evaluated the effect of intravaginal micronized P on pregnancy rates in clomiphene citrate and letrozole ovulation induction cycles in women with polycystic ovary syndrome

Women with PCOS who underwent ovulation induction with either clomiphene citrate (n = 90; CC 50-250 mg x 5 days) or letrozole (n = 31; L 5 mg x 5 days) were considered. After either intercourse or IUI, patients received intravaginal micronized P (200 mg twice daily) . In clomiphene cycles, clinical pregnancies were documented in 15.3% of cycles (19 of 124) when P was added , compared with 12.1% (11 of 91) whithout P .. In letrozole cycles, clinical pregnancies were documented in 21.1% of cycles (8 of 38) with P , compared with none (0 of 13) without P. Therefore,women with PCOS who used letrozole for ovulation induction had higher clinical pregnancy rates when using intravaginal P support. Luteal supplementation with P should be strongly considered in women with PCOS,especially in those using letrozole for ovulation induction [20].Considering that treatment with pulsatile GnRH infusion by the intravenous or subcutaneous route ,using a portatile pump, has been successfully used in patients with hypogonadotrophic hypogonadism , it was hypothesized a similar advantage in PCOS patients. However,until now the little experience in this field and the paucity of the Literature data hinder to prove or discard the value of this treatment [21] Polycystic ovary syndrome is often characterized by chronic oligo- or anovulation ,usually manifested as oligo- or amenorrhea, and hyperandrogenism. In addition, 30-40% of PCOS women showing glucose tolerance and a defect in the insulin signaling pathway seems to be implicated in the pathogenesis of insulin resistance. PCOS patients are subfertile as a consequence of such ovulatory disorders and often need drugs, such as clomiphene citrate or follicle-stimulating hormone, for ovulation induction, which increases the risk of multiple pregnancy and ovarian hyperstimulation syndrome. It was hypothesized that the administration of an isoform of inositol (myo-inositol), belonging to the vitamin B complex, would improve the insulin-receptor activity, restoring the normal ovulatory function. Twenty-five PCOS women of childbearing age with oligo- or amenorrhea were enrolled in a study.Ovulatory disorder due to PCOS was apparently the only cause of infertility; no tubal defect or deficiency of male semen parameters was found. Myo-inositol combined with folic acid 2 g twice a day was administered continuously. During an observation period of 6 months, ovulatory activity was monitored with ultrasound scan and hormonal profile, and the numbers of spontaneous menstrual cycles and eventually pregnancies were assessed. Twenty-two out of the 25 (88%) patients restored at least one spontaneous menstrual cycle during treatment, of whom 18 (72%) maintained normal ovulatory activity during the follow-up period. A total of 10 singleton pregnancies (40% of patients) were obtained. Nine clinical pregnancies were assessed with fetal heart beat at ultrasound scan. Two pregnancies evolved in spontaneous abortion. Myo-inositol is a simple and safe treatment that is capable of restoring spontaneous ovarian activity and consequently fertility in most patients with PCOS.This therapy did not cause multiple pregnancy [22]. To investigate the effects of treatment with Myo-inositol on circulating insulin, glucose tolerance, ovulation and serum androgens concentrations in women with the Polycystic Ovary Syndrome (PCOS) a study was performed.. Forty-two women with PCOS were treated in a double-blind trial with Myo-inositol plus folic acid or folic acid alone as placebo. In the group treated with Myo-inositol the serum total testosterone decreased from 99.5 ± 7 to 34.8 ± 4.3 ng/dl (placebo group: from 116. ± 15 to 109 ± 7.5 ng/dl; P = 0.003), and serum free testosterone from 0.85 ± 0.1 to 0.24 ± 0.33 ng/dl (placebo group: from 0.89 ± 0.12 to 0.85 ± 0.13 ng/dl; P = 0.01). Plasma triglycerides decreased from 195 ± 20 to 95 ± 17 mg/dl (placebo group: from 166 ± 21 to 148 ± 19 mg/dl; P = 0.001). Systolic blood pressure decreased from 131 ± 2 to 127 ± 2 mmHg (placebo group: from 128 ± 1 to 130 ± 1 mmHg; P = 0.002). Diastolic blood pressure decreased from 88 ± 1 to 82 ± 3 mmHg (placebo group: from 86 ± 1 to 90 ± 1 mmHg; P = 0.001). The area under the plasma insulin curve after oral administration of glucose decreased from 8.54 ± 1.149 to 5.535 ± 1.792 microU/ml/min (placebo group: from 8.903 ± 1.276 to 9.1 ± 1.162 microU/ ml/min; P = 0.03). The index of composite whole body insulin sensitivity (ISI comp) increased from 2.80 ± 0.35 to 5.05 ± 0.59 mg(-2)/dl(-2) (placebo group: from 3.23 ± 0.48 to 2.81 ± 0.54 mg(-2)/dl(-2); P < 0.002). 16 out of 23 women of Myo-inositol group ovulated (4 out of 19 in placebo group).Treatment of PCOS patients with Myo-inositol provided a decreasing of circulating insulin and serum total testosterone as well as an improvement in metabolic factors [23]. Three infertile patients with PCOS, submitted to oocytes' IVM without previous ovarian stimulation, were included in a study. During the procedure of oocytes' collection, each ovary was drilled from four to eight times.None of the patients got pregnant with the IVM technique.Evaluating the cases' follow-up, in seven months after the procedure, the three patients got pregnant without the help of techniques of assisted reproduction, which resulted in three births. Therefore,multiple drillings in the ovary of these patients with PCOS, during the process to collect oocytes, may have contributed to their pregnancy in the months following the procedure [24] To investigate the serum and follicular fluid concentrations of insulin resistance and homocysteine and their effect on IVF outcome,patients nonobese, nonhyperandrogenemic and, with polycystic ovary syndrome were compared with normal women Despite elevated serum insulin, HOMA-IR, and homocysteine levels, and their effects on oocyte numbers and maturation in PCOS patients, there were no differences in follicular parameters and clinical pregnancy rates between hyperinsulinemic and hyper homocysteinemic PCOS patients with respect to the control group [25]. The aim of another study was to develop a clinically useful predictive model of live birth with varying ovulation induction methods. Four prognostic models were proposed from a large multicenter randomized controlled infertility trial of 626 women with PCOS . This study was performed at Academic Health Centers in the United States, to predict success of ovulation, conception, pregnancy, and live birth, evaluating the influence of patients' baseline characteristics.Ovulation was induced with clomiphene, metformin, or the combination of both for up to six cycles or conception. The primary outcome of the trial was the rate of live births. Baseline free androgen index, baseline proinsulin level, interaction of treatment arm with body mass index, and duration in attempting conception were considered significant predictors in all four models. History of a prior pregnancy loss predicted ovulation and conception, but not pregnancy or live birth was obtained. A modified Ferriman Gallwey hirsutism score of less than 8 was predictive of conception, pregnancy, and live birth ; although it did not predict ovulation success. Age was a divergent predictor based on outcome; age greater than 34 predicted ovulation, whereas age less than 35 was a predictive factor for a successful pregnancy and live birth. Smoking history had no predictive value.Therefore, a live birth prediction chart developed from basic clinical parameters (body mass index, age, hirsutism score, and duration of attempting conception) may help physicians counsel and select infertility treatments for women with PCOS [26].In conclusion, clinical management of the PCOS have to be organized in regard to patient's age, history ,desire of pregnancy and medical staff experience [27]. Clomifene citrate is the first and the most used agent for inducing ovulation in patients affected by polycystic ovary syndrome (PCOS). About 60-85% of PCOS women ovulated under clomifene citrate, whereas the others were defined clomifene citrate-resistant. Frequent purpose is to play treatment strategies to induce ovulation in infertile PCOS patients with clomifene citrate resistance. Clomifene citrate and metformin association are a valid option for inducing ovulation in clomifene citrate-resistant PCOS patients. Surgical ovulation induction by laparoscopic ovarian drilling should be reserved to well selected cases. Excellent preliminary results are obtained using new drug formulations, such as aromatase inhibitors. In clomifene citrate-resistant PCOS patients, clomifene citrate and metformin combination with laparoscopic ovarian drilling, in selected cases, should be considered before gonadotropin administration. The efficacy of the other treatments must be confirmed in future well designed studies [28] .A randomized trial was performed in 126 PCOS women who had a history of infertility for at least an year and resistance to clomiphene citrate. The participants received metformin treatment or underwent to laparoscopic ovarian drilling (LOD).The results showed that the serum levels of testosterone and LH were lower after the treatments in both groups. The proportion of women with regular menstrual cycles increased to 35% in LOD and 49% in Met groups,respectively.Hirsutism decreased from 100% to 79.37% in both groups. While,the levels of follicle-stimulating hormone resulted unchanged after both treatments (29). Ovarian drilling was successfully employed without any surgical complications and the mean duration of follow-up time was 29.73 ± 10.64 months. In the follow-up period, 93.3% of the subjects were recorded to have regular cycles and 64.4% pregnancy rate was achieved, spontaneously. In choosing ovulation induction method in clomiphene resistant PCOS patients, LOD may avoid or reduce the risk of OHSS(ovarian hyperstimulation)and multiple pregnancy than gonadotrophins with the same success rate of conception. The high pregnancy rate, and economic aspect of the procedure offer an attractive management for patients with PCOS [30]. Until now,there was no evidence of a difference in the live birth rate and miscarriage rate in women with clomiphene-resistant PCOS undergoing LOD compared to gonadotrophin treatment. The reduction in multiple pregnancy rates in women undergoing LOD makes the option attractive. In addition,LOD is a suitable method especially for PCOS patients with the highest LH concentrations.However, there are ongoing concerns about long-term effects of LOD on ovarian function [31]. Ovulation induction is the principal infertility treatment for women with polycystic ovarian syndrome (PCOS). Among PCOS patients who are overweight or obese, weight loss is the most physiologic method of inducing ovulation. For women in whom weight loss is not possible, or for lean women with PCOS, clomiphene citrate is an effective first-line method of ovulation induction. In clomiphene-resistant women, alternative treatments include adjunctive metformin or dexamethasone, aromatase inhibitors, or ovarian drilling. If there is no pregnancy despite several cycles of successful ovulation induction, gonadotropin treatment should be considered, and where in vitro fertilization is recommended as the safest and most effective strategy [32]. Assisted

Polycystic Ovarian Syndrome: Symptoms and Clinical Manifestations 129

reproduction is preferable in PCOS women with a BMI of 30 kg/m² or less; however, obese women with polycystic ovarian syndrome show a trend toward poorer in vitro fertilization-embryo transfer outcomes than lean women with the same condition. In fact, the combination of PCOS and obesity seems to be worse than obesity alone [33,34] It seems that there is a trend toward lower implantation rates in obese patients with PCOS, but no other differences [35]. Although, these patients have more favorable IVF-embryo transfer cycle characteristics if they have a BMI in the lean rather than the obese range; clinical pregnancy rates and live birth rates are not significantly different [36].The purpose of another study was to examine the effects of polycystic ovary syndrome (PCOS) and body mass index (BMI) on selected indicators of IVF or intracytoplasmic sperm injection (ICSI) treatment success. This is a retrospective cohort study that was conducted using existing data on 69 IVF/ICSI treatment cycles undergone by PCOS women and an individually matched sample of 69 IVF/ICSI treatment cycles undergone by non-PCOS women at a fertility treatment centre. Results indicated that PCOS was directly associated with the number of oocytes retrieved.Irrespective of PCOS status, continuous BMI was inversely associated with total and mature oocytes retrieved. Multiple linear regression analyses indicated no significant effects of PCOS or continuous BMI on the number of mature oocytes fertilized per mature oocyte retrieved or inseminated. Similarly, multiple logistic regression analyses suggested no significant effect of PCOS and continuous BMI on the odds of pregnancy, miscarriage or live birth .Furthermore,categorical BMI did not influence process and outcome measures of IVF/ICSI treatment success. PCOS and continuous BMI appear to have distinct effects on early stages, but not on later stages,of IVF/ICSI treatment [37].In any case,there are few controlled trials upon which to base a pratical recommendation regarding in vitro maturation before IVF or ICSI for women with PCOS [35].In an attempt to examine whether body mass index may influence IVF outcome in polycystic ovary syndrome, patients undergoing ovarian stimulation with either gonadotrophin-releasing hormone (GnRH)-agonist or antagonist ,in 100 IVF/cycles. In both, agonist and antagonist groups, patients with BMI ≤ 25 kg/m² had a significantly higher fertilization rate compared with patients with BMI > 25 kg/m² (P < 0.02 and P < 0.01, respectively). Lean patients (BMI ≤ 25) undergoing ovarian stimulation using the GnRH-agonist, demonstrated the highest pregnancy rate. In conclusion, in this series of PCOS patients undergoing IVF embryo transfer cycles, ovarian stimulation utilizing the midluteal long GnRH-agonist suppressive protocol yielded a higher pregnancy rate in lean patients, probably due to its ability to lower the high basal LH milieu and its detrimental effect on oocyte quality and implantation potential(38).It was investigated the effect of pre-treatment with metformin in women with polycystic ovaries and at least one of the following criteria: hyperinsulinism, decreased SHBG levels or hirsutism, hyperandrogenaemia or elevated LH/FSH ratio.The results showed that pre-treatment with metformin prior to conventional IVF/ICSI in women with PCOS does not improve stimulation or clinical outcome. However, among normal weight PCOS women, pre-treatment with metformin tends to improve pregnancy rates [39].The Cochrane review 2009 found no evidence that metformin pre-treatment before ART improves live birth or pregnancy rates but the risk of ovarian hyperstimulation syndrome in PCOS women undergoing IVF/ICSI seems reduced [40] Low-dose aspirin is sometimes used to improve the outcome in women undergoing in vitro fertilization, despite inconsistent evidence of efficacy and the potential risk of significant side effects .The most appropriate time to commence this therapy and length of treatment required is also still to be determined. In any case,until now no significant difference was found in clinical pregnancy rate between treatment and control groups,based on the results from 1240 participants in seven studies [41]. In conclusion, women with PCOS undergoing in vitro fertilization (IVF) are at a substantial risk of ovarian hyperstimulation syndrome and this approach should be avoided if at all possible. If it is required these women may be suitable candidates for in vitro maturation of oocytes so avoiding ovarian hyperstimulation. Women with PCOS are potentially at increased risk of miscarriage and their pregnancies are at increased risk of developing gestational diabetes, pregnancy - induced hypertension and pre-eclampsia. Furthermore, the neonate has a significantly higher risk of admission to a neonatal intensive care unit and a higher perinatal mortality [42].In conclusion, women suffering from anovulatory infertility associated with PCOS could be successfully treated today if the management is based on gynaecological experience on the endocrinological field, consideration of the reproductive and metabolic characteristics of each patient and good knowledge of current international protocols .[43].

References

[1]   Stamets K, Taylor DS, Kunselman A, Demers LM, Pelkman CL, Legro RS. A randomized trial of the effects of two types of short-term hypocaloric diets on weight loss in women with polycystic ovary syndrome. *Fertil. Steril.* 2004 Mar;81(3):630-7.

[2]   Nelson SM, Fleming RF.The preconceptual contraception paradigm: obesity and infertility. *Hum. Reprod.* 2007 ;22(4):912-5.

[3]   Gosman GG,King WC,Schrope B,Steffen KJ,Strain GW,Courcoulas AP,Flum DR, Pender JR,Simhan HN.Reproductive health of women electing bariatric surgery. *Fertil. Steril.* 2009;[Epub ahead of print].

[4]   Pagidas K, Carson SA, McGovern PG, Barnhart HX, Myers ER, Legro RS, Diamond MP, Carr BR, Schlaff WD, Coutifaris C, Steinkampf MP, Cataldo NA, Nestler JE, Gosman G, Giudice LC; for the National Institute of Child Health and Human Development-Reproductive Medicine Network. Body mass index and intercourse compliance. *Fertil. Steril.* 2009 . [Epub ahead of print].

[5]   Meczekalski B, Podfigurna-Stopa A. The role of inhibins in functions and dysfunctions of female reproduction. Part I. *Pol. Merkur. Lekarski.* 2009 ;26(153):258-62.

[6]   La Marca A,Broekmans FJ,Volpe A,Fauser BC, Macklon NS;ESHRE. Anti-Mulleeian hormone(AMH) :what do we still need to know? *Hum. Reprod.* 2009;24(9):2264-75.

[7]   Sastre ME, Prat MO, Checa MA, Carreras RC.Current trends in the treatment of polycystic ovary syndrome with desire for children. *Ther. Clin. Risk Manag.* 2009; 5(2):353-60.

Polycystic Ovarian Syndrome: Symptoms and Clinical Manifestations 131

[8] Vanky E,Backe B,Carlsen SM. Sex ratio and pregnancy complications according to mode of conception in women with polycystic ovary syndrome. *Acta Obstet. Gynecol. Scand.* 2009; 88 11): 1261-6.

[9] Tang T, Lord JM, Norman RJ, Yasmin E, Balen AH. Insulin-sensitising drugs (metformin, rosiglitazone, pioglitazone, D-chiro-inositol) for women with polycystic ovary syndrome, oligo amenorrhoea and subfertility. *Cochrane Database Syst. Rev.* 2009 ;(4):CD003053.

[10] Dasari P, Pranahita G. The efficacy of metformin and clomiphene citrate combination compared with clomiphene citrate alone for ovulation induction in infertile patients with PCOS. *J. Hum. Reprod. Sci.* 2009 ;2(1):18-22.

[11] Farquhar C, Beck J, Boothroyd C, Hughes E.Clomiphene and anti-oestrogens for ovulation induction in PCOS. *Cochrane Database Syst. Rev.* 2009 Oct 7;(4):CD002249.

[12] Qublan HS, Al-Khaderei S, Abu-Salem AN, Al-Zpoon A, Al-Khateeb M, Al-Ibrahim N, Megdadi M, Al-Ahmad N.Metformin in the treatment of clomiphene citrate-resistant women with polycystic ovary syndrome undergoing in vitro fertilisation treatment: a randomised controlled trial. *J. Obstet. Gynaecol.* 2009 Oct;29(7):651-5.

[13] Motta AB. Mechanisms involved in metformin action in the treatment of polycystic ovary syndrome. *Curr. Pharm. Des*. 2009;15(26):3074-7.

[14] van Santbrink EJ, Fauser BC.Ovulation induction in normogonadotropic anovulation (PCOS). *Best Pract. Res. Clin. Endocrinol. Metab*. 2006 ;20(2):261-70.

[15] Gilbert C, Valois M, Koren G.Pregnancy outcome after first-trimester exposure to metformin: a meta-analysis. *Fertil. Steril.* 2006 ;86(3):658-63.

[16] Glueck CJ, Wang P, Goldenberg N, Sieve-Smith L.Pregnancy outcomes among women with polycystic ovary syndrome treated with metformin. *Hum. Reprod.* 2002 ; 17(11):2858-64.

[17] Eckmann KR,Kockler DR. Aromatase inhibitors for ovulation and pregnancy in polycystic ovary syndrome. *Ann. Pharmacother*. 2009: 43(7):1338-46.

[18] Badawy A,Abdel Aal I,Abulatta M. Clomiphene citrate or letrozole for ovulation induction in women with polycystic ovarian syndrome:a prospective randomized trial. *Fertil. Steril.* 2009;92(3):849-52.

[19] Abu Hashim H, Shokeir T, Badawy A.Letrozole versus combined metformin and clomiphene citrate for ovulation induction in clomiphene-resistant women with polycystic ovary syndrome: a randomized controlled trial. *Fertil. Steril.* 2009. [Epub ahead of print].

[20] Montville CP, Khabbaz M, Aubuchon M, Williams DB, Thomas MA. Luteal support with intravaginal progesterone increases clinical pregnancy rates in women with polycystic ovary syndrome using letrozole for ovulation induction. *Fertil. Steril.* 2009 . [Epub ahead of print].

[21] Bayram N,van Wely M,van der Veen F.Pulsatile gonadotrophin releasing hormone for ovulation induction in subfertility associated with polycystic ovary syndrome. *Cochrane Database Syst. Rev.* 2004; (1): CD000412. 23(12):700-3.

[22] Papaleo E,Unfer V, Baillargeon JP, De Santis L, Fusi F,Brigante C, Marelli G, Cino I, Redaelli A, Ferrari A.Myo-inositol in patients with polycystic ovary syndrome: a novel method for ovulation induction. *Gynecol. Endocrinol*. 2007;

[23] Costantino D, Minozzi G, Minozzi E, Guaraldi C. Metabolic and hormonal effects of myo-inositol in women with polycystic ovary syndrome: a double-blind trial. *Eur. Rev. Med. Pharmacol. Sci.* 2009 ;13(2):105-10.

[24] Frantz N,Ferreira M,Hoher M,Bos-Mikich A.Spontaneous pregnancies after ovarian puncture for in vitro maturation in women with the polycystic ovary syndrome. *Rev. Bras. Ginecol. Obstet.* 2009;31(3): 138-41.

[25] Nafiye Y, Sevtap K, Muammer D, Emre O, Senol K, Leyla M.The effect of serum and intrafollicular insulin resistance parameters and homocysteine levels of nonobese, non hyperandrogenemic polycystic ovary syndrome patients on in vitro fertilization outcome. *Fertil. Steril.* 2009 . [Epub ahead of print].

[26] Rausch ME, Legro RS, Barnhart HX, Schlaff WD, Carr BR, Diamond MP, Carson SA, Steinkampf MP, McGovern PG, Cataldo NA, Gosman GG, Nestler JE, Giudice LC, Leppert PC, Myers ER, Coutifaris C; Reproductive Medicine Network. Predictors of pregnancy in women with polycystic ovary syndrome. *J. Clin. Endocrinol. Metab.* 2009; 94(9):3458-66.

[27] Mourali M, Fkih C, Essoussi-Chikhaoui J, Ben Hadj HA, Binous N, Ben Zineb N. Polycystic ovary syndrome with infertility. *Tunis Med.* 2008 ;86(11):963-72.

[28] Palomba S, Falbo A, Zullo F. Management strategies for ovulation induction in women with polycystic ovary syndrome and known clomifene citrate resistance. *Curr. Opin. Obstet. Gynecol.* 2009 . [Epub ahead of print].

[29] Ashrafinia M, Hosseini R,Moini A,Eslami B,Asgari Z.Comparison of metformin treatment and laparoscopic ovarian diathermy in patients with polycystic ovary syndrome. *Int. J. Gynaecol. Obstet.* 2009; [Epub ahead of print].

[30] Api M, Görgen H, Cetin A. Laparoscopic ovarian drilling in polycystic ovary syndrome. *Eur. J. Obstet. Gynecol. Reprod. Biol.* 2005 Mar 1;119(1):76-81.

[31] Farquhar C. ,Liford RJ,Marjoribanks J,Vandekerckhove P.Laparoscopic drilling by diathermy or laser for ovulation in anovulatory polycystic ovary syndrome. *Cochrane Database Syst. Rev.* 2007 ;(3):CD001122.

[32] Guzick DS. Ovulation induction management of PCOS. Clin Obstet Gynecol. 2007 ;50(1):255-67. Zain MM, Norman RJ. Impact of obesity on female fertility and fertility treatment. *Women Health (Lond.Engl.)* 2008;4(2):183-94.

[33] Wilkes S,Murdoch A, Obesity and female fertility:a primary care perspective. *J. Fam. Plann. Reprod. Health Care* 2009;35(3): 181-5.

[34] Hirschberg AL. Polycystic ovary syndrome.obesity and reproductive implications. *Womens Health (Lond.Engl.)* 2009; 5(5): 529-40.

[35] Siristatidis CS,Maheshwari A,Bhattacharya S. In vitro maturation in subfertile women with polycystic ovarian syndrome undergoing assisted reproduction. *Cochrane Database Syst. Rev.* 2009,(1): CD006606.

[36] McCormick B, Thomas M, Maxwell R, Williams D, Aubuchon M. Effects of polycystic ovarian syndrome on in vitro fertilization-embryo transfer outcomes are influenced by body mass index. *Fertil. Steril.* 2008 ;90(6):2304-9.

[37] Beydoun HA, Stadtmauer L, Beydoun MA, Russell H, Zhao Y, Oehninger S.Polycystic ovary syndrome, body mass index and outcomes of assisted reproductive technologies. *Reprod. Biomed. Online.* 2009 ;18(6):856-63.

[38] Orvieto R, Nahum R, Meltcer S, Homburg R, Rabinson J, Anteby EY, Ashkenazi J.Ovarian stimulation in polycystic ovary syndrome patients: the role of body mass index. *Reprod Biomed Online.* 2009 Mar;18(3): 333-6.

[39] Kjotrod SB,vON During V,Carlsen SM.Metformin treatment before IVF/ICSI in women with polycystic ovary syndrome;a prospective,randomized,double blind study. *Hum. Reprod.* 2004;19(6):1325-22.

[40] Tso LO, Costello MF, Albuquerque LE,Andriolo RB,Freitas V.Metformin treatment before and during IVF or ICSI in wonen with polycystic ovary syndrome. *Cochrane Database Syst. Rev.* 2009;15(2): CD006105.

[41] Poustie VJ,Dodd S,Drakeley AJ.Low-dose apirin for in vitro fertilisation. *Cochrane Database Syst. Rev.* 2007;17(4):CD004832.

[42] Hart R. PCOS and infertility. *Panminerva Med.* 2008;50(4):305-10.

[43] Homburg R.The management of infertility associated with polycystic ovary syndrome. *Reprod. Biol. Endocrinol.* 2003;1; 109.

Problems in Pregnant PCOS Women

Polycystic ovary syndrome is a main cause of infertility, particularly in high risk settings such as spontaneous abortions . There is an increasing body of evidence indicating that PCOS may have significant implications for pregnancy outcomes and long-term health of a woman and her offspring. Whether or not PCOS itself or the symptoms that coincide with PCOS, like obesity and fertility treatment, are responsible for these increased risks is a continuing matter of debate. Miscarriage rates, among women with PCOS, are believed to be increased compared with normal fertile women, although supporting evidence is limited. Pregnant women with PCOS experience a higher incidence of perinatal morbidity from gestational diabetes, pregnancy-induced hypertension, and preeclampsia. Their babies are at an increased risk of neonatal complications, such as preterm birth and admission at a neonatal intensive care unit. Pre-pregnancy, antenatal, and intrapartum care should be aimed at reducing these risks. The use of insulin sensitizing drugs to decrease hyperinsulinemic- insulin resistance has been proposed during pregnancy to reduce the risk of developing preeclampsia or gestational diabetes. Although, metformin appears to be safe, there are too few data from prospective, randomized controlled trials to support treatment during pregnancy [1].

Miscarriage

Women with PCOS who conceive either spontaneously or after ovulation induction seem to be at high risk of miscarriage. It was long believed that women who suffer with PCOS have a higher rate of miscarriage, suffering this loss at a rate of 45 to 50 percent as compared to the national rate of 15 to 25 percent for women who do not have this condition .However, many studies have investigated the prevalence of PCOS in recurrent miscarriage, the extent to which PCOS contributes remains highly uncertain. The majority of the studies performed in the past have used the polycystic ovary morphology alone to define PCOS and the results are extremely variable due to a variety of diagnostic and selection criteria used. Only a very small number of studies have investigated the prevalence of hyperandrogenaemia in recurrent miscarriage. Using the Rotterdam criteria, it was established that of 300 women who had recurrent miscarriage , 8.3-10% had PCOS.Therefore, the prevalence of PCOS in women with RM is considerably lower than has previously been accepted [2].Particularly, a Japanese study, based on Japanese criteria of PCOS classification,seems to deny the relation between a diagnosis of PCOS, PCO morphology, elevated LH, free testosterone or obesity and the subsequent miscarriage rate [3].Hence, there is an urgent need to reappraise the prevalence of PCOS in recurrent miscarriage using the Rotterdam criteria. Hyperandrogenaemia, obesity and hyperinsulinaemia are the most likely candidates as possible mechanisms by which PCOS could cause recurrent miscarriage; although further work is clearly needed. A study was performed with the aim to determine the incidence of an abnormal glucose tolerance test in patients with recurrent spontaneous abortion and whether metformin would safely reduce the rate of first trimester spontaneous abortions in patients without polycystic ovary syndrome as well as with PCOS and an abnormal glucose tolerance test. Patients with a history of recurrent spontaneous abortion and women with a history of normal full term pregnancy were considered. Metformin and placebo were given to women with an abnormal glucose tolerance test and who had recurrent spontaneous abortions.Twenty-nine of the patients in the group with recurrent spontaneous abortion were found to have an abnormal glucose tolerance test compared with just four (5.4%) patients in the normal pregnancy group.The abortion rate was significantly reduced after metformin therapy in patients without PCOS in comparison to the placebo group (15% vs. 55%).This study indicates an important link between an abnormal glucose tolerance test and a history of recurrent abortion.It was also found that metformin therapy improves the chances of a successful pregnancy in patients with an abnormal glucose tolerance test [4]. While,it has been showed that metformin has no effect on the abortion risk in PCOS patients when administered before pregnancy [5]. Another investigation explores the relationship between the spontaneous abortion and changes of estrogen (ER) and progesterone receptors(PR) in the endometrium of patients with PCOS. Thirty-two patients who suffered from PCOS combined with infertility were enrolled in a experimental group ; while 20 patients with tubal infertility were considered as control group.The expressions of ER and PR in the endometrium were observed by pathological examination and immunohistochemical staining. The expressions of ER and PR in the glands and interstitium of endometriun in the PCOS group were significantly lower than those of the tubal infertility group. The expressions of ER in the glands of endometrium in the spontaneous abortion group were significantly lower than those of the non-spontaneous abortion group, but there was no statistical difference between the two groups in the interstitium of endometrium. The expression of PR in the glands interstitium of endometrium showed no statistical difference between the spontaneous abortion group and the non-spontaneous abortion group. In conclusion,the decrease of ER and PR of endometrium in the PCOS patients, may be a reason for spontaneous abortion, and the cyclical irregularity of ER and PR in the PCOS patients seem to be another cause of spontaneous abortion [6]. Polycystic ovarian syndrome is associated with insulin-induced plasminogen activator inhibitor-1 (PAI-1) elevation. It is well known that thrombophilic states correlate with high miscariage rates; therefore, the link with PCOS has been hypothesized. However,a recent study aimed at looking for thrombophilic predisposition in PCOS women, compared with non-PCOS controls, seems to deny this hypothesis. The prevalence of antithrombin III, protein S and protein C deficiencies, as well as factor V Leiden, prothrombin G20210A factor and methylene tetrahydrofolate reductase (MTHFR) mutations, was compared between two different groups of women, one with PCOS (n = 30) and one without PCOS (n = 45). There was no evidence that the genetic analysis for factor V Leiden or prothrombin factor differed between the two samples.The odds ratio (OR) of bearing a mutation on the MTHFR gene was 1.2-fold higher in women with PCOS than in women without. Although, this difference is not statistically significant and,it might indicate only a slightly higher prevalence of heterozygous genotypes in women with PCOS. In conclusion,molecular risk factors of hereditary thrombophilia do not show an increased prevalence in women with PCOS, in comparison with women in the general population. The existence of a possible trend towards higher prevalence of MTHFR mutation in women with PCOS needs further studies, particularly regarding homocysteine levels [7]. Another study investigated the effect of genetic polymorphisms in angiotensin-converting enzyme (ACE) and plasminogen activator inhibitor-1 (PAI-1) on the occurrence of spontaneous abortion (SA) in PCOS. Were considered for this study: 142 PCOS patients (83 women have a history of one or more unexplained SA, 59 women have successfully live births) and 107 healthy controls matched for age and body mass index . ACE D/I and PAI-1 4G/5G gene polymorphisms were performed. The D/D and/or 4G/4G genotype frequency, the D or 4G allelic frequency, the combination of the ACE D/D and PAI-1. 4G/5G, D/I and 4G/4G genotypes of PCOS patients with SA women were statistically higher than non-SA group (P<0.05). The 4G/4G or D/D genotype of PCOS with SA patients had significantly higher PAI-1 levels than non-SA women. The ACE D/I and PAI-1 4G/5G gene polymorphisms might represent risk factor in PCOS with SA. Homozygosity for ACE D or PAI-1 4G polymorphisms as well as compound carrier status are significant positive explanatory variables for PCOS patients with SA, which may result in increased PAI-1 concentrations and hypofibrinolysis contributing to early pregnancy loss [8]. Thrombophilia, hypofibrinolysis, and polycystic ovary syndrome (PCOS) are associated with recurrent pregnancy loss (RPL) and spontaneous abortion (SA) alone and concurrently.The efficacy and safety of combined enoxaparin-metformin was prospectively assessed in women with PCOS with one or more previous SA, thrombophilia, and/or hypofibrinolysis.Twenty-four white women with PCOS were studied; 23 with previous pregnancies, seven with RPL of unknown etiology (≥ three consecutive pregnancy losses <20 weeks' gestation), two with two consecutive SA, 13 with one SA, and one with one live birth (HELLP syndrome). Prospectively, metformin (1.5 to 2.55 g/day) was administered before and throughout gestation, with concurrent enoxaparin (60 mg/day) throughout gestation. The 24 cases differed from 93 normal white female controls for the factor V Leiden mutation, 17% vs. 2%, , and for the 4 G4G mutation of the plasminogen activator inhibitor-1 (PAI-1) gene (46% vs. 24%). The patients also differed from 44 normal white female controls for high levels (> 21.1 U/mL) of the PAI-1 gene product, plasminogen activator inhibitor activity (PAI-Fx) (33% vs. 8%), and for high factor VIII (>150%) (22% vs. 0%). Of the 24 women, 23 had 65 previous pregnancies without metformin or enoxaparin,with 18 live births, 46 SA(71%), and one elective abortion.On metformin- enoxaparin, the same 23 women had 26 current pregnancies (28 fetuses), with 20 live births, two normal pregnancies 13 weeks or longer, and six SA (21%), 3.4-fold lower than previous gestations (p<.0001).There were no adverse maternal or fetal therapy effects.Enoxaparin-metformin reduces pregnancy loss in women with PCOS with one or more previous SA, who also have thrombophilia and/or hypofibrinolysis [9]. Since hypercoagulability might result in recurrent miscarriage, anticoagulant agents could potentially increase the live-birth rate in subsequent pregnancies in women with either inherited thrombophilia or unexplained recurrent miscarriage [10]. Polycystic ovary syndrome , thrombophilia, and hypofibrinolysis are associated with recurrent pregnancy loss (RPL) and spontaneous abortion (SA). In 28 Caucasian women, 21 women with PCOS (4 with previous thrombosis, 18 with 1 SA or more, and 20 with 1 coagulation disorder or more),and 7 women with coagulation disorders-thrombi,the prospective treatment with enoxaparin-metformin or enoxaparin alone would successfully and safely promote healthy live births compared with previous untreated pregnancies. In 21 women with PCOS, metformin (1.5-2.55 g/day) was given before and during pregnancy with concurrent enoxaparin (60 mg/day).Of 21 PCOS women, 19 women had 40 previous untreated pregnancies, 7 had live births (18%), 3 had elective abortions (ABs) (8%), and 30 had SA (75%).On enoxaparin-metformin, these 19 women had 24 pregnancies, 20 live births (83%),and 4 SA(17%); the SA rate was 4.4-fold lower than previous untreated pregnancies.Two women with PCOS without previous pregnancies , but with previous thrombosis, had 2 pregnancies on enoxaparin-metformin and 2 live births. Of the 7 women with coagulation disorders-thrombi, 4 had 15 previous pregnancies without enoxaparin, with 6 live births (40%), 8 SA (53%), and 1 elective AB (7%).On enoxaparin, these 4 women had 4 pregnancies, with 4 (100%) live births (P = 0.005). The other 3 women with coagulation disorders-thrombi had 4 pregnancies on enoxaparin with 4 live births. No adverse maternal-fetal side effects were reported on enoxaparin alone or enoxaparin-metformin. In conclusion,this clinical trial shows that the association Enoxaparin-metformin reduces pregnancy loss in women with PCOS-coagulation disorders and in women with coagulation disorders-thrombi [11]. It was reported that polycystic ovaries are more frequently seen in women with recurrent pregnancy loss but the presence of PCO on ultrasound did not predict the outcome in subsequent pregnancies. Homburg has shown that miscarriage rates after ovulation induction or IVF is decreased when women are pretreated with a GnRH-agonist such as Synarel, Lupron or Zoladex [12].The association between polycystic ovary syndrome and recurrent miscarriage (RM) has been long established, but the relative importance of this condition as a cause of RM is far from clear..In spite of the common use of progestogen , there is no evidence to support its routine use to prevent miscarriage in early to mid-pregnancy.However, there seems to be evidence of benefit in women with a history of recurrent miscarriage [13].

Hyperinsulinemia may be a contributing factor in the higher rate of miscarriage [14]. Elevated levels of insulin interfere with the normal balance between factors promoting blood clotting and those promoting breakdown of the clots. Increases in plasminogen activator inhibitor activity (PAI) associated with high insulin levels may result in increased blood clotting at the interface between the endometrium and the placenta. This could lead to placental insufficiency and miscarriage.There is not definitive large consensus to indicate whether pregnancy outcomes are improved using insulin-lowering medications or whether pregnancy outcomes are better in those who continue metformin throughout the pregnancy or those who discontinue. In the meantime, it seems that use of metformin to manage non-insulin dependent diabetes during pregnancy can be accomplished safely [15,16].Some studies reported that women who conceive following metformin, have an unacceptably high (>30%) risk of miscarriage[17]. However, the risk of miscarriage is increased in those patients with a prior history of miscarriage and those with high LH, high androgen levels, hyperinsulinemia or elevated PAI-F [18]. Initial findings of current clinical trials suggest a decreased risk of miscarriage if metformin is continued throughout the pregnancy. At present,there is insufficient data to routinely advise continuation of metformin during pregnancy. As an alternative in continuing metformin therapy, those women with increased risk of abnormal blood clotting may benefit from baby aspirin, folate supplementation and low dose heparin therapy [1].

Pregnancy Complications in PCOS Women

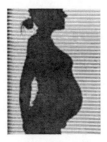

Although,PCOS is a major cause of infertility, its etiology remains unknown and its treatment difficult. A retrospective analysis.found that of the 2270 infertility patients evaluated, 1057(46,59%) had PCOS. Of the PCOS patients, 914 were considered for this study.and 814 of those came for treatment.The overall pregnancy rate was 48.40% (394/814).

The pregnancy rate per cycle with timed intercourse was 44.77% (47/105), 17.09% (286/1673) with intrauterine insemination (IUI), 29.82% (51/171) with in vitro fertilization (IVF) and 22.22% (10 /45) with frozen embryo transfer (FET).The maximum number of pregnancies (85.29%, 284/333) were achieved in the first three treatment cycles.The abortion rate was 19.01% (73/384) and the incidence of ectopic pregnancy was 5.47% (21/384). Complications seen were in the form of ovarian hyperstimulation (OHSS), retention cyst on day two and multiple pregnancies in 11.71% (228/1946) of the total treatment cycles. Therefore,:most PCOS symptoms could be adequately controlled or eliminated with proper diagnosis and treatment.Thus, ovulation induction protocols and treatment modalities must be balanced for optimal results [19]. Polycystic ovary syndrome is an endocrine dysfunction closely associated with insulin resistance and obesity, which predisposes to pregnancy complications. Particularly, gestational diabetes mellitus (GDM) is defined as glucose intolerance that has its onset or is first recognized during pregnancy .GDM occurs in 2-5% of all pregnancies, although the majority of women with GDM regain normal glucose tolerance postpartum. Women with history of GDM are at a substantially increased risk of developing type 2 diabetes later in the life ; in fact, they demonstrate abnormalities in both insulin secretion and function which resembles those with type 2 diabetes [20]. Indeed, it has been suggested that both GDM and type 2 diabetes are the same disorder .There are some metabolic similarities between women with history of gestational diabetes mellitus (GDM) and women with polycystic ovary syndrome; so, it has been postulated that there may be shared etiopathological factors between these conditions[21,22,23]. It is important to follow - up the patients who became pregnant after diet, exercise and metformin treatment intervention during the whole pregnancy [24]. Seventy pregnant PCOS women and forty normal pregnant (NP) women of similar age and with singleton pregnancies were included in a study. During gestational ages 10-16 and 22-28 weeks, a 2h, 75 g oral glucose tolerance test (OGTT) was performed with measurement of glucose and insulin in each sample. No differences were found in duration of gestation, weight gain during pregnancy, or systolic and diastolic blood pressure between PPCOS and NP women. There were significant differences in body mass index at the initiation and in the third trimester of pregnancy between both groups. The incidence of gestational diabetes was significantly higher (p <0.01) in the PCOS group (35.2%) compared to the control group (5.0%) [25]. Gestational diabetes mellitus (GDM) is a type of diabetes that presents during pregnancy and usually disappears shortly after a woman gives birth (26). GDM appears to be common, independent of maternal weight [26,27,28]. Better recognition of the risk factors of GDM, combined with more universal screening for the disease in many countries, has led to the increased detection of GDM along with other forms of pregestational diabetes. Women presenting for GDM screening were randomised to GR1 [1-hour, 50-g glucose screen (GS) ± 3-hour, 100-g oral glucose tolerancetest (OGTT)], GR2 (50-g GS ± 2-hour, 75-g OGTT) or GR3 (2-hour, 75-g OGTT Among women in the two-step method groups diagnosed with GDM, 39% of the GR1 and 61% of the GR2 groups were diagnosed at the first step by GS ≥ 10.3 mmol/l, according to the Canadian Diabetes Association recommendations, contributing to a lower total cost in these groups.The GDM prevalence was similar (3.7%,3.7% and 3.6%, respectively). Finally, careful consideration should be given to an internationally recommended method of universal screening for GDM which minimises the burden and cost for individual women and the health care system, yet provides diagnostic efficacy.The two-step method (GS ± OGTT) accomplished this better than the one-step method (75-g OGTT)(22) It is uncertain whether treatment of mild gestational diabetes mellitus improves pregnancy outcomes. A study evaluated women who were in the 24th to 31st week of gestation and who met the criteria for mild gestational diabetes mellitus (abnormal oral glucose-tolerance test but fasting glucose level below 95 mg per deciliter) .These were randomly assigned to usual prenatal care or dietary intervention, self-monitoring of blood glucose, and insulin therapy, if necessary .The results showed that although treatment of mild gestational diabetes mellitus did not significantly reduce the frequency of a composite outcome that included stillbirth or perinatal death and several neonatal complications, it did reduce the risks of fetal overgrowth, dystocia, cesarean delivery, and hypertensive disorders.[28].There is a growing evidence that GDM significantly increases the risk of a number of short- and long-term adverse consequences for the fetus and mother, the most significant of which is a predisposition to the development of metabolic syndrome and Type 2 diabetes. The prevalence of small for gestational age (SGA) infants tended to be higher in the PCOS group. During pregnancy, 2h glucose and insulin were significantly higher in PPCOS than in NP women. PCOS mothers showed a higher prevalence of gestational diabetes and SGA newborns, which cannot be attributed to the weight gain during pregnancy, and seems to be more related to the BMI at the initiation of pregnancy, and to the PCOS condition of the mother. Significantly more women with both GDM and PCOS had pregnancy-induced hypertension/ preeclampsia (15.9% vs. 3.9%). Women with GDM and PCOS tended to have more preterm deliveries (25.0%vs. 11.8%).

Recent data have shown that PCOS is associated with an increased rate of adverse pregnancy outcomes.A recent, retrospective study determined the frequency and contributors to preterm delivery (PTD, <37 weeks) among 1018 women with PCOS. The PTD rate was 19% overall and 67% for multiple gestation pregnancy. Among 908 singleton deliveries, 116 (13%) had PTD (21% delivered at <28 wks, 15% at 28-31.9 wks, and 65% at 32-36.9 wks). Causes of singleton PTD included preterm labor (41%) and incompetent cervix (10%), with the remainder due to hypertensive complications (20%), preterm premature rupture of membranes (15%), fetal placental concerns (9%) and intrauterine fetal demise (5%) resulting in iatrogenic or inevitable delivery. The singleton PTD rate was higher among nulliparous women (15% vs 10%, p=0.03). Half of singleton pregnancies conceived using fertility medications (including assisted reproduction) but PTD rates did not differ between these two groups.Considering that Preterm births account for 35% of US health care spending for infants and 10% of spending for children. Future studies should investigate mechanisms leading to PTD and potential areas of intervention to reduce adverse pregnancy outcomes in PCOS women [29]More infants of women with GDM and PCOS required phototherapy treatment for hyperbilirubinemia (25.0% vs.7.9%) [30]. Gestational diabetes mellitus (GDM) was significantly more frequent in the PCOS group than in the other groups (20% vs. 3.6% ; P<0.01). Preterm birth was more frequent in the PCOS group than in control group (20% vs. 6.9%; P<0.05), whereas mean length of gestation was not different.The higher occurrence of adverse outcomes may be, at least partly, related to a higher weight gain during pregnancy in PCOS group with respect to the other groups . Women affected by PCOS carry an increased risk of adverse pregnancy outcomes [31] An interesting study evaluated twenty women with and 24 without GDM for two years after delivery. Clinical features, blood biochemistry, and hormonal profile were compared between two groups. Ovarian morphology was studied via abdominal ultrasonography. The prevalence of PCOS was higher in the GDM group than that in the non-GDM group (45% vs.25%); however, the difference was not statistically significant. The GDM group had a higher prevalence of overweight, central obesity, hirsutism, irregular menses, and PCOS than did the women in the non-GDM group. The serum levels of fasting blood sugar, hemoglobin A1C, lipid profiles, and insulin were also higher in the GDM group. Testosterone levels tended to be higher in the GDM group; significantly, free testosterone index (Figure 1)[32]

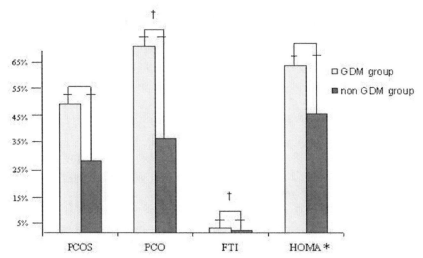

Figure 1. Comparison of PCOS and PCO morphology and FTI and HOMA between the case group (history of GDM) and control group (without history of GDM)

Gestational hypertension and gestational diabetes mellitus are the most frequent obstetric disorders during pregnancy. The rates of both disorders are expected to increase as a result of delayed pregnancy at a later maternal age, the epidemic of obesity and the increased frequency of using assisted reproductive technology in these women.. Pregnancies complicated one or both of these disorders are also associated with adverse consequences for the mother and infant, acute and long-term. The objective of a review was to describe the association between gestational hypertension and gestational diabetes, and to discuss approaches to management and summarize long-term consequences of gestational hypertension [33].In conclusion, mothers with both disorders should be monitored more carefully and counseled regarding their increased risk of both maternal and fetal complications .Among 29 PCOS women who received metformin, gestational diabetes developed during one of 29 pregnancies (3.44%) versus nine of 30 pregnancies (30%) without metformin. All babies born in the metformin group had normal birth weight ,while in the control group 4 babies(13.33%) were large for date. In PCOS, use of metformin throughout pregnancy is associated with a nine fold reduction of gestational diabetes [34].Systematic review and meta-analysis of observational studies allowed to consider five thousand two hundred ninety-three pregnant women (721 women with PCOS and 4,572 normal). Data showed that women with PCOS have significantly higher risk for the development of GDM as compared with women without PCOS [35]. Polycystic ovary syndrome (PCOS) and gestational diabetes mellitus are both characterized by an increase in insulin resistance.The goal could be to measure insulin resistance and parameters of low-grade inflammation in non-diabetic, non-hyperandrogenic ovulatory women with previous GDM and in non-diabetic women with classic PCOS,characterized by hyperandrogenism and oligo/anovulation. Twenty women with PCOS, 18 women with previous GDM and 19 controls, all matched according to body mass index ,were evaluated.. Fasting blood samples were drawn in all women 3-6 days after spontaneous or dydrogesterone-induced withdrawal bleeding. Body fat distribution was assessed using dual-energy X-ray absorptiometry in all women. After adjusting for age and percent body fat, measures of insulin resistance such as SHBG and adiponectin concentrations were decreased and central obesity was increased in women with PCOS and pGDM compared with controls (p < 0.05). Parameters of low-grade inflammation such as serum tumor necrosis factor-alpha and highly sensitive C-reactive protein concentrations, white blood cell and neutrophil count were increased only in women with PCOS compared with BMI-matched controls[36].Certain markers of insulin resistance are increased in both women with PCOS and women with pGDM, while low-grade inflammation is increased only in PCOS. PCOS and GDM might represent specific phenotypes of one disease entity with an increased risk of cardiovascular disease, whereby women with PCOS demonstrate an augmented cardiovascular risk profile [37]. The purpose of the present study was to examine long-term reproductive outcome and ovarian reserve in an unselected population of women with polycystic ovary syndrome (PCOS). A total of 91 patients with confirmed PCOS and 87 healthy controls were included in the study. Patients had been diagnosed between 1987 and 1995 and at the time of the follow-up, subjects were 35 years of age or older. Among women who had attempted a pregnancy, 86.7% of PCOS patients and 91.6% of controls had given birth to at least one child. Among PCOS patients who had given birth, 73.6% had done so following a spontaneous conception.Mean ovarian volume and the number of antral follicles in PCOS patients were significantly greater than in control women (P < 0.001). PCOS patients also had higher serum concentrations of anti-Müllerian hormone and lower follicle-stimulating hormone levels. Most women with PCOS had given birth, and the rate of spontaneous pregnancies was relatively high. Together with the ultrasound findings and the hormonal analyses, this finding could imply that PCOS patients have a good fecundity, and an ovarian reserve possibly superior to women with normal ovaries [38].Polycystic ovary syndrome is the most frequent cause of female infertility with an estimated prevalence of 6-10% in premenopausal women. Due to its long-term metabolic and cardiovascular consequences, it sometimes poses a severe health problem. Visceral obesity and subsequent insulin resistance represent the core pathophysiology of PCOS, clearly suggesting that measures to reduce abdominal obesity should be pursued.   Although, the cases of severe obesity in infertile PCOS women may be quickly solved only after laparoscopic gastric banding. In addition ,after this bariatric surgery , glucose levels normalised completely. Therefore, the gastric banding should be performed based on the body mass index, the metabolic disorders, and the wish of the patient to become pregnant [39]. It is therefore advisable that they be screened at 12 weeks of pregnancy for diabetes and thyroid disease . Moreover, all women with PCOS should be given a glucose tolerance test between 24-28 weeks of pregnancy. More than half the women with gestational diabetes turn out to have PCOS when tested after they had delivered. Pre-eclampsia is a serious complication of late pregnancy characterised by a sudden increase in blood pressure, excessive weight gain, swelling and protein in the urine. It requires immediate medical attention. Insulin resistance is a known risk factor for pre-eclampsia. Women with PCOS are particularly at risk during their first pregnancy.

References

[1]   Boomsma CM, Fauser BC, Macklon NS.Pregnancy complications in women with polycystic ovary syndrome. *Semin. Reprod. Med.* 2008 ;26(1):72-84.

[2] Cocksedge KA, Saravelos SH, Metwally M, Li TC.How common is polycystic ovary syndrome in recurrent miscarriage? *Reprod. Biomed. Online.* 2009 Oct;19 (4): 572-6.

[3] Sugiura-Ogasawara M,Sato T,Suzumori N,Kitaori T,Humagai K,Ozaki Y.The polycystic ovary syndrome does not predict further miscarriage in Iapanese couples experiencing recurrent miscarriages. *Am. J. Reprod. Immunol.* 2009;61(1): 62-7.

[4] Zolghadri J, Tavana Z, Kazerooni T, Soveid M, Taghieh M.Relationship between abnormal glucose tolerance test and history of previous recurrent miscarriages, and beneficial effect of metformin in these patients: a prospective clinical study. *Fertil. Steril.* 2008 ;90(3):727-30.

[5] Palomba S,Falbo A,Orio F.Jr,Zurlo F. Effect of preconceptional metformin on abortion risk in polycystic ovary syndrome: a systematic review and meta-analysis of randomized controlled trials. *Fertil. Steril.* 2009; 92(5): 1646-58.

[6] Shi XB, Zhang J, Fu SX.Spontaneous abortion and changes of estrogen receptors and progesterone receptors in the endometria of patients with polycystic ovary syndrome. *Zhong Nan Da Xue Xue Bao Yi Xue Ban.* 2008 ;33(6):518-22.[Article in Chinese].

[7] Tsanadis G, Vartholomatos G, Korkontzelos L, Avgoustatos F, Kakosimos G, Sotiriadis A, Tatsioni A, Eleftheriou A, Lolis D. Polycystic ovarian syndrome and thrombophilia. *Human Reproduction* 2002;17(2): 314-319.

[8] Sun L, Lv H, Wei W, Zhang D, Guan Y.Angiotensin-converting enzyme D/I and plasminogen activator inhibitor-1 4G/5G gene polymorphisms are associated with increased risk of spontaneous abortions in polycystic ovarian syndrome. *J. Endocrinol. Invest.* 2009 Jul 28. [Epub ahead of print].

[9] Glueck CJ, Wang P, Goldenberg N, Sieve L. Pregnancy loss, polycystic ovary syndrome, thrombophilia, hypofibrinolysis, enoxaparin, metformin. *Clin. Appl. Thromb. Hemost.* 2004 Oct;10(4):323-34.

[10] Kaandorp S,Di Nisio M, Goddijn M, Middeldorp S. Aspirin or anticoagulants for treating recurrent miscarriage in women without antiphospholipid syndrome. *Cochrane Database Syst. Rev.* 2009; 21(1): CD004734.

[11] Ramidi G, Khan N, Glueck CJ, Wang P, Goldenberg N.Enoxaparin-metformin and enoxaparin alone may safely reduce pregnancy loss. *Transl. Res.* 2009 ;153(1):33-43.

[12] Homburg R. Polycystic ovary syndrome: induction of ovulation. *Ballieres Clinical Endocrinologys and Metabolism* 1996; 10:281-292.

[13] Haas DM,Ramsey PS.Progestogen for preventing miscarriage. *Cochrane Database Syst. Rev.* 2008; 16(2): CD003511.

[14] Utiger RD. Insulin and the polycystic ovary syndrome. *New England J. Medicine* 1996, 335:657658.

[15] Coetzee EJ, Jackson WP. The management of non-insulin-dependent diabets during pregnancy. *Diabetes Res. Clin. Pract.* 1985-86;1:281-287.

[16] Velazquez EM, Mendosa S, Hamer T, Sosa F, Glucck CJ. Metformin therapy in women with polycystic ovary syndrome reduces hyperinsulinemia, insulin resistance, hyperandrogenemia, and systolic blood pressure, while facilitating menstrual regularity and pregnancy. *Metabolism* 1994,43:647-655.

[17] Glueck CJ, Wang P, Fontaine R, Tracy T, Sieve-Smith L. Metformin-induced resumption of normal menses in 39 of 43 (91%) previously amenorrheic women with polycystic ovary syndrome. *Metabolism* 1999; 48:1-10.

Polycystic Ovarian Syndrome: Symptoms and Clinical Manifestations   143

[18] Tulppala M, Stenman UH, Cacciatore B, Ylikorkala O. Polycystic ovaries and levels of gonadotropins and androgens in recurrent miscarriage: preliminary experience of 500 consecutive cases. *Hum. Reprod.* 1994;9:1328-32.

[19] Rajashekar L,Krishna D,Patil M.Polycystic ovaries and infertility: Our experience. *J. Hum. Reprod.* 2008;1(2):65-72.

[20] Lanzone A, Caruso A, Di Simone N, et al.Polycystic ovary disease.A risk factor for gestational diabetes? *Reprod. Med.* 1995; 40: 312- 6.

[21] Wortsman J, de Angeles S, FutterweitW, et al. Gestational diabetes and neonatal macrosomia in the polycysticovary syndrome. *J. Reprod. Med.* 1991;36: 659 -61.

[22] Lesser KB, Garcia FA. Association between polycystic ovary syndrome and glucose intolerance during pregnancy. *J. Matern. Fetal Med.* 1997; 6: 303- 7.

[23] Lo JC, Feigenbaum SL, Escobar GJ, et al. Increased prevalence of Gestational Diabetes Mellitus among women withdiagnosed Polycystic Ovary Syndrome. *Diabetes Care* 2006; 29: 1915-720.

[24] Reece EA.The fetal and maternal consequences of gestational diabetes mellitus. *J. Matern. Fetal Neonatal.Med.* 2010 [Epub ahead of print].

[25] Villarroel AC, Echiburú B, Riesco V, Maliqueo M, Cárcamo M, Hitschfeld C, Sánchez F, del Solar MP, Sir-Petermann T.Polycystic ovary syndrome and pregnancy : clinical experience [Article in Spanish] *Rev. Med. Chil.* 2007 ;135(12):1530-8.

[26] Meltzer SJ,Snyder J,Penrod JR,Nudi M, Morin L.Gestational diabetes mellitus screening and diagnosis: a prospective randomized controlled trial comparing costs of one-step and two-step methods. *BJOG 2010* [Epub ahead of print].

[27] Holte, J., Gennarelli, G., Wide, L. et al. High prevalence of polycystic ovaries and associated clinical, endocrine, and metabolic features in women with previous gestational diabetes mellitus. *J. Clin. Endocrinol. Metab.* 1998; 83: 1143–1150.

[28] Paradisi, G., Fulghesu, A.M., Ferrazzani, S. et al. (1998) Endocrino-metabolic features in women with polycystic ovary syndrome during pregnancy. *Hum. Reprod.* 1998;. 13: 542–546.

[29] Yamamoto M, Feigenbaum SL,Crites Y, Escobar G.J , Ferrara A,. Lo J.C. Preterm delivery in pregnant women with polycystic ovarian syndrome (PCOS). Fertil. Steril. 2010 :94(4):S 197.

[30] Landon MB,Spong CY,Thom E,Carpenter MW,Ramin SM et al.A multicenter randomized trial of treatment for mild gestational diabetes. *N. Engl. J. Med.* 2009 Oct 1;361(14):1339-48.

[31] Alshammari A,Hanley NiA,Tomlinson G,Feiq DS Does the presence of polycystic ovary syndrome increase the risk of obstetrical complications in women with gestational diabetes? *J. Matern. Fetal Neonatal. Med.* 2009; [Epub ahead of print]

[32] Tehrani M , Parvizi M1, Moghadan A, , Heshmat R1, nejad-Khas S.,Golchin M1 The prevalence of polycystic ovary syndrome in Iranian women withgestational diabetes: a pilot study. *Iranian Journal of Diabetes and Lipid Disorders*; 2009; 57-64.

[33] Altieri P, Gambineri A,Prontera O,Cionci G,Franchina M,Pasquali R.Maternal polycystic ovary syndrome may be associated with adverse pregnancy outcomes. *Eur. J. Obstet. Gynecol. Reprod. Biol.* 2010; [Epub ahead of print].

[34] Sibai BM,Ross MG. Hypertension in gestational diabetes mellitus: Pathophysiology and long-term consequences. *J. Matern.Fetal Neonatal. Med.* 2010 [Epub ahead of print].

[35] Begum MR,Khanam NN,Quadir E,Ferdous J,Begum MS, Begum A. Prevention of gestational diabetes mellitus by continuing metformin therapy throughout pregnancy in women with polycystic ovary syndrome. *J. Obstet. Gynaecol. Res.* 2009; 35(2): 282-6.

[36] Toulis KA, Goulis DG, Kolibianakis EM, Venetis CA, Tarlatzis BC, Papadimas I.Risk of gestational diabetes mellitus in women with polycystic ovary syndrome: a systematic review and a meta-analysis. *Fertil. Steril.* 2009 ;92(2):667-77.

[37] Thomann R, Rossinelli N, Keller U, Tirri BF, De Geyter C, Ruiz J, Kränzlin M, Puder JJ.Differences in low-grade chronic inflammation and insulin resistance in women with previous gestational diabetes mellitus and women with polycystic ovary syndrome. *Gynecol. Endocrinol.* 2008 ; 24(4):199-206.

[38] Hudecova M, Holte J, Olovsson M, Sundström Poromaa I.Long-term follow-up of patients with polycystic ovary syndrome: reproductive outcome and ovarian reserve. *Hum. Reprod.* 2009 ;24(5): 1176-83.

[39] Stroh C, Hohmann U, Lehnert H, Manger T. PCO syndrome--is it an indication for bariatric surgery? *Article in German Zentralbl Chir.* 2008 ;133(6):608-10.

Dermatologic Aspects

Hyperandrogenism in women can be caused by various conditions, the most prevalent of which is polycystic ovary syndrome. PCOS affects 5-10% of reproductive-aged women and is one of the most common female endocrine disorders.Women with PCOS show a range of signs and symptoms,and face increased risks of reproductive,metabolic, psychologic, cardiovascular and neoplastic sequelae, particularly if the condition is left unrecognized or untreated. The clinical definition of PCOS has changed in recent years and includes as one of its cardinal criteria the dermatologic manifestations of hyperandrogenism, chiefly hirsutism , acne and androgenetic alopecia.Acanthosis nigricans, a cutaneous sign of hyperinsulinemia, may also be present.[1] These dermatologic features may provide early clinical clues to recognition of PCOS, and treatment of these cutaneous conditions may improve the patient's quality of life restoring the psychological well-being.The effects of androgen on pilosebaceous unit in the skin can vary by anatomic location, producing pathophysiologic effects on hair growth and differentiation, sebaceous gland size and activity, and follicular keratinization. A recent study pointed out as total testosterone was not significantly different among patients with hirsutism, alopecia, or acne, and did not significantly correlate with hirsutism score. Hirsutism as oligo-amenorrhea is one of the most sensitive symptoms of hyperandrogenism, and no androgenic parameter alone may consent to identify all cases of hyperandrogenism [2] In conclusion, acne and androgenic alopecia seem to be not good markers for the hyperandrogenism in PCOS.While, hirsutism appears to be strongly related with hyperandrogenism and metabolic abnormalities in PCOS women[3].Treatments for the dermatologic conditions of hyperandrogenism include lifestyle modification, oral contraceptives, antiandrogens, insulin-sensitizing medications as well as non-hormonal therapies directed toward specific dermatologic conditions [4].

Acne

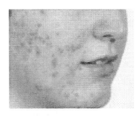

Acne vulgaris is the most common skin disorders affecting more than 40 million people in the United States ,more than half of whom are women older than 25 years of age [5,6,7]. It is characterized by noninflammatory follicular papules or comedones and by inflammatory papules , pustules, and nodules in its more severe forms. Acne lesions are commonly located on the face, neck, chest, upper back, and upper arms..Although severe acne is inflammatory, acne can also manifest in noninflammatory forms. This disorder occurs most commonly during adolescence, affecting more than 89% of teenagers,and frequently continues into adulthood .For most people, acne diminishes over time and tends to disappear,or decrease, after one reaches one's early twenties. There is,however, no way to predict how long it will take to disappear entirely,and some individuals will carry this condition well into their thirties, forties and beyond [8,9]. The multifactorial pathogenesis of acne results still not fully known but it is believed to be related in part to the interaction of sebaceous hyperplasia, follicular hyperkeratinization, proliferation of Propioni-bacterium acnes, inflammation and immune reaction [10,11,12,13] . Large individual variations in the response to normal or elevated androgens suggests considerable differences in local androgen metabolism and androgen receptor-mediated activities,which may partly be related to genetic disposition.Some studies have shown the importance of genetic factors in the pathogenesis of acne but the role of heredity on acne severity and response to treatment remains unclear [14].

While,the role of androgens is well established and their action is mediated by the androgen receptors. The amino-terminal domain of the receptor, is required for transcriptional activation and contains a region of polyglutamine encoded by CAG trinucleotide repeats. In humans, the number of CAG repeats is polymorphic.[15,16].Recently. some studies have shown an association between this polymorphism and acne together with other androgens influence diseases, such as androgenetic alopecia. Other genetic studies have shown a relationship between polymorphisms in the Human cytochrome P-450 1A1 gene (CYP1A1) and acne. The cytochrome P-450 1A1 is one of the most active enzymes involved in retinoids metabolism. Retinoids are morphogenic for the sebaceous gland. In a recent study it has been signalled in acne patients a high frequency of the thymine-to-cytosine (T-to-C) transition situated at position 6235 creating an additional cleavage site for MspI. In order to improve the treatment of patients, prognostic factors of acne severity and evolution must be studied.

Systematic assessment of the severity of acne continues to challenge the clinician. Acne is a pleomorphic disorder of variable course and anatomical distribution. Hormonal etiology can be very distinctly visible in the steroid androgenic premenstrual,menopausal acne as well as in juvenile acne and acne neonatorum[17].Most of acnes may be related to an idiopathic skin hyperandrogenism due to in situ enzyme activity and androgen receptor hypersensitivity as also noted in idiopathic hirsutism. The presence of acne in women may lead to a diagnosis of functional hyperandrogenism , either polycystic ovarian syndrome or non-classical 21-

hydroxylase deficiency. Plasma level assays for testosterone, delta 4 androstenedione and 17 OH progesterone and ovarian echography are necessary to determine the possibility for an ovarian or adrenal hyperandrogenism [18]. Women suffering from acne scarring may have psychological consequences, such as reduced self-esteem and, according to several studies , depression and in some cases suicide. Acne usually appears during adolescence, when people already tend to be most socially insecure. Early and aggressive treatment is therefore advocated by some to lessen the overall impact to individuals [19]. Oral contraceptives , particularly those containing chlormadinone acetate or drospirenone, have proven useful for the treatment of androgen disorders of the skin [20,21]. The mechanisms of action by which oral contraceptives correct skin androgen levels include inhibition of 5 alpha-reductase and androgen receptor activity. Along with this, treatment with low dose spironolactone can have anti-androgenetic properties, especially in patients with polycystic ovarian syndrome. If a pimple is large and/or does not seem to be affected by other treatments, a dermatologist may administer an injection of cortisone directly into it, which will usually reduce redness and inflammation almost immediately.Other available treatments are: topical bactericidals (benzoyl peroxide cream, triclosan,chlorhexidine gluconate, azeleic acid) ; topical (erythromycin , clindamycin,tetracycline) and oral antibiotics (erythromycin or tetracycline antibiotics);topical and oral(isotretinoin) retinoids;microdermabrasion, phototherapy, lasertherapy. A combination of treatments can greatly reduce the amount and severity of acne in many cases. Those treatments that are most effective tend to have greater potential for side effects and need a greater degree of monitoring, so a step-wise approach is often taken. Particularly, however, isotretinoin over a period of 4-6 months can induce long-term resolution of acne ,it can also induce liver damage and increase of triglycerides .In addition,this drug also causes birth defects if women become pregnant while taking it or take it while pregnant. For this reason, female patients are required to use effective method of birth control or abstinence, while on the drug. A vaccine against inflammatory acne has been tested successfully in mice, but it is not certain that it would work similarly in humans [22,23].There are a number of treatments that have been proven effective on acne but the: first is the hygiene. In fact, proper washing and skin care can help to remove bacteria and oils which cause acne.

References

[1] Essah PA, Wickham EP 3rd, Nunley JR, Nestler JE .Dermatology of androgen-related disorders Clin Dermatol. 2006 ;24(4):289-98. 5.George George R,Clarke S,Thiboutot D.Hormonal therapy for acne. *Semin. Cutan. Med. Surg.* 2008;27(3): 188-196.

[2] Karrer-Voegeli S, Rey F, Reymond MJ, Meuwly JY, Gaillard RC, Gomez F. Androgen dependence of hirsutism, acne, and alopecia in women: retrospective analysis of 228 patients investigated for hyperandrogenism. *Medicine (Baltimore).* 2009 ;88(1):32-45.

[3] Ozdemir S, Ozdemir M, Görkemli H, Kiyici A, Bodur S. Specific dermatologic features of the polycystic ovary syndrome and its association with biochemical markers of the metabolic syndrome and hyperandrogenism. *Acta Obstet. Gynecol. Scand.* 2009; 10. [Epub ahead of print].

Polycystic Ovarian Syndrome: Symptoms and Clinical Manifestations   147

[4]   Lee AT,Zane LT. Dermatologic manifestations of polycystic ovary syndrome. *Am. J. Clin. Dermatol.* 2007;8(4):201-19.

[5]   George R,Clarke S,Thiboutot D.Hormonal therapy for acne. *Semin. Cutan. Med. Surg.* 2008; 27(3):188-196.

[6]   White MG. Recent findings in the epidemiologic evidence, classification, and subtypes of acne vulgaris. *J. Am. Acad. Dermatol.* 1998; 39: S34-7.

[7]   Schafer T, Nienhaus A, Vieluf D, Berger J, Ring J. Epidemiology of acne in the general population: the risk of smoking. *Br. J. Dermatol.* 2001; 145: 100-4.

[8]   James WD "Clinical practice. Acne". *N. Engl. J. Med.* 2006; 352 (14): 1463–72.

[9]   Anderson, Laurence Looking Good, the Australian guide to skin care, cosmetic medicine and cosmetic surgery. AMPCo. Sydney. 2006.

[10] Holland KT, Aldana O, Bojar RA, Cunliffe WJ, Eady EA, Holland DB, Ingham E, McGeown C, Till A, Walters C. Propionibacterium acnes and acne. *Dermatology* 1998; 196: 67-8.

[11] Burkhart CG, Burkhart CN, Lehmann PF. Acne: a review of immunologic and microbiologic factors. *Postgrad. Med. J.* 1999; 75: 328-31.

[12] Olutunmbi Y,Paley K, English JC 3rd.Adolescent female acne: etiology and management. *J. Pediatr. Adolesc. Gynecol.* 2008;21(4):171-6.

[13] Ingham E, Walters CE, Eady EA, Cove JH, Kearney JN, Cunliffe WJ. Inflammation in acne vulgaris: failure of skin micro-organisms to modulate keratinocyte interleukin 1a production in vitro. *Dermatology* 1998; 196: 86-8.

[14] Oberemok SS, Salita AR. Acne vulgaris, I: pathogenesis and diagnosis. *Cutis* 2002; 70:101-5.

[15] Imperato-McGinley J, Gautier T, Cai LQ, Yee B, Epstein J, Pochi P. The androgen control of sebum production. Studies of subjects with dihydrotestosterone deficiency and complete androgen insensitivity. *J. Clin. Endocrinol. Metabol.* 1993; 76: 524-8.

[16] Thiboutot D, Gilliland K, Light J, Lookingbill D. Androgen metabolism in sebaceous glands from subjects with and without acne. *Arch. Dermatol.* 1999; 135: 1041-5.

[17] Bergler –Czop B,Brzezinska - Wcisto L. Hormonal factors in etiology of common acne. *Pol. Merkur. Lekarski* 2004;16(95):490-2 B.

[18] Faure M.Management of acne in adolescents.Arch.Pediatr.2007;14(9):1152-6 Faure M. Acne and hormones. *Rev. Prat.* 2002;52(8):850-3.

[19] Goodman G . "Acne and acne scarring - the case for active and early intervention". *Aust. Fam. Physician* 2006;35 (7): 503–4.

[20] Raudrant D, Rabe T.Progestogens with antiandrogenic properties. Drugs 2003;63:463-92.

[21] Sabatini R,,Orsini G,Cagiano R,Loverro G.Noncontraceptive benefits of two combined oral contraceptives with antiandrogenic properties among adolescents.Contraception 2007; 76:342-347.

[22] Kim J "Acne vaccines: therapeutic option for the treatment of acne vulgaris?". *The Journal of Investigative Dermatology* 2008; 128 (10): 2353–4.

[23] Farrar MD, Howson KM, Bojar RA, et al. (June 2007). "Genome sequence and analysis of a Propionibacterium acnes bacteriophage". *Journal of Bacteriology* 189 (11): 4161- 7

Hair Problems in PCOS-Women

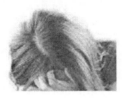

Androgenetic Alopecia

Female pattern hair loss (FPHL) is a clinical problem that is becoming more common in women [1]. Androgenetic alopecia is the term used to describe both male and female pattern baldness and is the most common cause of hair loss in women. It is estimated that it affects as many as 50% of men. The prevalence in women is reported to be up to 20% prior to menopause, while it increases to more than 40% after that, and, according to some, it may affect as many as 75% of women older than 65 years. Almost all subjects have some degree of androgenetic alopecia [2]. The hair loss usually begins between the ages of 12 and 40 years and is frequently insufficient to be noticed. However, visible hair loss occurs in approximately one half of all persons by the age of 50 years. In women, hairstyling may mask early hair loss [3]. It has been known that around 40% of women by age 50 show signs of hair loss and less than 45% of women actually reach the age of 80 with a full head of hair. Hair loss in women is most often very gradual, with the rate accelerating during pregnancy and at menopause. It is more often cyclical than in men, with seasonal changes that reverse themselves, and it is more easily affected by hormonal changes, medical conditions, and external factors. Hormone imbalance can also play an important role in the manifestation of androgenetic alopecia and as the cause for excessive hair loss. Women after menopause may have a net drop in the androgen antagonist estrogen and are much more susceptible to the onset of pattern baldness or female balding. Women who produce high levels of androgens as those who suffer from polycystic ovary syndrome result more susceptible to hair loss. Alopecia can be divided into disorders in which the hair follicle is normal but the cycling of hair growth is abnormal and disorders in which the hair follicle is damaged. In FPHL, there is diffuse thinning of hair on the scalp due to increased hair shedding or a reduction in hair volume, or both. It is normal to lose up to 50-100 hairs a day. Another condition called chronic telogen effluvium also presents with increased hair shedding and is often confused with FPHL. Hair growth occurs in three phases: one, the anagen, or active growth phase; two, the catagen, or transition phase; and three, the telogen, or dormant, resting phase. When dealing with pattern baldness, the anagen phase is obviously the most desirable of the three. Hair loss condition is characterized by progressive shortening of the anagen phase and prolongation of the telogen phase. As hair loss progresses, the follicle spends more and more time in the telogen phase, and less and less in the anagen phase. The hair thus becomes finer, as well as shorter and less pigmented. Eventually, it becomes much like the baby fine vellus hairs that are seen elsewhere on the body, and around the periphery of the scalp. This is often in evidence in area where most of the strong terminal hair has been lost; the bald area has soft, fine downy hair which provides essentially no coverage.Therefore, agents that may increase the anagen phase may be of benefit in pattern baldness, or androgenetic alopecia. It is important to differentiate between these conditions as management for both conditions differ. The diagnosis is usually based on a thorough history and a focused physical examination.

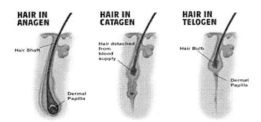

Telogen effluvium is diffuse hair loss caused by any condition or situation that shifts the normal distribution of follicles in anagen to a telogen-predominant distribution [4].Women with this disorder usually note an increased number of loose hairs on their hairbrush or shower floor. Daily loss may range from 100 to 300 hairs. If hair loss is at the lower end of the range, it may be inapparent. Telogen effluvium may unmask previously unrecognized androgenetic alopecia. In some patients, selected laboratory tests or punch biopsy may be necessary .As alopecia can be devastating for women, the management should include an assessment for psychologic effects [5,6].

Pathogenesis

There are a number of reasons to explain why hair loss in women presents differently than in men, although some factors are still not completely understood. The most important reason for difference in hair loss pattern is the difference in steroid metabolism; the metabolism of hormones, hormones which play an important role as the cause of hair loss both in women and men. The incidence is generally considered to be greater in males than females, although some evidence suggests that the apparent differences in incidence may be a reflection of different expression in males and females. This is an extremely common disorder that affects roughly 50% of men and perhaps as many women older than 40 years. As many as 13% of premenopausal women reportedly have some evidence of androgenetic alopecia. However, the incidence increases greatly in women following menopause.The incidence and the severity of androgenetic alopecia tend to be highest in white men, second highest in Asians and African Americans, and lowest in Native Americans and Eskimos. Almost all patients have an onset prior to age 40 years, although many of the patients, both male and female, show evidence of the disorder by age 30 years. This genetically determined disorder is progressive through the gradual conversion of terminal hairs into indeterminate hairs and finally to vellus hairs. Patients have a reduction in the terminal-to-vellus hair ratio, normally at least 2:1. Following miniaturization of the follicles, fibrous tracts remain. Patients with this disorder usually have a typical distribution of hair loss. The onset is gradual. Men present with gradual thinning in the temporal areas, producing a reshaping of the anterior part of the hairline For the most part, the evolution of baldness progresses according to the

Norwood/Hamilton classification of frontal and vertex thinning.Women usually present with diffuse thinning on the crown. Bitemporal recession does occur in women but usually to a lesser degree than in men. In general, women maintain a frontal hairline [7]. Androgenetic alopecia, or hair loss mediated by the presence of the androgen dihydrotestosterone, is the most common form of alopecia in men and women. The number and distribution of androgen receptors in the hair follicles, the enzymes 5 alpha reductase type I and II, and the local concentrations of dihyrotestosterone around hair follicles are the factors which are responsible for male androgenetic alopecia. It is presumed that in women there are additional factors which come into play such as the concentration of Cytochrome P-450-aromatase near hair follicles as well as the distribution of androgen receptor proteins. The cytochrome enzyme metabolizes androgens to estrogens, and modifies the ratio of androgens to estrogens by having a protective role by antagonizing the effects of androgens. Hair follicles contain androgen receptors. In the presence of androgens, genes that shorten the anagen phase are activated, and hair follicles shrink or become miniaturized. With successive anagen cycles, the follicles become smaller and nonpigmented vellus hairs replace pigmented terminal hairs. Differing concentrations of androgen metabolizing enzymes and androgen receptors have been identified in hair follicles from women compared to men.The concentration of Cytochrome P-450-aromatase is six times higher in women's frontal hair follicles compared to men's frontal hair follicles. Women also have around 3 times less alpha-5-reductase typeI or type II enzyme in their frontal hair follicles compared to men. Conversely, androgen receptor content in frontal hair follicles from men are 40% higher than for hair follicles from women. These differences between men and women most likely account for the overt clinical differences in patterns of hair loss [8]. In women, the thinning is diffuse, but more marked in the frontal and parietal regions. Even persons with severe androgenetic alopecia almost always have a thin fringe of hair frontally. Women with androgenetic alopecia do not have higher levels of circulating androgens. However, they have been found to have higher levels of 5α-reductase , more androgen receptors, and lower levels of cytochrome P450 [9] Most women with androgenetic alopecia have normal menses, normal fertility, and normal endocrine function, including gender-appropriate levels of circulating androgens. Therefore, an extensive hormonal work-up is unnecessary. The majority of women affected by FPHL do not underly to hormonal abnormalities. However a few women with FPHL are found to have excessive levels of androgens. These women tend also to suffer from acne, irregular menses and excessive facial and body hair. These symptoms are characteristic of PCOS although the majority of women with PCOS do not experience hair loss. Less often, congenital adrenal hyperplasia may be responsible. If a woman has irregular menses, abrupt hair loss, hirsutism,or acne recurrence, an endocrine evaluation is appropriate. In this situation, total testosterone, free testosterone, dehydroepiandrosterone sulfate, and prolactin levels should be obtained. Because the hair loss in androgenetic alopecia is an aberration of the normal hair cycle, it is theoretically reversible. Advanced androgenetic alopecia, however, may not respond to treatment. Women with androgenetic alopecia generally lose hair diffusely over the crown. This produces a gradual thinning of the hair rather than an area of marked baldness. The part is widest anteriorly. The frontal hairline is often preserved in women with this disorder, whereas men note a gradual recession of the frontal hairline early in the process. It is not uncommon to have accelerated phases of hair loss for 3-6 months, followed by periods of stability lasting 6-18 months.Without medication, it tends to progress in severity over the next few decades of life. This is essentially a cosmetic disorder; however, males with androgenetic alopecia seem to have an increased incidence of myocardial infarction [5].

Causes

Androgenetic alopecia is considered to be a dominantly inherited disorder with variable penetrance and expression. However, it may be of polygenic inheritance. In 2008, 95 families were studied genetically, and the locus with strongest evidence for linkage to androgenetic alopecia was the 3q26 site on the X chromosome.Androgen is necessary for progression of the disorder, as it is not found in males castrated prior to puberty. The progression of the disorder is stopped if postpubertal males are castrated. According to the American Academy of Dermatology, it's a growing problem, affecting some 30 million women in the United States with some forms of loss occurring at earlier ages, and being seen in increasing numbers.

Treatment

The preferred treatment is topical (Minoxidil 2%) because more effective. However, Minoxidil is not recommended for use in persons younger than 18 years Topical tretinoin (Retin-A) therapy as an adjunct to Minoxidil may be advised . In fertile women with androgenetic alopecia who require hormonal contraception, it is important to select a pill containing a progestin with antiandrogenic properties , such as norgestimate ,chlormadinone, drospirenone [10]. When hair loss is extensive, hair transplantation provides a more cosmetically effective outcome [11,12]

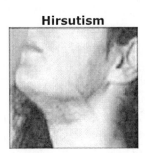

Hirsutism

Hirsutism affects 2 to 10% of women between the ages 18 to 45.[8]. It is defined as an excessive and increased hair growth in women, in locations where the occurrence of terminal hair normally is minimal or absent. Such male-pattern growth of terminal body, hair usually occurs in androgen-stimulated locations, such as the face, chest, and areolae.Hirsutism is often associated with other signs of androgen excess as acne, androgenetic alopecia, chronic anovulation and virilisation. Although the terms hirsutism and hypertrichosis often are used interchangeably, hypertrichosis actually refers to excess hair,terminal or vellus, in areas that are not predominantly androgen dependent.Hirsutism is often associated with measurably elevated androgen levels, but not in all cases Androgens in women arise from the ovary and adrenal glands, and peripherally from skin and fat. The most common cause of hirsutism is polycystic ovarian syndrome [13].Patients with "idiopathic" hirsutism have normal ovulatory cycles and androgen levels [14] .Whether a patient is hirsute often is difficult to judge because hair growth varies among individual women and across ethnic groups. What is considered hirsutism in one culture may be considered typical in another. Generally, women from the Mediterranean and the Indian subcontinent have more facial and body hair than do women from East Asia, sub-Saharan Africa, and northern Europe. Dark-haired, darkly pigmented individuals of either sex tend to be more hirsute than blond or fair-skinned persons. Hirsutism is a symptom rather than a disease and may be a sign of a more serious medical condition , especially if it develops well after puberty.It is usually an idiopathic condition, but some cases are explained by endocrine disturbances, including PCOS, the non-classic late-onset variant of congenital adrenal hyperplasia, hyperprolactinemia, and hormone-secreting adrenal or ovarian tumors. PCOS is numerically much the most important of these. In Unites States hirsutism is common and is estimated to occur in 1 in 20 women of reproductive age. Idiopathic hirsutism is common in certain groups, for example Euro-Asian people, and some degree of hirsutism is common in postmenopausal women, due to decrease in estrogen levels.Patients with hirsutism and insulin resistance are more likely to be obese and to have acanthosis nigricans as well.

Pathogenesis

The cause of hirsutism can be either an increased level of androgens or an oversensitivity of hair follicles to androgens. Androgens such as testosterone stimulate hair growth, increase size and intensify the pigmentation of hair. Central overproduction of androgen, increased peripheral conversion of androgen, decreased metabolism, and enhanced receptor binding are each potential causes of hirsutism. For circulating testosterone to exert its stimulatory effects on the hair follicle, it first must be converted into its more potent follicle-active metabolite, dihydrotestosterone. The enzyme, 5-alpha-reductase, which is found in the hair follicle, performs this conversion. Other symptoms may be associated with a high level of androgens as acne, irregular menstrual periods, deepening of the voice and increased muscle mass. Increased availability of free testosterone is linked to SHBG levels decrease in response to the exogenous androgens or in certain disorders that affect androgen levels, such as polycystic ovary syndrome. The amount of free testosterone,the biologically active androgen that, after conversion to dihydrotestosterone, causes hair growth is regulated by SHBG. Growing evidence implicates high circulating levels of insulin in women to the development of hirsutism. This theory is consistent with the observation that obese women , presumably insulin resistant and hyperinsulinemic, are at high risk of becoming hirsute. Further, treatments that lower insulin levels will lead to a reduction in hirsutism. It is speculated that insulin, at high enough concentration, stimulates the ovarian theca cells to produce androgens. Insulin resistance has been linked to hirsutism and occurs in 50% ot the women with PCOS. Patients with insulin resistance are more likely to be obese and to have acanthosis nigricans as well. The term HAIR-AN has been used to describe the combination of hyperandrogenism, insulin resistance, and acanthosis nigricans. Similarly, the acronym SAHA has applied to the combination of seborrhea, acne, hirsutism, and androgenetic alopecia. There may also be an effect of high levels of insulin to activate the insulin-like growth factor-I (IGF-1) receptor in those same cells. Again, the result is increased androgen production.

Classification

Hirsutism may occur in both congenital(rare familial disorders) and acquired forms, the latter being of importance as a manifestation of internal disease (paraneoplastic) . The following may be some of the conditions that may increase in women the normal level of androgens :

- Polycystic ovary syndrome
- Cushing's disease
- Tumours in the ovaries or adrenal gland
- Certain medications
- Congenital adrenal hyperplasia
- Insulin resistance
- Stromal Hyperthecosis - in postmenopausal women
- Obesity

PCOS is the more frequent cause of hirsutism. Virilization is minimal, and hirsutism is often prominent. Characteristic features include menstrual irregularities, dysmenorrhea, occasional glucose intolerance and hyperinsulinemia, and, often, obesity. The hyperinsulinemia is believed to hyperstimulate the ovaries to producing excess androgens. Women with PCOS may show other cutaneous manifestations of androgen excess in addition to hirsutism, such as recalcitrant acne, acanthosis nigricans, and alopecia on the crown area of the scalp . Hirsutism may also be seen in women with the following ovarian conditions, most of which are associated with virilization: luteoma of pregnancy ,arrhenoblastoma, Leydig cell tumors , hilar cell tumors, thecal cell tumor. More used method of evaluating hirsutism is the Ferriman-Gallwey score which gives a score based on the amount and location of hair growth on a woman. It involves grading 9 regions of the body on a scale of 0 to 4, depending on the extent of cover by terminal hair. The areas assessed include upper lip, chin, chest, upper lower back, upper-lower abdomen, upper arm and thighs.Maximum score is 36. Mild hirsutism is defined as a score 8 to 12, moderate 13 to 18, and severe >19. The scoring system is helpful in evaluating response to therapy[15].

Diagnosis

It is important to consider:

1) age at onset of hirsutism, familial history,past medical history ,drugs use
2) signs amd symptoms
3) physical examination

4) laboratory measurement of serum hormone levels (FSH, LH, free and total testosterone , androstenedione, DHEAS, TSH,prolactin).
5) Imaging: Pelvic ultrasonography, CT, or both should be done to rule out pelvic or adrenal cancer, particularly when a pelvic mass is appreciated, when the total testosterone level is > 200 ng/dL (> 100 ng/dL in postmenopausal women), or when the DHEAS level is > 7000 ng/dL (> 4000 ng/dL in postmenopausal women). However, the majority of patients with elevated DHEAS have adrenal hyperplasia rather than adrenal carcinoma.

Patients with signs of Cushing's syndrome or an adrenal mass on imaging studies should have 24-h urine cortisol levels measured. Pituitary, ovarian, and adrenal tumors are important, but rare causes of hirsutism, although history and examination are important. Laboratory investigation is essential in women with moderate to severe, sudden onset or rapidly progressing hirsutism. Identification of the underlying etiology does not alter management, but detects patients at risk for infertility, diabetes,cardiovascular disease and endometrial carcinoma [16].

Treatment

The disorder is treated considering the cause. Treatment for hirsutism itself is unnecessary if the patient does not find the excess hair cosmetically objectionable.However, this disorder is generally of cosmetic and psychological concern. Nonandrogen-dependent excess hair growth, such as hypertrichosis, is treated primarily with physical hair removal methods. Patients with androgen-dependent hirsutism require a combination of hair removal and medical antiandrogen therapy. Hirsutism resulting from androgen excess usually requires long-term therapy because the source of excess androgen rarely can be eliminated permanently. Hormonal treatments include:hormonal contraceptives containing progestins with antiandrogenic properties , antiandrogenic drugs as finasteride, flutamide,spironolactone; insulin sensitizers and triptorelin [17,18,19,20].

References

[1] Camacho-Martinez FM. Hair loss in women. *Semin. Cutan. Med. Surg.* 2009; 28 (1):19-32.
[2] Tosti A, Piraccini BM. Androgenetic alopecia. *Int. J. Dermatol.* 1999;38(suppl 1):1–7.
[3] Sperling LC, Mezebish DS. Hair diseases. *Med. Clin. North Am*. 1998;82:1155–69.
[4] Paus R, Cotsarelis G. The biology of hair follicles. *N. Engl. J. Med.* 1999;341:491–7.
[5] Cash TF, Price VH, Savin RC. Psychological effects of androgenetic alopecia on women: comparisons with balding men and with female control subjects. *J. Am. Acad. Dermatol.* 1993;29: 568–75.
[6] Girman CJ, Hartmaier S, Roberts J, Bergfeld W, Waldstreicher J. Patient-perceived importance of negative effects of androgenetic alopecia in women. *J. Womens Health Gend. Based Med.* 1999; 8:1091–5.

[7] Shapiro J, Wiseman M, Liu H. Practical management of hair loss. *Can. Fam. Physician.* 2000; 46: 1469–77.
[8] Neithardt AB, Barnes RB. The diagnosis and management of hirsutism. *Semin. Reprod. Med.* 2003; 21:285-93.
[9] Drake LA, Dinehart SM, Farmer ER, Goltz RW, Graham GF, Hordinsky MK, et al. Guidelines of care for androgenetic alopecia. American Academy of Dermatology. *J. Am. Acad. Dermatol.* 1996;35(3 pt 1):465–9.
[10] Yip L, Sinclair R. Antiandrogen therapy for androgenetic alopecia. *Expert Rev. Dermatol.* 2006; 1(2):261-9.
[11] Price VH. Treatment of hair loss. *N. Engl. J. Med.* 1999;341:964–73.
[12] Avram MR. Hair transplantation in women. *Semin. Cutan. Med. Surg.* 1999;18:172–6.
[13] Somani N, Harrison S, Bergfeld WF. The clinical evaluation of hirsutism. *Dermatol. Ther.* 2008; 21(5): 376- 91.
[14] Aziz R, Carmina E, Sawaya ME. Idiopathic hirsutism. *Endocr. Rev.* 2000; 21:347-62.
[15] Ferriman D, Gallwey JD. Clinical assessment of body hair growth in women. *J. Clin. Endocrinol. Metab.* 1961; 21:144.
[16] Legro RS, Kunselman AR, Dodson WC, Dunaif A. Prevalence and predictors of risk for type 2 diabetes mellitus and impaired glucose tolerance in polycystic ovary syndrome: a prospective, controlled study in 254 affected women. *J. Clin. Endocrinol. Metab.* 1999; 84:165-9.
[17] Azziz R. The evaluation and management of hirsutism. *Obstet .Gynecol.* 2003; 101:995-1007.
[18] Heiner JS, Greendale GA, Kawakami AK, Lapolt PS, Fisher M, Young D, et al. Comparison of a gonadotropin-releasing hormone agonist and a low dose oral contraceptive given alone or together in the treatment of hirsutism. *J. Clin. Endocrinol. Metab.* 1995; 80:3412-8.
[19] Bertoli A, Fusco A, Magnani A, Marini MA, Di Daniele N, Gatti S, et al. Efficacy of low-dose GnRH analogue (Buserelin) in the treatment of hirsutism. *Exp. Clin. Endocrinol. Diabetes* 1995; 103:15-20.
[20] Hunter MH, Carek PJ. Evaluation and treatment of women with hirsutism. *Am. Fam. Physician* 2003; 67:2565-72.

Acanthosis Nigricans

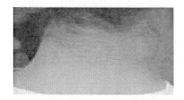

Acanthosis nigricans (AN) is a rare, poorly defined disorder characterized by abnormal hyperpigmentation and hyperkeratosis of the skin, mainly of skin fold regions, such as of the neck, groin, axillae and umbilicus. Involvement of other areas occurs as well. Acrochordons are commonly associated and predominantly affect the axillae, groins, submammary region, back and sides of the neck. The neck is involved 93% to 99% of the time [1,2]. The surface of the lesions may be warty, eathery or papillomatous.More subtle or otherwise atypical presentations are common in the medical experience and may be overlooked or misdiagnosed.Involvement of the scalp may have a tinea amiantacea appearance [3]. Involvement over joints appears quite common, including the elbow, knees and knuckles. Well-defined hyperkeratotic plaques may occur,even on the face and palms [4].Hyperinsulinemia, a consequence of insulin resistance that occurs associated with obesity, stimulates the formation of these characteristic plaques [5,6,7]. Nonetheless , AN is not a skin disease but a sign of an underlying condition or disease. It has a well established association with obesity [8,9] .

History of Acanthosis Nigricans

Addison observed a case of acanthosis nigricans (AN) before 1885 but misdiagnosed it as Addison disease. Hence, the first documented case was reported in 1889 in Germany by Paul Gerson Unna, who called acanthosis nigricans this disease.While, the first studies on this field were performed in 1890 and 1891 by Sigmund Pollitzer and Vítězslav Janovský [10].Later, Helene Ollendorff Curth classified AN as benign, malign and pseudoacanthosis introducing the concept of syndrome. In 1976, Kahn et al in Boston published their landmark study in which the association between acanthosis nigricans and insulin resistance was first described. Particularly Kahn, considering the clinical features of the observed cases, supported two unique clinical syndromes: Type A, a syndrome in younger females with signs of virilization or accelerated growth, in whom the receptor defect may be primary, and Type B, a syndrome in older females with signs of an immunologic disease, in whom circulating antibodies to the insulin receptor are found [11].In 2000, the American Diabetes Association established acanthosis nigricans as a formal risk factor for the development of diabetes in children.This condition may be inherited or may be associated with endocrine abnormality, obesity, use of drugs, or internal malignancy [12,13].

Epidemiology

AN tipically occurs in subjects younger than age 40; however, the hereditary subtype frequently affects children.Children with this condition are 1.6 to 4.2 times as likely as those without it to have hyperinsulinemia [14,15].When seen in individuals older than age 40, AN is commonly associated with an internal malignancy, usually adenocarcinoma, and most commonly of the gastrointestinal (GI) tract or uterus; less commonly of the lung, prostate, breast, or ovary. Acanthosis nigricans of the oral mucosa or tongue is highly suggestive of a neoplasm, especially of the GI tract[16]. It was estimated that only 2 of 12,000 patients with cancer have signs of AN. Approximately 61.3% of the cases are diagnosed simultaneously with cancer manifestation, while 17.6% of malignant AN cases predate the diagnosis of malignancy. The disease is much more common in people with darker pigmentation. Prevalence in white is 1 to 5.5%, but in African Americans is higher :13.3% [17].It is interesting to report that in native American population,a study showed 34.2% of Cherokee patients aged 5-40 years with AN with an increase of 73% of those patients with diabetes [14,18]. AN tends to affect males and females equally[19]. However, when considering that hyperandrogen insulin resistance acanthosis nigricans (HAIR-AN) subtype affects females, it must be recognized that obese females with high androgen levels are at an increased risk as compared to males [20] . The posterior neck of an unselected population of 1412 children of the public schools of Galveston, Texas, was examined . Acanthosis nigricans was present in 7.1% of the 1,412 children , with a definite correlation with certain races. The skin lesion was equally distributed between boys and girls and was most common among children with severe obesity. The condition was present in two of 440 white non-Hispanics, 19 of 343 Hispanics, and 80 of 601 blacks examined. The fasting plasma insulin concentrations measured in some of these children and in previously evaluated subjects, strongly correlated with the presence and severity of the acanthosis nigricans skin lesions [19] . Similar prevalence was found by Haffner et al considering the three ethnic groups: non-Hispanic whites 5.0%, Hispanics 5.5%, and African-Americans 13.3%, respectively [21] Another study on 481 obese women showed that of the 80.7% cases of AN, 66.9% of this group had white skin, whereas 86.1% and 90.6% of the patients had a mulatto and black skin type,respectively [22]. Native Americans also have been shown to have an increased risk, which correlates with their increased risk of diabetes [18].

Classification

There are two important types of acanthosis nigricans:

A. BENIGN ACANTHOSIS NIGRICANS

1) Hereditary benign acanthosis nigricans: runs in family, usually no malignancy associated.
2) Endocrinal acanthosis nigricans: Caused by Endocrine disturbances
3) Pseudo acanthosis nigricans: Associated with obesity
4) Drug - induced acanthosis nigricans: nicotinic acid , hormonal treatment, insulin, etc

B. MALIGNANT ACANTHOSIS NIGRICANS
- Associated with internal malignancy

Although classically described as a sign of internal malignancy, this is very rare. Benign types, sometimes described as "pseudoacanthosis nigricans "are much more common. Acanthosis nigricans may be also divided into the following types [13]:

- Acanthosis nigricans type I
- Acanthosis nigricans type II
- Acanthosis nigricans type III

Acanthosis nigricans associated with malignancy ,also known as "Acanthosis nigricans type I", is the malignant type of acanthosis nigricans that may either precede (18%), accompany (60%), or follow (22%) the onset of an internal cancer.[23]. Malignancy-associated acanthosis nigricans is usually rapid in onset and may be accompanied by skin tags, multiple seborrheic keratoses, or tripe palms [24]. Familial acanthosis nigricans,also known as "Acanthosis nigricans type II", is a rare type of acanthosis nigricans which is seen in birth or in early childhood. The clinical features tend to worsen during puberty. It has an autosomal dominant inheritance pattern and is not associated with any increase in cancer risk [23,24,7,25].Acanthosis nigricans associated with obesity, insulin-resistant states, and endocrinopathy ,also known as "Acanthosis nigricans type III" is the most common variety of acanthosis nigricans, presenting with a grayish, velvety thickening of the skin on the sides of the neck, axillae, and groins [23]. AN associated with endocrine dysfunction is more insidious in its onset,is less widespread, and the patients are often obese.Obesity is highly related, as is insulin resistance and diabetes mellitus. Flier et al stated that patients who present with AN should be worked up for diabetes mellitus, as most have either clinical or subclinical insulin resistance [26]. Also,Mukhtar et al showed that hyperinsulinemia and obesity are both independently positively correlated with AN. In a study on 675 middle school students from New Mexico,18.9% were found to have AN. The estimated hyperinsulinemia prevalence in this population was 8.9%, and 47% of the students with AN were obese and had increased insulin levels [15].The HAIR-AN type typically presents in a young girl with signs of increased androgen levels, clinically manifested by insulin resistance and pubic hair development before the age of 8 years old [27]. Based on the predisposing conditions, acanthosis nigricans has been divided into 7 types [28]:

- Obesity-associated acanthosis nigricans
- Syndromic acanthosis nigricans (hyperinsulinemia,Cushing's syndrome, PCOS, Lipodystrophy)
- Benign acanthosis nigricans or acral acanthotic anomaly
- Drug-induced acanthosis nigricans (insulin, nicotinic acid, systemic corticosteroids, hormonal treatments)
- Hereditary benign acanthosis nigricans (AN inherited as an autosomal dominant trait)
- Malignant acanthosis nigricans
- Mixed type acanthosis nigricans (when two or more types of AN are present in a patient)

Curth et al describes four main types with different etiologies and clinical presentations (29)

1. malignancy associated
2. hereditary
3. endocrinopathy associated
4. drug induced.

Some cases are idiopathic, with unknown cause. Brown et al showed that in 90 AN cases, 20 patients had endocrine disease, 17 had a malignancy, six had inherited causation, two had nicotinic-acid-induced AN, and the rest of the cases were idiopathic [30].The most prevalent form is idiopathic , but the most common form associated with a diagnosable condition is Type III, or endocrinopathy AN [31].Generalized AN does not represent a specific type, and it can be seen as a variant or rare manifestation of certain types of AN [32].

Pathogenesis

Studies of insulin receptors on circulating monocytes suggested that the insulin resistance in these patients was due to a marked decrease in insulin binding to its membrane receptors. When these patients were fasted, there was a fall in plasma insulin but no increase in insulin binding, suggesting that the receptor defect was not secondary to the hyperinsulinemia [11]. Acanthosis nigricans most likely is caused by factors that stimulate epidermal keratinocyte and dermal fibroblast proliferation. In the benign form of acanthosis nigricans, the factor is probably insulin or an insulin-like growth factor (IGF) that incites the epidermal to cell proliferation [7]. Other proposed mediators include tyrosine kinase receptors (epidermal growth factor receptor [EGFR] or fibroblast growth factor receptor [FGFR])[33]. At high concentrations, insulin may exert potent proliferative effects via high-affinity binding to IGF-1 receptors. In addition, free IGF-1 levels may be elevated in obese patients with hyperinsulinemia, leading to accelerated cell growth and differentiation [34,35]. However, more direct evidence for abnormal tyrosine kinase receptor signalling in AN has been provided by studies of craniosynostosis and skeletal dysplasia syndromes with AN, which have identified activating mutations in fibroblast growth factor receptors. Familial and syndromic forms of acanthosis nigricans have been identified [36]. Many syndromes share common features, including obesity, hyperinsulinemia, and craniosynostosis.These have been subdivided into insulin resistance syndromes and fibroblast growth factor defects. Insulin-resistance syndromes include those with mutations in the insulin receptors (leprechaunism, Rabson-Mendenhall syndrome), peroxisome proliferator-activated receptor gamma (as type1 diabetes with acanthosis nigricans and hypertension),1-acylglycerol-3-phosphate Oacyltransferase-2 orseipin(Berardinelli-Seip syndrome), lamin A/C (Dunnigan syndrome), and Alstrom syndrome gene [37]. Fibroblast growth factor defects include activating mutations in FGFR2 (Beare -Stevenson syndrome), FGFR3 (Crouzon syndrome with acanthosis nigricans, thanatophoric dysplasia , severe achondroplasia with developmental delay, and acanthosis nigricans [SADDAN])[38,39,40].Familial cases of acanthosis nigricans with no other syndromic findings have also been linked to FGFR mutations [36].Perspiration or friction may also play a contributory role, as suggested by the predilection of acanthosis nigricans for body folds. In malignant acanthosis nigricans, the stimulating factor is hypothesized to be a substance secreted either by the tumor or in response to the tumor. Transforming growth factor (TGF)-alpha is structurally similar to epidermal growth factor and is a likely candidate.TGF-alpha and epidermal growth factor have both been found in gastric adenocarcinoma cells, and EGFR expression has been identified in skin cells within acanthosis nigricans lesions. Reports of urine and serum TGF-alpha levels normalizing after surgical tumor removal exist,with subsequent regression of skin lesions[41]. Exogenous medications also have been implicated as etiologic factors, including insulin injections, likely due to activation of IGF receptors[42].It was reported as palifermin(recombinant keratinocyte growth factor used to decrease mucositis with chemotherapy and stem cell transplantation) may induces transient but dramatic acanthosis nigricans-like lesions, presumably due to activation of the FGFR [42,43,44].Of interest, ectopic acanthosis nigricans has been described in a syndromic patient who required skin grafting from the groin for syndactyly repair, with delayed acanthosis nigricans formation at the graft sites [45,29,30,31] .AN can also be associated with autoimmune diseases such as systemic lupus erythematous and scleroderma, often preceding the development of the disease. Long-term follow-up for all AN patients is recommended[46].

Histologic Findings

Histopathology reveals hyperkeratosis, papillomatosis, with minimal or no acanthosis or hyperpigmentation. The dermal papillae project upward as finger-like projections, with occasional thinning of the adjacent epidermis

Despite the term "Acanthosis",the amount of acanthosis,or thickening of the stratum spinosum,is generally mild [47]. Pseudohorn cysts may be present. Clinical dyschromia is secondary to the hyperkeratosis and not to increased melanocytes or increased melanin deposition. Dermal inflammatory infiltrate composed of lymphocites, plasma cells, or neutrophils may be present but is generally minimal or nonexistent. In conclusion, acanthosis is often not really present, so acanthosis nigricans is often a misnomer in many cases. Mucosal acanthosis nigricans reveals epithelial hyperkeratosis and papillomatosis along with parakeratosis. AN associated with hyperandrogenism is slightly different histologically. The papillary dermis contains glycosamino-glycans from hyaluronic acid, not found in other subtypes of AN [48].Acanthosis nigricans can occur with psoriasis, though the frequency of this combination is unknown.Lesions of psoriasis in patients with acanthosis nigricans may exhibit verrucous hyperkeratosis. Both conditions may occur separately or together in the same patient. Histologically, psoriasis and acanthosis nigricans are easily differentiated. by biopsy. In Acanthosis the epidermis is papillomatous (undulates) and pigmented ("nigricans"). The changes of acanthosis nigricans are manifest by a mammillated, acanthotic epidermis with orthohyperkeratosis ,and there is no significant inflammatory infiltrate Psoriasis is also characterized by epidermal thickening, but in contrast to acanthosis nigricans, this thickening occurs by elongation of the rete ridges and is associated with parakeratosis and with a superficial perivascular infiltrate.

Treatment

A doctor can diagnose acanthosis nigricans by doing a medical history and physical exam. There is no specific acanthosis nigricans treatment. In fact,because acanthosis nigricans itself usually only causes changes to the appearance of the skin, no particular treatment is needed. Treatment of the lesions of acanthosis nigricans is for cosmetic reasons only. In any case, it is very important to get checked for type 2 diabetes and other possible causes. The skin changes often get better with the improved diet and exercise that treat or help prevent diabetes. Fish oil supplements may also be recommended. Dermabrasion or laser therapy may help reduce the thickness of certain affected areas..Other treatments of acanthosis nigricans include the antibiotic creams,.retinoids., taken orally or used in a cream., topical corticosteroid creams. Other treatments to improve skin appearance, involving alpha hydroxy acid, and salicylic acid, may be helpful in some people. Sometimes, most effective treatment is obtained through weight loss and exercise. Eating a healthy diet can help reduce circulating insulin and can lead to improvement, and occassionally resolution, of the skin problem. Agents that improve insulin sensitivity present attractive candidates for the treatment of individuals with severe insulin resistance. Metformin has been shown to improve glycemia in patients with the type B syndrome or lipoatrophic diabetes but did not improve the insulin resistance in patients with myotonic dystrophy [49]. More recently, troglitazone, a thiazolidinedione that improves insulin sensitivity in NIDDM, was shown to improve insulin resistance in patients with Werner's syndrome and is currently being studied in individuals with other syndromes of severe insulin resistance, including the HAIR-AN syndrome [50]. Furthermore, administration of vanadate or vanadium salts to patients with NIDDM has led to improvement in glycemic profile and peripheral insulin resistance although the roles of these compounds in patients with severe insulin resistance remain unclear.[49,51]. Limited data suggest an improvement in insulin sensitivity in response to administration of phenytoin to patients with the type A syndrome [49]. Additionally, functional activation of a mutant IR, obtained from a patient with the Rabson-Mendenhall syndrome , by a monoclonal antibody in vitro led to improved IR autophosphorylation and glycogen synthesis in vitro, raising hopes that such therapy may benefit patients with severe insulin resistance [52]. Some studies suggested improvement in insulin sensitivity of patients with lipodystrophic diabetes in response to administration of bezafibrate or dietary supplementation with -3 fatty acid-rich fish oil, possibly by interfering with Randle's cycle Finally, immunosuppressants and plasmapheresis have been tried in some patients with the type B syndrome with beneficial results [48,53, 49, 54]

Conclusion

The cause for acanthosis nigricans is still not clearly defined but it appears caused by hyperinsulinemia, a consequence of insulin resistance that occurs associated with obesity .The association of acanthosis nigricans with hyperinsulinemia has led to consider a possible further association with type 2 diabetes. The natural history of acanthosis nigricans with respect to type 2 diabetes has not been determined, but evidence suggests the former may be a risk factor for the latter.[18,2,35] Type 2 diabetes mellitus has reached epidemic proportions in the United States, affecting 20.8 million people, or 7% of the population. [55] As the frequency and degree of obesity increase in the population, a concomitant increase in acanthosis nigricans can be expected. These patients have hyperinsulinemia and may be at greater risk of consequent atherosclerotic cardiovascular disease. It has long been observed that diabetes mellitus is associated with severe atherosclerotic cardiovascular disease. Tight control of blood glucose improves the microvascular components of diabetic vasculopathy but is relatively ineffective at controlling the atherosclerosis of large vessels, including coronary and carotid disease. It is speculated that hyperinsulinemia may be an important contributor to the atherosclerotic large vessel associated with diabetes mellitus. [2] It is essential for dermatologists to recognize all presentations of acanthosis nigricans to identify patients at risk for associated medical conditions. Since the subset of obese patients with acanthosis nigricans have hyperinsulinemia and may be at greater risk for atherosclerotic cardiovascular disease,the dermatologist has an important role in identifying the subset of obese patients with acanthosis nigricans. A readily apparent, rapidly identifiable physical examination marker identifying patients at increased risk for type 2 diabetes could stimulate discussions of lifestyle modifications in the primary care setting..

References

[1] Burke JP, Hale DE, Hazuda HP, Stern MP.A quantitative scale of acanthosis nigricans. *Diabetes Care*. 1999;22(10):1655-1659.

[2] Stuart CA, Gilkison CR, Smith MM, et al. Acanthosis nigricans as a risk factor for non-insulin dependent diabetes mellitus. *Clin. Pediatr*.1998;37(2):73-79.

[3] Azizi E, Trau H, Schewach-Millet M, Rosenberg V, Schneebaum S, Michalevicz R. Generalized malignant acanthosis nigricans. *Archives of Dermatology*, 1980, 116 (4): 381.

[4] Hazen PG, Carney JF, Walker AE, Stewart JJ. Acanthosis nigricans presenting as hyperkeratosis of the palms and soles. *J. Am. Acad. Dermatol.* 1979;1(6):541-4.

[5] Davidson MB. Clinical implications of insulin resistance syndromes. *Am. J. Med.* 1995;99(4):420-6.

[6] Moller DE, Flier JS. Insulin resistance--mechanisms, syndromes, and implications. *New England Journal of Medicine*, 1991 26, 325(13):938-48.

[7] Cruz PD Jr, Hud JA Jr. Excess insulin binding to insulin-like growth factor receptors: proposed mechanism for acanthosis nigricans. *Journal of Investigative Dermatology* 1992; 98(6 Suppl):82-5.

[8] Brickman WJ, Binns HJ, Jovanovic BD, Kolesky S, Mancini AJ, Metzger BE. Acanthosis nigricans: a common finding in overweight youth. *Pediatr. Dermatol.* 2007;24(6):601-6.

[9] Hud JA Jr, Cohen JB, Wagner JM, Cruz PD Jr. Prevalence and significance of acanthosis nigricans in an adult obese population. *Arch. Dermatol.* 1992; 128 (7): 941-4.

[10] Pollitzer S. In Unna PG,Morris M,Besner E et al. International Atlas of rare skin disorders. London HK Lewis and Co 1890;10:1-3.

Polycystic Ovarian Syndrome: Symptoms and Clinical Manifestations 163

[11] Kahn CR, Flier JS, Bar RS, Archer JA, Gorden P, Martin MM, Roth J. The syndromes of insulin resistance and acanthosis nigricans. Insulin-receptor disorders in man. *N. Engl. J. Med.* 1976 1;294 (14):739-45.

[12] Hurwitz S. Acanthosis nigricans. In: Hurwitz S,ed. Clinical Paediatric Dermatology,2nd ed Philadelphia: *WB Saunders*, 1993: 675-676.

[13] Levine N. Acanthosis nigricans. In: Schachner LA, Hansen RC, eds. Paediatric Dermatology, 1st ed. New York: Churchill Livingstone,1988: 1146-1150.

[14] Stoddart ML, Blevins KS, Lee ET, Wang W, Blackett PR. Association of acanthosis nigricans with hyperinsulinemia compared with other selected risk factors for type 2 diabetes in Cherokee Indians: theCherokee Diabetes Study. *Diabetes Care*. 2002;25(6): 1009-1014. 11.

[15] Mukhtar Q, Cleverley G, Voorhees RE, McGrath JW. Prevalence of acanthosis nigricans and its association with hyperinsulinemia inNew Mexico adolescents. *J. Adolesc. Health.* 2001;28(5):372-376.

[16] Schnopp C, Baumstark J.Oral acanthosis nigricans.N.Engl.J.Med.2007;357: 9-10. 17.Nguyen TT, Keil MF, Russell DL, et al. Relation of acanthosis nigricans to hyperinsulinemia and insulin sensitivity in overweight African American and white children. *J. Pediatr.* 2001;138 (4): 474-80.

[17] Stuart CA, Smith MM, Gilkison CR, Shaheb S, Stahn RM. Acanthosis Nigricans among Native Americans: an indicator of high diabetes risk. *Am. J. Public Health.* Nov 1994;84(11):1839-42.

[18] Stuart CA, Pate CJ, Peters EJ. Prevalence of acanthosis nigricans in an unselected population. *Am. J. Med.* 1989; 87 (3):269-72.

[19] Barbieri RL,Ryan KJ. Hyperandrogenism, insulin resistance,and acanthosis nigricans syndrome : a common endocrinopathy with distinct pathophisiologic features. *Am. J. Obstet. Gynecol.* 1983; 147:90-101.

[20] Haffner SM, D'Agostino R, Saad MF, Rewers M, Mykkänen L, Selby J, Howard G, Savage PJ, Hamman RF, Wagenknecht LE, et al.Increased insulin resistance and insulin secretion in nondiabetic African-Americans and Hispanics compared with non-Hispanic whites. The Insulin Resistance Atherosclerosis Study. *Diabetes*. 1996 ;45(6):742-8.

[21] Araujo LMB, Porto MV, Netto EM, Ursich MJ. Association of acanthosis nigricans with race and metabolic disturbances in obese women. *Braz. J. Med. Biol. Res.* 2002 Jan;35(1):59-64. \

[22] James W,Berger T, Elston D. Andrews' Diseases of the Skin: *Clinical Dermatology.* (10th ed.). Saunders (2005).

[23] Rapini, R P, Bolognia, Jorizzo, J. L. Dermatology 2007; Vol. 2 . St. Louis: Mosby. Rapini.

[24] Sinha S, Schwartz RA. Juvenile acanthosis nigricans. *J. Am. Acad. Dermatol.* 2007;57(3): 502-8.

[25] Flier JS. Metabolic importance of acanthosis nigricans. *Arch. Dermatol.* 1985 ;121 (2):193-4.

[26] Esperanza LE,Fenske NA.Hyperandrogenism, Insulin Resistance, and Acanthosis Nigricans (HAIR-AN) Syndrome: Spontaneous remission in a 15 year old girl. *J. Am. Acad. Dermatol.* 1996 ; 34(5 Pt 2):892-7.

[27] Schwartz RA.Acanthosis nigricans. *J. Am. Acad. Dermatol.* 1994; 311-19.

[28] Curth HO. Classification of acanthosis nigricans. *Int. J. Dermatol.* 1976 ;15(8):592-3.

[29] Brown J, Winkelmann RK. Acanthosis Nigricans: A study of 90 cases. *Medicine*. 1968; 47(1): 33-51.

[30] Robson KJ, Piette WW. Cutaneous manifestations of systemic disease. *Med. Clin. North Am.* 1998 ;82(6):1359-79.

[31] Blume-Peytavi U, Speiker T, Reupke H,Orfanos CE.Generalized Acanthosis nigricans with vitiligo. *Acta Derm.Venereol.* 1996; 76:377-380.

[32] Logié A,Dunois-Larde C,Rosty C.Activating mutations of the tyrosine kinase receptor FGFR3 are associated with benign skin tumors in mice and humans . *Hum. Mol. Genet.* 2005;14(9): 1153- 1160.

[33] Torley D, Bellus GA, Munro CS. Genes, growth factors and acanthosis nigricans. *Br. J. Dermatol.* 2002;147(6):1096-101.

[34] Burke JP, Duggirala R, Hale DE, Blangero J, Stern MP. Genetic basis of acanthosis nigricans in Mexican Americans and its association with phenotypes related to type 2 diabetes. *Hum. Genet.* 2000;106(5):467-72.

[35] Berk DR, Spector EB, Bayliss SJ. Familial acanthosis nigricans due to K650T FGFR3 mutation. *Arch. Dermatol.* 2007;143(9):1153-6.

[36] Musso C , Cochran E, Moran SA, et al. Clinical course of genetic diseases of the insulin receptor (type A and Rabson-Mendenhall syndromes): a 30-year prospective. *Medicine (Baltimore).* 2004; 83(4):209-22.

[37] Przylepa KA,Paznekas W,Zhang M,Golabi M,Bias w, Bamshad MJ et al. Fibroblast growth factor receptor mutations in Beare-Stevenson cutis gyrata syndrome. *Nat. Denet.* 1996;13:492-4.

[38] Wilkes D,Rutland P,Pulleyn LJ,Reardon W,Moss C,Ellis JP et al. A recurrent mutation,ala391 glu,in the transmembrane region of FGFR3 causes Crouzon syndrome and acanthosis nigricans. *J. Med.Genet.* 1996;33:744-8.

[39] Bellus GA,Bamshad MJ,Przylepa KA,Dorst J,Lee RR,Hurko O et al.Severe achondroplasia with developmental delay and acanthosis nigricans (SADDAN):phenotypic analysis of a new skeletal dysplasia caused by a Lys650Met mutation in fibroblast growth factor receptor 3. *Am. J. Med.Genet.* 1999; 85: 53-65.

[40] Krawczyk M, Mykala-Ciesla J, Kolodziej-Jaskula A. Acanthosis nigricans as a paraneoplastic syndrome. Case reports and review of literature. *Pol. Arch. Med. Wewn.* 2009; 119(3):180-3.

[41] Lane SW, Manoharan S, Mollee PN. Palifermin-induced acanthosis nigricans. *Intern. Med. J.* Jun 2007;37(6): 417-8.

[42] Geffner ME, Golde DW. Selective insulin action on the skin, ovary, and heart in insulin resistance states. *Diabetes Care.* 1988 Jun;11(6):500-5.

[43] Mailler-Savage EA, Adams BB. Exogenous insulin-derived Acanthosis nigricans. *Arch. Dermatol.* 2008; 144 (1):126-7.

[44] Wu JC, Cunningham BB. Ectopic acanthosis nigricans occurring in a child after syndactyly repair. *Cutis.* 2008 ; 81(1):22-4.

[45] Sturner RA, Denning S, Marchase P. Acanthosis nigricans and autoimmune reactivity. *JAMA.* 1981 Aug 14;246(7):763-5.

[46] Rogers DL.Acanthosis nigricans.Semin. *Dermatol.* 1991;10:160-3.

[47] Wortsman J, Matsuoka LY, Kupchella CE, Gavin Jr 3rd, Dietrich JG. Glycosaminoglycan deposition in the acanthosis nigricans lesions of the polycystic ovary syndrome. *Arch. Intern. Med.* 1983 ;143(6):1145-8.

Polycystic Ovarian Syndrome: Symptoms and Clinical Manifestations   165

[48] Mantzoros CS, Moses AC. Treatment of severe insulin resistance. In: Azziz R, Nestler JE, Dewailly D, eds. Androgen excess disorders in women, Philadelphia: Lippincott Raven; 1997; 247–255.

[49] Izumino K, Sakamaki H, Ishibashi M, et al. Troglitazone ameliorates insulin resistance in patients with Werner's syndrome. *J. Clin. Endocrinol. Metab*. 1997; 82:2391.

[50] Goldfine AB, Simonson DC, Folli F, Patti ME, Kahn CR. Metabolic effects of sodium metavanadate in humans with insulin-dependent and noninsulin-dependent diabetes mellitus: in vivo and in vitro studies. *J. Clin. Endocrinol. Metab*. 1995;80:3311–3320.

[51] Krook A, Soos M, Kumar S, Siddle K, O'Rahilly S. Functional activation of mutant human insulin receptor by monoclonal antibody. *Lancet*. 1996;347:1586–1590.

[52] Panz VR, Wing JR, Raal FJ, Kedda MA, Joffe BI. Improved glucose tolerance after effective lipid-lowering therapy with bezafibrate in a patient with lipoatrophic diabetes mellitus: a putative role for Randle's cycle in its pathogenesis? *Clin. Endocrinol.* (Oxf). 1997; 46:365–368.

[53] Mantzoros CS, Flier JS. Insulin resistance: the clinical spectrum. In: Mazzaferi E, ed. Advances in endocrinology and metabolism. St. Louis: Mosby-Year Book; 1995 ; vol 6:193–232.

PCOS and Depression

Polycystic ovary syndrome,the leading cause of anovulatory infertility that affects up to 20% of the reproductive age-women, is a complex disorder of genetic and environmental determination but still unknown origin. Besides of infertility, PCOS women may complain of menstrual disturbances, obesity symptoms, acne and hirsutism that are well known causes of psychological distress [1,2]. Therefore, PCOS women show a significant increase of psychological disturbances and decrease of sexual satisfaction when compared with healthy controls. Depression is a prominent characteristic of women who have polycystic ovary syndrome.

Causes of Depression in PCOS Women

Part of the depression stems from the emotional difficulty of being infertile, overweight, too hairy, or having acne, hair loss or some other disturbing symptoms. However, the primary cause of depression in PCOS appears to be hormonal in nature.A number of studies have shown a connection between a negative mood and elevated androgens such as testosterone.In one interesting study,there was a correlation between the most intense depression and testosterone levels slightly above normal, but not when testosterone was low or extremely high [3].Of course, depression is not limited to elevated testosterone. Depression has also been associated with insulin resistance and depressed thyroid function. Disturbed LH levels and rhythms have been found in depressed women compared to women who are not depressed [4].Abnormal estrogen and cortisol are additional hormonal factors connected to depression. Furthermore,it seems that women with mixed anxiety-depression disorder have high levels of homocysteine in the follicular and luteal phase , and they have higher blood homocysteine levels as compared to healthy women. Women with PCOS commonly have elevated homocysteine levels. Normally, homocysteine is broken down and made harmless. However, a poor diet that is deficient in calcium and B vitamins, and drugs such as metformin can help to elevate homocysteine [5,6]. All of the above factors for depression are common in PCOS women. Many women with PCOS often experience depression, anxiety and other mood-related disorders. A question that often arises is whether depression and anxiety are a result of having the symptoms of PCOS or whether they are caused by the hormone imbalance related to PCOS. A study conducted at the University of Chicago Hospital Department of Medicine linked slightly elevated free testosterone (FT) levels with increased rates of mood-related disorders. The study looked at 27 women with PCOS and elevated FT levels and 27 women without PCOS and normal ranges of FT levels.The results of the study show that women with slightly elevated levels of FT were more likely to be depressed than women with normal or very elevated levels of FT. This is a rather interesting finding because it showed how FT can have a negative effect on mood at slightly elevated levels but not have much of an effect at extremely elevated levels. One thought was that women with extremely elevated levels of FT become accustomed to the high levels and their bodies adjust accordingly [7,8]. Although more research is needed to determine the exact causes of this link, there are studies that link depression to diabetes. Therefore, in PCOS, depression may be related to Insulin Resistance. It also could be a result of the hormonal imbalances and the cosmetic symptoms of the condition, such as acne, hair loss and other symptoms of PCOS. Women with diabetes, who have twice the risk of developing depression, showed improvement in depressive instances when they received education and treatment for Insulin Resistance. Patients with depression and other affective disorders should be regularly screened for Insulin Resistance. While, there has been a tendency in the medical community to view depression only as a mental illness, there is growing evidence that the imbalance of glucose and insulin in the blood stream plays a far more serious role than previously thought. Current knowledge advises physicians to be aware that depression may be a symptom of the hormone imbalance found in women with PCOS [9]. Treatments aimed at treating the cause of PCOS and balancing hormone levels may help many women relieve their depression and anxiety along with other symptoms of PCOS, which can range from infertility and excess facial hair to skin conditions, like acne and brown patches and male pattern baldness. Studies have shown that a multifaceted approach is necessary to address the symptoms .The treatment may be based on a single pharmaceutical or even a combination of them, which will not eradicate or reverse these conditions.It is bad enough for women to suffer with the pain,but for women who have baldness, excessive hair growth or acne it can become devastating. Many women become depressed and self conscious because of their looks [9]. A lot of women will have anxiety attacks when they have to go out in public.They prefer to stay at home most of the time because of the fear of ridicule and rejection.Their depression and anxiety only gets worse and some may even have suicidal thoughts.In the meantime, it seems that overweight / obesity and hirsutism, but not the presence of acne, may significantly impair the quality of life. Indeed, PCOS features regarding the physical aspect more than others can lead to psychological problems [7,9,10,11].Body image is strongly associated with depression,even after controlling body mass. Particularly,it was evaluated that body dissatisfaction and education may explain 66% of the variance in depression among PCOS women [12]. The majority of patients with PCOS exhibit subclinical levels of psychological disturbances; however, psychiatric disease may be undetected in a proportion of these women. In any case, emotional distress together with obesity lead to large decrease in quality of life in PCOS [13] .In the former time, little attention has focused on psychological correlates of this frequent disorder but now is clear that PCOS is associated with several mental health problems: including depression and anxiety, body dissatisfaction,eating disorders,reduced sexual satisfaction and lowered health-related quality of life [14]. Women with PCOS seem to be at risk for depressive disorders compared with controls.The overall risk of depressive disorders in women with PCOS is 4.23, independent of obesity and infertility. Compared with the nondepressed PCOS women,the depressed PCOS women have a higher body mass index and evidence of insulin resistance [15]. Unexpectedly,several investigations have showed that women with unfulfilled desire to conceive compared with women without wish for a child reveal no impact on mood ,quality of life and emotional status. Therefore, reduced sexual satisfaction and self-worth could be induced by partnership status and not by infertility [16]. Objective phenotypic severity of hyperandrogenic symptoms seems to increase the risk of eating disorders and obesity seems to be the most prevalent cause of mental distress; whereas,other features such as hirsutism and infertility are less well defined as major factors .However, in PCOS women with facial hirsutism, an important prevalence of psychological problems was reported (36.3%)[10].Clinicians treating women with PCOS should be aware that these women are at high risk for affective and anxiety disorders as well as suicide attempts. In fact,suicide attempts are seven times more common in the PCOS women than in the controls [15,16]. In conclusion,women with PCOS have higher lifetime incidence of depressive episodes,social phobia and eating disorders than women without PCOS Women with PCOS need to remember to take care of their mental health too.The increased health risks (diabetes, endometrial cancer, cardiac issues) in addition to embarrassing physical symptoms make it easy to become overwhelmed, lonely and depressed. Several trials have found that women with PCOS and/or infertility are often more likely to suffer from depression and anxiety. The experience over the years with women who have PCOS is that many suffer from anxiety and depression and more than half of PCOS sufferers were affected by at least one mental health disorder. Forty percent battled depression, 15 percent struggled with panic disorders, and binge-eating disorder was a problem for 23 percent.[17]. The number and severity of mood disorders seems to increase over time. Researchers recommended that doctors aggressively pursue diagnosis and treatment for acne and weight issues as it has been found that the hirsutism, acne and weight excess associated with PCOS contribute to emotional problems. In fact,, these physical symptoms can increase depression and social anxiety. It may be hypothesized that many women also suffer from depression due to the fatigue, infertility issues and frustration that come along with PCOS. Worsened quality of life, anxiety and depression in young women with PCOS is related to BMI. Risk perception is appropriately high in PCOS, yet perceived risks of future metabolic complications are less common than those related to weight gain and infertility [18]. A better understanding of the symptoms is needed to identify and alleviate anxiety symptoms in this vulnerable group [19].

References

[1] Eggers S,Kirchengast S.The polycystic ovary syndrome-a medical condition but also an important psychosocial problem. *Coll. Antropol*. 2001;25(2): 673- 85.

[2] Bishop SC,Basch S,Futterweit W. Polycystic ovary syndrome,depression,and affective disorders. *Endocr. Pract*. 2009;15(5): 475-82.

[3] Weiner CL, Primeau M, Ehrmann DA.Androgens and mood dysfunction in women: comparison of women with polycystic ovarian syndrome to healthy controls. *Psychosom. Med*. 2004 ;66(3):356-62.

[4] Grambsch P,Young EA, Meller WH Pulsatile luteinizing hormone disruption in depression. *Psychoneuroendocrinology* 2004 Aug;29(7):825-9.

[5] Rasgon NL, Rao RC, Hwang S, Altshuler LL,Elman S, Zuckerbrow-Miller J, Stanley G. Korenmanet SG. Depression in women with polycystic ovary syndrome: clinical and biochemical correlates, *J. Affect Disord*. 2003 May;74(3):299-304.

[6] Tallova J.Tomandl J Bicikova M , Hill M, Changes of plasma total homocysteine levels during the menstrual cycle, in depressive women. *Eur. Clin. Invest*. 1999; 33(3): 268-72.

[7] Hahn S,Janssen OE,Tan S,Pleger K,Schedlowski M,Kimmig R,Benson S,Balamitsa E,Elsenbruch S.Clinical and psychological correlates of quality of life in polycystic ovary syndrome. *Eur. J. Endocrinol*. 2005;153(6): 853-60.

[8] Benson S,Hahn S,Tan S,Mann K,Janssen OE,Schedlowski M,Elsenbruch S.Prevalence and implications of anxiety in polycystic ovary syndrome:results of an internet-based survey in Germany. *Hum. Reprod*. 2009;24(6): 1446-51.

[9] Himelein MJ, Thatcher SS. Depression and body image among women with polycystic ovary syndrome. *J. Health Psychol*. 2006;11(4): 613-25.

[10] Elsenbruch S,Benson S,Hahn S,Tan S,Mann K,Pleger K, Kimming R,Janssen OE. Determinants of emotional distress in women with polycystic ovary syndrome. *Hum. Reprod*. 2006;21(4): 1092-9.

[11] Himelein MJ,Thatcher SS. Polycystic ovary syndrome and mental health: a review. *Obstet. Gynecol, Surv*. 2006;61(11):723-32.

[12] Hollinrake E,Abreu A,Maifeld M,Van Voorhis BJ,Dokras A. Increased risk of depressive disorders in women with polycystic ovary syndrome. *Fertil. Steril*. 2007; 87(6): 1369-76.

[13] Tan SH, Hahn S, Benson S,Janssen OE,Dietz T,Kimmig R,Hesse-Hussain J,Mann K, Schedlowski M,Arck PC,Elsenbruch S. Psychological implications of infertility in women with polycystic ovary syndrome. *Hum. Reprod*. 2008; 23(9): 2064-71.

[14] Morgan J,Scholtz S,Lacey H,Conway G.The prevalence of eating disorders in women with facial hirsutism: an epidemiological cohort study. *Int. J. Eat. Disord*. 2008;41(5):427-31.

[15] Hollinrake E,Abreu A,Maifeld M, Van Voorhis BJ, Dokras A. Increased risk of depressive disorders in women with polycystic ovary syndrome. *Fertil. Steril*. 2007;87(6):1369-76.

[16] Mansson M,Holte J,Landin-Wilhelmsen K,Dahlgren E,Johansson A,Landen M.Women with polycystic ovary syndrome are often depressed or anxious: a case control study. Psychoneuroendocrinology 2008;33(8):1132-8.

[17] Kerchner A,Lester W,Stuart SP,Dokras A.Risk of depression and other mental health disorders in women with polycystic ovary syndrome: a longitudinal study. *Fertil. Steril.* 2009;91(1):207-12.

[18] Moran L, Gibson-Helm M,Teede H, Deeks A. Polycystic ovary syndrome: a biopsychosocial understanding in young women to improve knowledge and treatment options. *J. Psychosom. Obstet. Gynaecol.* 2010; [Epub ahead of print].

[19] Jedel E, M. Waern M, D. Gustafson D, Landén M.,Eriksson E,Holm G., Nilsson L., Lind A.K., Janson P.O , Stener-Victorin E.Anxiety and depression symptoms in women with polycystic ovary syndrome compared with controls matched for body mass index. *Human Reproduction* 2010 25(2):450-456.

Impaired Glucose Tolerance and type 2 Diabetes in PCOS women

Polycystic ovary syndrome is associated with hyperinsulinemia, insulin resistance (IR), increased risk of glucose intolerance, and type 2 diabetes [1]. Not surprising, women with PCOS are more likely to develop gestational diabetes [2]. Ovarian effects of increased insulin are described in women with diabetes mellitus, obesity, syndromes of extreme insulin resistance and PCOS [3]. Insulin resistance (IR), defined as a diminished effect of a given dose of insulin on glucose homeostasis, is a highly prevalent feature of women with PCOS. IR is closely associated with an increase in truncal-abdominal fat mass, elevated free fatty acid levels, increased androgens, particularly free testosterone through reduced SHBG levels, and anovulation.In addition,in women with PCOS and severe insulin resistance, insulin sensitivity appears to be the major determinant of adiponectin levels rather than adiposity. Low adiponectin levels may predict women with PCOS who are at high risk for developing type 2 diabetes [4].Adiponectin is an adipocytokine with insulin-sensitizing and suggested antiatherosclerotic properties. PCOS per se is not associated with decreased levels of plasma adiponectin. However, circulating adiponectin is independently associated with the degree of IR in PCOS women and, may contribute to the development and/or maintenance of insulin resistance, independent from adiposity [5].Lower adiponectin levels were observed more in PCOS group than in control women, and these differences were probably due to higher prevalence of IGT in these cases [6].In the insulin-resistant patients with normal glucose tolerance, most of the hyperinsulinaemia is probably due to secondarily increased insulin secretion and decreased insulin degradation.However,a component of the increased first-phase insulin release is not due to measurable insulin resistance. Notably, this is also found in lean women with normal insulin sensitivity, and is not reversed after weight reduction, in contrast to the findings for insulin resistance. Obese women with PCOS are more insulin resistant than non-obese controls, suggesting that obesity and PCOS exert independent effects on insulin resistance. Weight loss restores insulin sensitivity only in some, and insulin resistance is described also in nonobese PCOS subjects[7,8].IR in PCOS is more prominent in anovulatory women than equally hyperandrogenemic women with regular menses [8,9].Therefore, it seems that only those with the endocrine syndrome of hyperandrogenism and chronic anovulation appear to be insulin resistant and at high risk for glucose intolerance[8,10,11]. Ovulatory women with the polycystic ovary morphology seem to be not insulin resistant[8] Besides insulin-resistance, some of these women also have alterations in beta-cell function [12,13,14].Resistance to insulin-stimulated glucose uptake is present in the majority of patients with impaired glucose tolerance(IGT) or non-insulin-dependent diabetes mellitus (NIDDM) and in approximately 25% of nonobese individuals with normal oral glucose tolerance. In these conditions,deterioration of glucose tolerance can only be prevented if the beta-cell is able to increase its insulin secretion and maintain a state of chronic hyperinsulinemia .Insulin resistance and β-cell dysfunction are both known to precede the development of glucose intolerance and type 2 DM [15].Thus, PCOS women would be predicted to be at an increased risk for type 2 DM. Dunaif et al.have originally reported that up to 40% of obese PCOS women had impaired glucose tolerance or frank type 2 DM, when the WHO criteria are used.[10]. These prevalence rates are substantially higher than those found in a major population-based studies in women of similar age (10 %)[16]. Both disorders, insulin resistance and beta-cell-dysfunction, are recognized as major risk factors for the development of type 2 diabetes [12,13,14,15,16]. Long-term studies, evaluating the glucose-insulin system in women affected by PCOS, have shown a higher incidence of glucose intolerance, including both impaired glucose tolerance and type 2 diabetes, compared to age and weight matched control populations. The risk of glucose intolerance among PCOS subjects seems to be approximately 5 to 10 fold higher than normal and appears not limited to a single ethnic group. Moreover, the onset of metabolic anomalies in PCOS women has been reported to occur at an earlier age than in the normal population , approximately 18-36 years [10,11]. However, other risk factors such as obesity, a positive family history of type 2 diabetes and hyperandrogenism may contribute to increasing the diabetes risk in PCOS [16]. Although glucose is the major regulator of insulin secretion by pancreatic beta cells, its action is also modulated through hormones secreted by intestinal endocrine cells which stimulate glucose-induced insulin secretion ,very potently after nutrient absorption.These hormones, called incretins are major regulators of postprandial glucose homeostasis. The main gluco-incretins are GIP (gastric inhibitory polypeptide or glucose-dependent insulinotropic polypeptide) and GLP-1 (glucagon-like polypeptide-1). GIP accounts for about 50% of incretin activity, and the rest may be due to GLP-1 which is produced by proteolytic processing of the preproglucagon molecule in intestinal L cells. Contrary to GIP, the incretin effect of GLP-1 is maintained in non-insulin-dependent diabetic patients [17]. The impaired GIP effect seems to have a genetic background, but could be aggravated by the diabetic state. Several GLP-1 analogues are currently in clinical development and the reported results are,so far, encouraging [18]. Disturbances in the secretion of the incretin hormones glucose-dependent insulinotropic polypeptide (GIP) and glucagon-like peptide 1 (GLP-1) have been observed in states with impaired glucose regulation (19). Increased total GIP and lower late phase active GLP-1 concentrations during OGTT characterize PCOS women with higher C-peptide secretion in comparison with healthy controls, and may be the early markers of a pre-diabetic state. In normal subjects, the incretin hormones glucagon-like peptide-1 (GLP-1) and glucose-dependent insulinotropic polypeptide (GIP) are responsible for 70% of the insulin response during a meal; but in diabetic subjects and other insulin-resistant conditions, the incretin effect is impaired..Metformin increases GIP and GLP-1 in lean women with PCOS , and a similar trend was seen in the obese women; although GIP secretion is attenuated in obese women with PCOS (20). NIDDM commonly occurs among women with polycystic ovary syndrome

[21,22]. In addition to hyperinsulinemia and insulin-resistance, altered first-phase insulin secretion, impaired glucose tolerance, dyslipidemia, hypertension and impaired fibrinolysis have also been described in PCOS [10,23,24] Dyslipidemia, diabetes and obesity are all potent cardiovascular risk factors that tend to cluster in women with polycystic ovary syndrome [25,26]. Metabolic disorders in patients with PCOS cannot be explained solely by the presence of obesity. In fact, insulin resistance is associated with dyslipidemia, independent of obesity.[7,27].In any case, this cluster of metabolic disturbances places women with PCOS at a high risk for the development of cardiovascular disease and diabetes and implies that the PCOS by itself may not be considered just a hyperandrogenic disorder, exclusively related to young and fertile age women, but a syndrome which may have some health implications later in life. In the past decade it became apparent that the syndrome is also associated with metabolic disturbances. Burghen and colleagues in 1980, first reported that women with PCOS had higher basal and glucose-stimulated insulin levels than weight-matched controls [9].It is a very important affirmation; in fact, now it has been accepted that hyperinsulinemia,a frequent finding in PCOS women, may suggest the insulin resistance Subsequently, other studies worldwide demonstrated that hyperinsulinemia and insulin-resistance are common features of a large number of patients affected by PCOS [28,29,30].Family studies have indicated a genetic susceptibility to PCOS [1,21]. Several clinical trials have shown a high frequency of impaired glucose tolerance (IGT) and non-insulin dependent diabetes mellitus (NIDDM) in women with polycystic ovarian syndrome.[22].

1999 WHO Diabetes criteria - Interpretation of Oral Glucose Tolerance Test								
Glucose levels	NORMAL		IFG		IGT		DM	
Venous Plasma	Fasting	2hrs	Fasting	2hrs	Fasting	2hrs	Fasting	2hrs
(mmol/l)	<6.1	<7.8	≥ 6.1 & <7.0	<7.8	<7.0	≥7.8	≥ 7.0	≥11.1
(mg/dl)	<100	<140	≥100 & <126	<140	<126	≥140	≥126	≥200

IGF= impaired fasting glycaemia, IGT= impaired glucose tolerance, DM= diabetes mellitus

It is important to consider that the American Diabetes Association (ADA) criteria, applied to fasting glucose, significantly underdiagnosed diabetes compared to the WHO criteria (Legro 1999)[31]. The prevalence and natural history of NIDDM precursor, impaired glucose tolerance (IGT), is less well known. In fact, little is known about the change in glucose tolerance that occurs over a period of several years in women with PCOS.This problem was investigated in 122 women with clinical and hormonal evidence of PCOS at the University of Chicago. All women had a standard oral glucose tolerance test (OGTT) with measurement of glucose and insulin levels. A subset of 25 women were subsequently restudied with the aim of characterizing the natural history of glucose tolerance in PCOS. Glucose tolerance was abnormal in 55 (45%) of the 122 women: 43 (35%) had IGT and 12 (10%) had NIDDM at the time of initial study. The women with NIDDM differed from those with normal glucose tolerance in that they had a 2.6-fold higher prevalence of first-degree relatives with NIDDM (83 vs. 31%, P < 0.01) and were significantly more obese (BMI 41.0 ± 2.4 vs. 33.4 ± 1.1 kg/m², P < 0.01). For the entire cohort of 122 women, there was a significant correlation between fasting and 2-h glucose After a mean follow-up of 2.4 ± 0.3 years, 25 women had a second OGTT. The glucose concentration at 2 h during the second glucose tolerance test was significantly higher than the 2-h concentration during the first study (161 ± 9 vs. 139 ± 6 mg/dl, P < 0.02). The prevalence of IGT and NIDDM in women with PCOS is substantially higher than expected when compared with age- and weight-matched populations of women without PCOS. The conversion from IGT to NIDDM is accelerated in PCOS. The fasting glucose concentration does not reliably predict the glucose concentration at 2 h after an oral glucose challenge, particularly among those with IGT, the subgroup at highest risk for subsequent development of NIDDM. In conclusion, women with PCOS should periodically have an OGTT and must be closely monitored for deterioration in glucose tolerance [30].Another study prospectively considered 254 PCOS women, aged 14–44 yr. A 75-g oral glucose challenge was administered after a 3-day 300-g carbohydrate diet and an overnight fast with 0 and 2 h blood samples for glucose levels. Diabetes was categorized according to WHO criteria. The prevalence of glucose intolerance was: 31.1% and 7.5% of diabetes. In nonobese PCOS women (body mass index, <27 kg/m2), 10.3% IGT and 1.5% diabetes were found. The prevalence of glucose intolerance was significantly higher in PCOS than in control women values [31]. This evaluation permit some considereations: 1)PCOS women are at significantly increased risk for IGT and type 2 diabetes mellitus at all weights and at a young age; 2) the similarity of prevalence rates in different populations of PCOS women, may suggest that PCOS may be a more important risk factor than ethnicity or race for glucose intolerance in young women . A recent Chinese study analyed 257 PCOS patients after OGTT (75 g oral glucose tolerance test). The authors found ,according to the WHO criteria, that 69.3% had normal glucose tolerance,30.7 % abnormal glucose metabolism with 26.1% of them presenting impaired glucose tolerance (IGT) and 4.7 diabetes mellitus(DM)[32].It was affirmed that insulin resistance is independent of obesity in PCOS [33].In spite of this,several studies showed that IGT is significantly frequent only in overweight/ obese PCOS women than in healthy controls [34]. It has been suggested that a family history of diabetes worsens insulin secretion and glucose tolerance in PCOS [35]. Consistent with this hypothesis, it was shown that a first degree relative with diabetes was associated with an increased risk of glucose intolerance in PCOS women. However, the prevalence of glucose intolerance in PCOS, even in those women without a first degree relative with diabetes, was still much greater than that reported in the general U.S. population and was significantly higher than that in control women [16,34,35]. In any case, the factors associated with glucose intolerance in PCOS, age, BMI, waist/hip ratios, and family history of diabetes, were identical to those in other populations [16,21,35,36,37]. The origin of insulin resistance in PCOS, which in recent years has become established as feature of this syndrome, is still a matter of debate. Molecular causes of insulin resistance have been identified as an excessive phosphorylation of serine residues of the insulin receptor, mutations in insulin receptor gene or insulin receptor substrate-1 (IRS-1), a cellular adenosine depletion, a deficiency in peroxisome proliferator-activated receptor gamma (PPAR-gamma) and a defect at the glucose transport level [10,38,39] . Obesity, which is frequently associated with PCOS, seems to amplify the degree of insulin resistance [40]. Although insulin resistance has been described to affect obese, it affects also most normal-weight PCOS women Some studies have demonstrated that obese women, particularly those with the abdominal obesity phenotype, are more insulin resistant than their normal-weight counterpart . Obesity may contribute to determine the insulin resistant state in PCOS in a number of ways. In particular, several metabolites , free fatty acids and lactate, as well as tumor necrosis factor-alpha (TNF-alpha) and leptin, whose production rate increases in the obesity state, directly affect the peripheral action of insulin [3,14,33,41,42,43,44,45,46,47]. An underlying genetic defect conferring insulin resistance and perhaps ß-cell dysfunction interacts with environmental factors worsening insulin resistance [21,22,35,48]. ß-cell function worsens, and glucose intolerance supervenes [22,35,48]. Cross-sectional studies have shown a high frequency of impaired glucose tolerance (IGT) and non-insulin dependent diabetes mellitus (NIDDM) in women with polycystic ovarian syndrome (PCOS). A study evaluated sixty-seven women with PCOS receiving a 75 g glucose tolerance test with measurement of lipids at baseline and at follow-up after an average time of 6.2 years. All women followed prospectively had normal glucose tolerance (54 women) or IGT (13 women) at the start of the study. Change in glycaemic control from baseline was frequent, with 5/54 (9%) of normoglycaemic women at baseline developing IGT and a further 4/54 (8%) moving directly from normoglycaemic to NIDDM. For women with IGT at baseline, 7/13 (54%) had NIDDM at follow-up. Body mass index at baseline was an independent significant predictor of adverse change in glycaemic control..Therefore, women with PCOS, particularly those with a high BMI, should be reviewed regularly with respect to IGT or NIDDM, as the frequency of impaired glycaemic control is high, and the rate of conversion from normal glucose tolerance to IGT or NIDDM, or from IGT to NIDDM is substantial [49]. Another important study considered 50 859 infertile women at high risk, 2.0% were newly diagnosed with diabetes, 3.4% had IGT, and 10.8% had previously diagnosed diabetes. These estimates emphasize the high rates of IGT (13.4%) and NIDDM (16.4%) observed in the present study. Although, this study precluded from follow-up, patients with NIDDM at baseline, and the observed changes were achieved over a relatively short period of 6.2 years. This investigation also confirmed that obesity is a strong predictor of deteriorating glucose metabolism. Obese PCOS women had a 10-fold increase in their risk of suffering from IGT or NIDDM compared with normal weight (BMI <25 kg/m2) PCOS women. Even those moderately obese PCOS women (BMI 25–30 kg/m2) still had an approximately 7-fold increase. It is concluded that women with PCOS presenting for infertility care have a high frequency of hyperinsulinaemia and NIDDM, which is associated with a high concomitant incidence of deterioration in glycaemic control over 6 years. Routine assessment of glucose tolerance should occur in women with PCOS, particularly those with a high BMI (30,49,50). In conclusion, PCOS women have profound insulin resistance independent of obesity , that is secondary to a unique, apparently genetic, disorder of insulin action [33,38,39,51].

Treatment

In the former time, the medical approach to PCOS focused on the symptom care,.particularly on the improvement of hirsutism and on the restoration of ovulation. However, the knowledge that hyperinsulinemia and insulin resistance are implicated in the pathogenesis of the syndrome, and that these metabolic alterations have important implications for long-term health, induced many investigators to evaluate therapeutic strategies to control these disorders..Exercise and weight loss are important ways of reversing insulin resistance and associated metabolic disturbances. In obese women with PCOS even partial weight loss may in fact reduce glucose-stimulated insulin levels and improve insulin sensitivity [52,53,54].To improve hyperinsulinemia and insulin resistance, several insulin sensitizers drugs have been used in the management of PCOS. Metformin is widely used for the treatment of type 2 diabetes. Its mechanisms of action include a reduction of hepatic glucose production and an increase of sensitivity of peripheral tissue to insulin, without significant effects on beta-cell insulin production. Therefore, metformin can reduce peripheral insulin concentrations and improve glucose tolerance and metabolism recovering menses and fertility[55,56].Recently, a 6-month controlled study investigated the effect of combined metformin administration and hypocaloric diet on insulin other than androgens and fat distribution in a group of abdominally obese women with PCOS A more consistent decrease of serum insulin, of visceral fat and testosterone levels was observed after metformin administration when compared to placebo[54]. Another class of insulin-sensitizing agents, the thiazolidinediones, selective ligands for PPAR-gamma, a member of the nuclear receptor superfamily of ligand-activated transcription factors, have become available for the treatment of insulin resistant states. It is found that administration of troglitazone improved total body insulin sensitivity and lowered circulating insulin levels in obese PCOS women [57,58].

Among other insulin-sensitizing agents, the potential use of D-chiro-inositol, which may serve as a precursor for inositol glycan mediators of insulin signal transduction, is currently under investigation. Controversy still exists about the effects of combined hormonal contraceptive on glucose-insulin metabolism in PCOS. Some studies showed no effect and others a worsening of insulin sensitivity [59,60]. A recent prospective study compared a group of women with PCOS treated with long-term oestrogen-progestagen therapy, with or without hypocaloric diet, with a non-treated group. The results revealed that, contrary to the latter, the treated group had no changes in glucose tolerance and fasting or glucose-stimulated insulin levels after a ten-year follow-up [61]. The different results obtained in the available studies might be related, at least in part, to the different preparation administered and, particularly, to the different dosage of oestradiol content. In fact, studies performed in ovariectomized rats treated with different doses of 17-beta-estradiol showed that low concentrations of 17-beta-estradiol were able to up-regulate the IRS-1 and increase insulin sensitivity, both in muscle and adipose tissue ; whereas, high concentrations of 17-beta-estradiol down-regulated IRS-1 [62]. In summary, dietary-induced weight loss and the use of insulin-sensitizers could be viewed as a potential strategy for controlling the metabolic alteration and preventing the increased susceptibility to develop diabetes in obese PCOS women. However, this question needs to be verified by appropriate long-term intervention studies. Moreover, disparate effects of estrogen-progesterone compounds may be related to both patient selection and the type and amounts of steroid administered.

References

[1] Yildiz BO, Yarali H, Oguz H, Bayraktar M.Glucose intolerance, insulin resistance, and hyperandrogenemia in first degree relatives of women with polycystic ovary syndrome. *J. Clin. Endocrinol. Metab.* 2003 May;88(5):2031-6.

[2] Lanzone A, Caruso A, Di Simone N, DeCarolis S, Fulgheus AM, Mancuso S.Polycystic ovary disease. A risk for gestational diabetes?. *J. Reprod. Med.* 1995:40:312-6.

[3] Poretsky L, Cataldo NA, Rosenwaks Z and Guidice L. The Insulin-related regulatory system in health and disease. *Endocrine Reviews* 1999; 20: 535-82.

[4] Sepilian V, Nagamani M. Adiponectin levels in women with polycystic ovary syndrome and severe insulin resistance. *J. Soc. Gynecol. Investig.* 2005 Feb;12(2):129-34.

[5] Spranger J, Möhlig M, Wegewitz U, Ristow M, Pfeiffer AF, Schill T, Schlösser HW, Brabant G, Schöfl C.Adiponectin is independently associated with insulin sensitivity in women with polycystic ovary syndrome. *Clin. Endocrinol.* (Oxf). 2004 Dec;61(6):738-46.

[6] Sieminska L, Marek B, Kos-Kudla B, Niedziolka D, Kajdaniuk D, Nowak M, Glogowska-Szelag J.Serum adiponectin in women with polycystic ovarian syndrome and its relation to clinical, metabolic and endocrine parameters. *J. Endocrinol. Invest.* 2004 Jun;27(6):528-34.

[7] Chang RJ, Nakamura RM, Judd HL, Kaplan SA. Insulin resistance in nonobese patients with polycystic ovarian disease. *J. Clin. Endocrinol. Metab.* 1983; 57:356–359.

[8] Robinson S, Kiddy D, Gelding SV, et al. 1993 The relationship of insulin insensitivity to menstrual pattern in women with hyperandrogenism and polycystic ovaries. *Clin. Endocrinol.* (Oxf) 1993; 39:351–355.

[9] Burghen GA, Givens JR, Kitabchi AE. Correlation of hyperandrogenism with hyperinsulinism in polycystic ovarian disease. *J. Clin. Endocrinol. Metab.* 1980; 50:113-6.

[10] Dunaif A. Insulin resistance and polycystic ovary syndrome: mechanisms and implications for pathogenesis. *Endocr. Rev.* 1997; 18: 774–800.

[11] Dunaif A, Graf M, Mandeli J, Laumas V, Dobrjansky A. Characterization of groups of hyperandrogenic women with acanthosis nigricans, impaired glucose tolerance, and/or hyperinsulinemia. *J. Clin. Endocrinol. Metab.* 1987;65:499–507.

[12] O'Meara NM, Blackman JD, Ehrmann DA, et al. 1993 Defects in beta-cell function in functional ovarian hyperandrogenism. *J. Clin. Endocrinol. Metab.* 76:1241–1247 21.

[13] Ehrmann DA, Sturis J, Byrne MM, Karrison T, Rosenfield RL, Polonsky KS. 1995 Insulin secretory defects in polycystic ovary syndrome. Relationship to insulin sensitivity and family Interpretation of OGTT results. *J. Clin. Invest.* 1995; 96:520–527.

[14] Dunaif A, Finegood DT. Beta-cell dysfunction independent of obesity, and glucose intolerance in the polycystic ovary syndrome. *J. Clin. Endocrinol. Metab.* 1996; 81:942-7.

[15] Reaven GM. Role of insulin resistance in human disease. *Diabetes* 1988;37(12); 1595-1607.

[16] Harris MI, Hadden WC, Knowler WC, Bennett PH Prevalence of diabetes and impaired glucose tolerance and plasma glucose levels in U.S. population aged 20–74 yr. *Diabetes*.1987; 36:523–534.

[17] Thorens B. Glucagon-like peptide-1 and control of insulin secretion. *Diabete Metab*. 1995 Dec;21(5):311-8.

[18] Vilsbøll T, Holst JJ. Incretins, insulin secretion and Type 2 diabetes mellitus. *Diabetologia*. 2004 Mar;47(3):357-66.

[19] Vrbikova J, Hill M, Bendlova B, Grimmichova T, Dvorakova K, Vondra K, Pacini G.Incretin levels in polycystic ovary syndrome. *Eur. J. Endocrinol.* 2008 Aug;159(2):121-7.

[20] Svendsen PF, Nilas L, Madsbad S, Holst JJ Incretin hormone secretion in women with polycystic ovary syndrome: roles of obesity, insulin sensitivity, and treatment with metformin. *Metabolism.* 2009 May;58(5):586-93.

[21] Warram JH, Martin BC, Krolewski AS, Soeldner JS, Kahn CR. Slow glucose removal rate and hyperinsulinemia precede the development of type II diabetes in the offspring of diabetic parents. *Ann. Intern. Med.* 1990;113(909): 915-19.

[22] Lillioja S, Mott D, Spraul M, et al. Insulin resistance and insulin secretory dysfunction as precursors of non-insulin-dependent diabetes mellitus. *N. Engl. J. Med.* 2003; 329:1988 -1992.

[23] Pelusi B,Gambineri A,Pasquali R. Type 2 diabetes and the polycystic ovary syndrome. *Minerva Ginecol.* 2004; 56(1): 41-51.

[24] Dahlgren E, Johansoon S, Lindstedt G, Kautsson F, Oden A, Jonson PO, et al. Women with polycystic ovary syndrome wedge resected in 1956 to 1965: a long term follow up focusing on natural history and circulating hormones. *Fertil. Steril.* 1992; 57:505-13.

[25] Talbott E, Guzick D, Clerici A, Berga S, Detre K, Weiner K, kuller L. Coronary heart disease risk factors in women with polycystic ovary syndrome. *Arterioscler. Tromb. Vasc. Biol.* 1995; 15:821-6.

[26] Kalra A., Nair S., Rai L. Association of obesity and insulin resistance with dyslipidemia in Indian women with polycystic ovarian syndrome. *Indian J. Medical Sciences* 2006; 60(11): 447- 453.

[27] Shoupe D, Kumar DD, Lobo RA. 1983 Insulin resistance in polycystic ovary syndrome. *Am. J. Obstet. Gynecol.* 147:588–592.

[28] Pasquali R, Venturoli S, Paradis R, Capelli M, Parenti M, Melchionda N. 1982 Insulin and C-peptide levels in obese patients with polycystic ovaries. *Horm. Metab. Res*. 14 284–287.

[29] Flier JS, Eastman RC, Minaker KL, Matteson D, Rowe JW. 1985 Acanthosis nigricans in obese women with hyperandrogenism. Characterization of an insulin-resistant state distinct from the type A and B syndromes. *Diabetes.* 34:101–107.

[30] Ehrmann DA,Barnes RB,Rosenfield RL,Cavaghan MK,Imperial J. Prevalence of impaired glucose tolerance and diabetes in women with polycystic ovary sindrome. *Diabetes Care* 1999; 22(1): 141-6.

[31] Legro RS,Kunselman AR,Dodson WC, Dunaif A. Prevalence and predictors of risk for type 2 diabetes mellitus and impaired glucose tolerance in polycystic ovary syndrome:a prospective, controlled study in 254 affected women. *J. Clin. Endocrinol. Metab.* 1999; 84(1): 165-9.

[32] Ho W,Hu WH,Qiao J,Wang LN,Zhao CY.Characteristics of abnormal glucose tolerance in patients with polycystic ovary syndrome. *Zhonghua Yi Xue Za Zhi* 2009;89(29):2053-5.

[33] Dunaif A, Segal KR, Futterweit W, Dobrjansky A. 1989 Profound peripheral insulin resistance, independent of obesity, in polycystic ovary syndrome. *Diabetes* 1989;38:1165–1174.

[34] Harris MI, Flegal KM, Cowie CC, et al.Prevalence of diabetes, impaired fasting glucose, and impaired glucose tolerance in U.S. adults. *Diabetes Care.*1998; 21:518–524.

[35] Haffner SM. 1995 Risk factors for non-insulin-dependent diabetes mellitus. *J. Hypertens. Suppl.* 13:S73–S76.

[36] Eriksson J, Franssila-Kallunki A, Ekstrand A, et al. Early metabolic defects in persons at risk for noninsulin-dependent diabetes. *N. Engl. J. Med.* 1989; 321:337–343.

[37] Vrbikova J,Fanta M,Cibula D,Vondra K,Bendlova B.Impaired glucose metabolism in women with polycystic ovary syndrome. *Gynecol. Obstet. Invest.* 2009; 68(3):186-90.

[38] Dunaif A, Xia J, Book CB, Schenker E, Tang Z. Excessive insulin receptor serine phosphorylation in cultured fibroblasts and in skeletal muscle. A potential mechanism for insulin resistance in the polycystic ovary syndrome. *J. Clin. Invest.* 1995; 96:801–810.

[39] Ciaraldi TP, el-Roeiy A, Madar Z, Reichart D, Olefsky JM, Yen SSC. Cellular mechanisms of insulin resistance in polycystic ovarian syndrome. *J. Clin. Endocrinol. Metab.* 1992; 75:577–583.

[40] Franks S. Polycystic ovary syndrome. *N. Eng. J. Med.* 1995; 333:853-61.

[41] Holte J. Disturbances in insulin secretion and sensitivity in women with the polycystic ovary syndrome. *Bailliers Clin. Endocrinol. Metab.* 1996; 10:221-47.

[42] Dunaif A, Sorbara L, Delson R, Green G. Ethnicity and polycystic ovary syndrome are associated with independent and additive decreases in insulin action in Caribbean-Hispanic women. *Diabetes* 1993; 42:1462-8.

[43] Holte J, Bergh T, Gennarelli G, Wide L. The independent effects of polycystic ovary syndrome and obesity on serum concentrations of gonadotropins and sex steroids in premenopausal women. *Clin. Endocrinol.* (Oxf) 1994; 41:473-81.

[44] Morin-Papunen LC, Vauhkomen I, Koivumen RM, Rouokomen A, Tapanaimen JS. Insulin sensitivity, insulin secretion, and metabolic and hormonal parameters in healthy women and women with polycystic ovary syndrome. *Hum. Reprod.* 2000; 15:1266-74.

[45] Morales AJ, Laughlin GA, Batzow T, Maheshwari H, Baumann G, Yen SC. Insulin, somatotropic, and luteinizing hormone axes in lean and obese women with polycystic ovary syndrome: common and distinct features. *J. Clin. Endocrinol. Metab.* 1996; 81:2854-64.

[46] Micic D, Macut DJ, Popovic V, Sumarac-Dumanovic M, Kendereski A, Colic M, et al. Leptin levels and insulin sesitivity in obese and non-obese patients with polycystic ovary syndrome. *Gynecol. Endocrinol.* 1997; 11:315-20.

[47] Grulet H, Heeart AC, Delemer B, Gross A, Sulmont V, Leutenegger M, Caron J. Roles of LH and insulin resistance in lean and obese polycystic ovary syndrome. *Clin. Endocrinol.* (Oxf) 1993; 38:621-6.

[48] DeFronzo RA. 1997 Pathogenesis of type 2 diabetes: metabolic and molecular implications for identifying diabetes genes. *Diabetes Rev.* 5:177–269.

[49] Norman RJ,Masters L, Milner CR, Wang JX, Davies MJ. Relative risk of conversion from normoglycaemia to impaired glucose tolerance or non-insulin dependent diabetes mellitus in polycystic ovarian syndrome. *Human Reproduction* 2001;16,(9): 1995-1998.

[50] Welborn.T.A,Reid C.M,.Marriott, G.Australian Diabetes Screening Study: impaired glucose tolerance and non- insulin-dependent diabetes mellitus. *Metabolism* 1997: 46, 35–39.

[51] Dunaif A, Segal KR, Shelley DR, Green G, Dobrjansky A, Licholai T.Evidence for distinctive and intrinsic defects in insulin action in polycystic ovary syndrome. *Diabetes* 1992; 41:1257–1266.

[52] Pasquali R,Casimirri F. The impact of obesity on hyperandrogenism and polycystic ovary syndrome in premenopausal women. *Clin. Endocrinol.* (Oxf) 1993; 39:1-16.

[53] Kiddy DS, Hamilton-Fairley D, Bush A, Short F, Anyaoku V, Reed MJ, Franks S. Improvement in endocrine and ovarian function during dietary treatment of obese women with polycystic ovary syndrome. *Clin. Endocrinol.* (Oxf) 1992; 36:105-11.

[54] Pasquali R, Gambineri A, Biscotti D, Vicennati V, Gagliardi L, Colitta D, et al. Effect of long term treatment with metformin added to hypocaloric diet on body composition, fat distribution, and androgen and insulin levels in abdominally obese women with and without the polycystyc ovary syndrome. *J. Clin. Endocrinol. Metab.* 2000; 85:2767-74.

[55] Velazquez EM, Mendoza S, Hamer T, Sosa F, Glueck CJ. Metformin therapy in polycystic ovary syndrome reduces hyperinsulinemia, insulin resistance, hyperandrogenemia, and systolic blood pressure, while facilitating normal menses and pregnancy. *Metabolism* 1994; 43:647-54.

[56] Nestler JE, Jakubowicz DJ. Decreases in ovarian cytochrome P450c17alpha activity and serum free testosterone after reduction of insulin secretion in polycystic ovary syndrome. *N. Engl. J. Med.* 1996; 335:617-23.

[57] Dunaif A, Scott D, Finegood D, Quintana B, Whitcomb R. The insulin sensitising agent troglitazone improves metabolic and reproductive abnormalities in the polycystic ovary syndrome. *J. Clin. Endocrinol. Metab.* 1996; 81:3299-306.

[58] Ehrmann DA, Scheneider DJ, Sobel BE, Cavaghan MK, Imperial J, Rosenfield RL, Polonsky KS. Troglitazone improves defects in insulin action, insulin secretion, ovarian steroidogenesis and fibrinolysis in women with polycystic ovary syndrome. *J. Clin. Endocrinol. Metab.* 1997; 82:2108-16.

[59] Armstrong VL, Wiggam MI, Ennis CN, Sheridan B, Traub AI, Atkinson AB, Bell PM. Insulin action and insulin secretion in polycystic ovary syndrome treated with ethinyloestradiol/cyproterone acetate. *QJM* 2001; 94:31-7.

[60] Korytkowski MT, Mokan M, Horwitz MJ, Berga SL. Metabolic effects of oral contraceptives in women with polycystic ovary syndrome. *J. Clin. Endocrinol. Metab.* 1995; 80:3327-34.

[61] Pasquali R, Gambineri A, Anconetani B, Vicennati V, Colitta D, Caramelli E, et al. The natural history of the metabolic syndrome in young women with the polycystic ovary syndrome and the long-term effect oestrogen-progestagen treatment. *Clin. Endocrinol.* (Oxf) 1999; 50:517-27.

[62] Gonzalez C, Alonso A, Gruseo NA, Diaz F, Esteban MM, Fernandez S, Patterson AM. Effect of treatment with different doses of 17-beta estradiol on insulin receptor substrate-1 *Pancreas*(Online) 2001; 2:140-9.

In:Polycystic Ovarian Syndrome: An Enigmatic...
Editor: Rosa Sabatini

ISBN: 978-1-61761-853-6
©2011 Nova Science Publishers, Inc.

Chapter IV

Metabolic Syndrome in PCOS Women

Rosa Sabatini and Raffaele Cagiano***

*Expert Family Planning Service. Department of Obstetrics and Gynecology
**Department of Pharmacology and Human Physiology
Policlinico-University of Bari. Piazza Giulio Cesare 11.70124 Bari. Italy

The term "Metabolic syndrome" defines a cluster of abnormalities associated with increased risk for the development of type 2 diabetes and atherosclerotic vascular disease (heart disease, arterial disease and stroke).Metabolic syndrome (MS) is also known as metabolic syndrome X, syndrome X, insulin resistance syndrome, Reaven 's syndrome, and CHAOS (Coronary artery disease, Hypertension, Atherosclerosis, Obesity and Stroke). The current term "metabolic syndrome" was firstly used in 1947 by Jean Vague who observed that the upper body obesity could predispose to diabetes, atherosclerosis.gout and calculi [1]. After twenty years from this report, Avogaro described six obese women with diabetes mellitus, hyperlipoproteinemia hyperuricemia and hypertriglyceridemia , all of which improved when were subjected to a hypocaloric, low carbohydrate diet [2] .The year 1977 has been important for the metabolic syndrome history. In that period,in fact, Haller used this term for the association of obesity, diabetes mellitus, hyperlipoproteinemia, hyperuricemia and hepatic steatosis describing the additive risk factors for atherosclerosis; while, Singer described the association of obesity, gout, diabetes mellitus and hypertension with hyperlipoproteinemia [3,4].The next year, Phillips developed the concept that a constellation of abnormalities as glucose intolerance, hyperinsulinemia, hyperlipidemia , hypercholesterolemia , hypertension and hypertriglyceridemia could concur to myocardial infarction .In addition, Philips hypothesized that this cluster of disorders could be associated not only with heart disease, but also with aging, obesity and other clinical states being the sex hormonal status, a common linking factor [5,6] .In 1988,Gerald M.Reaven proposed the insulin resistance as the underlying factor and named "Syndrome X" the constellation of related abnormalities. Reaven did not include ''abdominal obesity'' as part of the condition , which was hypothesized, instead.[7].

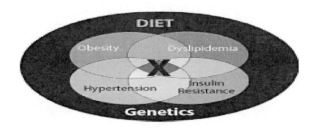

Hence,there are several definitions for the syndrome and this led to a lot of confusion and debates in the medical community. Currently,despite the heterogeneity, there is a conceptual agreement on the definition of metabolic syndrome but the cut-off values and the selection of diagnostic parameters are still conflicting. Diagnostic or definitive components of the syndrome , such as obesity and insulin resistance, should be considered separately from the associated-conditions (polycystic ovary, obstructive sleep apnea,microalbuminuria,non-alcoholic steatohepatitis...)of metabolic syndrome, during the course of diagnosis. The maintenance of the metabolic syndrome, as a diagnostic category, would still seem to be useful for an effective multiple cardiovascular risk prediction [8]. An agreement was found on the new guidelines at a joint meeting of ESHRE and ASRM in 2004. In any case, despite the controversy on the metabolic syndrome, it is widely accepted that individuals with multiple risk factors are at increased risk for cardiovascular diseases and diabetes, and the new term cardiometabolic risk is born. This word evolved from the understanding the cluster of established and emerging risk factors . The cluster of risk factors includes those associated with metabolic syndrome and other risk factors which contribute to cardiometabolic morbidity. The definition of cardiometabolic risk (CMR) represents the overall risk of developing type 2 diabetes and cardiovascular diseases , due to a cluster of risk factors. The risk factors include:

- Classical risk factors. Smoking, high LDL-cholesterol, hypertension, elevated blood glucose

- Recent risk factors. Abdominal obesity, insulin resistance, low HDL-cholesterol, high triglycerides, hyperuricemia, fibrinogen, microalbuminuria, PAI-1, ROS, NASH, Hcy and inflammatory markers.

- Cardiometabolic Risk Factors. Adiposity, elevated triglycerides, low HDL, elevated blood pressure, elevated blood glucose.

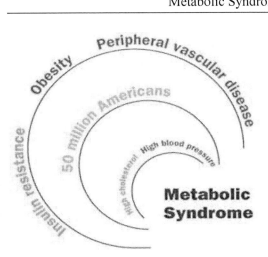

Three of the most commonly used definitions are validated by the World Health Organization (WHO), the National Cholesterol Education Program. Expert Panel on Detection, Evaluation, and Treatment of High Blood Cholesterol in Adults Treatment - Panel III (NCEPATPIII) and the International Diabetic Federation (IDF) criteria

Various groups have proposed similar definitions of the syndrome. Since the manifestations of MS are not uniform, most experts allowed to a "choice" from the list of components. In fact, to establish the diagnosis of MS, the US recommendation stipulates that "at least three" components must be present, whereas the World Health Organization (WHO) definition requires the presence of glucose/insulin abnormalities combined with more than two other factors.

Major definitions for Metabolic Sindrome

The World Health Organization criteria (WHO 1999):require presence of diabetes mellitus, impaired glucose tolerance, impaired fasting glucose or insulin resistance and two of the following :
- blood pression≥140/90 mmHg
- dyslipidemia:triglycerides≥ 1.695 nmol/L and high-density lipoprotein cholesterol(HDL-C)≤1.0 nmol/L(female)
- central obesity: waist : hip ratio>0.85(female),and/or Body mass index>30 kg/m²
- microalbuminuria: urinary albumin excretion ratio≥20 mg/min or albumin:creatinine ratio≥30 mg/g

The European Group for the Study of Insulin Resistance criteria (EGIR 1999)require insulin resistance defined as the top 25% of the fasting insulin values among non-diabetic individuals and two or more of the following:
- central obesity: waist circumference ≥80 cm(female)
- dyslipidemia: triglycerides≥2.0 nmol/L and/or HDL-C<1.0 nmol/L or treated for dyslipidemia
- hypertension : blood pressure ≥ 140/90 mmHg or antihypertensive medication
- fasting plasma glucose ≥6.1 nmol/L

The US National Cholesterol Education Program Adult Treatment Panel III (NCEP ATP III 2001) requires at least three of the following:
- central obesity: waist circumference ≥88 cm or 36 inches(female)
- triglyceridemia ≥ 1.695 nmol/L (150 mg/dl)
- dyslipidaemia: high-density lipoprotein cholesterol(HDL-C)≤ 50 mg/dl (female)
- blood pressure ≥ 130/85 mmHg
- fasting plasma glucose ≥ 6.1 nmol/L (110 mg/dl)

This relative vagueness of the definition underscored the main problems of MS research. It was hypothesized that the syndrome might have a single common pathophysiology, but its components could evolve with different speed as resulting in the various clinical pictures. However, it was equally postulated that MS might have different etiologies, but sharing a common intermediary mechanism. It was estimated that the prevalence of Metabolic Syndrome in women with PCOS is 33% by WHO,37% by NCEP-ATP and 40% by IDF criteria ,compared with 10% by NCEP-ATP and 13% by IDF in controls (P<.001) [9] .

The Metabolic Syndrome "Reloaded"

Metabolic syndrome (Syndrome X) "reloaded" is a unique clustering of clinical syndromes and metabolic derangements. In 1988 Reaven initially discussed the four major determinants consisting of Hypertension, Hyperinsulinemia, Hyperlipidemia (Dyslipidemia of elevated VLDL – triglycerides, decreased HDL-cholesterol, and elevated small dense atherogenic LDL-cholesterol) and Hyperglycemia or impaired glucose tolerance, impaired fasting glucose, or even overt type 2 diabetes mellitus (T2DM) and the central importance of insulin resistance and hyperinsulinemia. The important association of polycystic ovary syndrome, hyperuricemia, fibrinogen, CRP, microalbuminuria, PAI-1, and more recently reactive oxygen species (ROS), NASH, and the damaging oxidative potential of Hcy and endothelial dysfunction, all of which have contributed to a better understanding of this complicated   clustering   phenomenon.   ROS,   hyperuricemia,microalbuminuria, hyperhomocysteinemia, highly sensitive C-reactive protein (CRP), indicate the newer additions as giving rise to the new terminology '': Metabolic Syndrome Reloaded''[10] .

The Relationships between PCOS and MS

The metabolic syndrome and the polycystic ovary syndrome are distinct entities; although, they appear interrelated . PCOS is characterized by anovulaton, hyperandrogenism and polycystic ovaries but is also associated with insulin resistance (IR) and obesity. In women with PCOS, smoking was associated with statistically significant increased levels of fasting insulin and free testosterone (FT) and with a raised free androgen index (FAI) score, which resulted in aggravated scores on the homeostatic model for assessment of insulin resistance (HOMA-IR). However, no differences were observed between the smoking and nonsmoking groups with regard to the clinical parameters for hirsutism, acne, ovulatory function , or polycystic ovaries using the ultrasound criteria recommended according to the Rotterdam definition [11] Women with polycystic ovary syndrome (PCOS) have an increased prevalence of insulin resistance (IR) and related disorders. Currently,elevated serum levels of high sensitivity CRP (hs-CRP), interleukin-6 (IL-6) and tumor necrosis factor alpha (TNF-alpha) ,all reflecting a low-grade chronic inflammation , have been associated with several insulin-resistant states; they are useful cardiovascular risk markers. A study has investigated whether soluble inflammatory markers are altered in PCOS focusing on its relationship with obesity and indexes of insulin resistance. One hundred and eight women with PCOS and 75 healthy women were recruited. According to body mass index (BMI), patients were divided into two groups; group I (BMI < 27 kg/m²) and group II (BMI ≥ 27 Kg/m²).Serum levels of hs-CRP, IL-6, and TNF-alpha, lipid and hormone profiles were measured. From this study emerged that PCOS patients had increased levels of testosterone, luteinizing hormone (LH), androstendione, insulin level and HOMA index compared to healthy BMI matched controls. High-density lipoprotein (HDL) concentrations were significantly reduced in both, patient groups compared to their controls, while triglyceride levels were significantly increased in obese group compared to controls.There were no significant difference in serum inflammatory markers between women of the group I and their matched controls.Furthermore, there were highly significant positive correlation between hs-CRP and IL-6, hs-CRP and TNF-alpha and, also between IL-6 and TNF-alpha . These inflammatory markers significantly correlated with BMI and HOMA index. It seems that BMI and HOMA indexes could be predictors of IL-6 levels ; while, BMI was the only predictor of hs-CRP levels and TNF-alpha levels. Therefore, evidence suggests that PCOS and obesity induce an increase in serum inflammatory cardiovascular risk markers. The precise mechanisms underlying these associations require additional studies to clarify the state of the cardiovascular system in women with PCOS compared with controls in large numbers of patients in order to determine the relative contribution of different factors, including insulin resistance, androgen status and BMI [12]. It was evaluated the level of high sensitive serum C-reactive protein (HS-CRP) levels in patients affected by normoinsulinemic polycystic ovary syndrome (PCOS) without metabolic syndrome and the relationship between HS-CRP and other cardiovascular risk factors such as obesity and serum lipids. A total of 52 normoinsulinemic PCOS women without metabolic syndrome and 48 normoandrogenic ovulatory women were enrolled in this study. Endocrine screening, including FSH, LH, total testosterone, free testosterone, sex hormone-binding globulin, dehydroepiandrosterone sulfate, low-density lipoprotein (LDL), high-density lipoprotein (HDL), total cholesterol (TC) and triglyceride (TG),has been considered . Normal insulin sensitivity was defined on the basis of fasting serum glucose and insulin levels, and serum insulin response to an oral glucose tolerance test and homeostatic model of insulin resistance. HS-CRP was assessed spectrophotometrically. The results showed that PCOS patients had increased HS-CRP compared to the control group (P < 0.0001) and, that HS-CRP was positively correlated with body mass index (BMI) ,waist-to-hip ratio (WHR) , LDL,TC and TG , and negatively correlated with HDL .In this study, it was also reported a strong association between HS-CRP and PCOS status (P < 0.0001) .In conclusion, elevated HS-CRP was associated with cardiovascular risk factors in normoinsulinemic PCOS without metabolic syndrome [13]. The circulating follistatin and high-sensitivity C-reactive protein (hsCRP) concentrations were significantly higher in 155 Taiwanese women with polycystic ovary syndrome than in 37 healthy controls..Follistatin and hsCRP levels in the PCOS and control groups were significantly correlated but independent from obesity and insulin resistance [14]. Therefore,women with polycystic ovary syndrome have chronic low-level inflammation that can increase the risk of atherogenesis. Circulating proatherogenic inflammatory mediators as interleukin-6 (IL-6), soluble intercellular adhesion molecule-1 (sICAM-1),monocyte chemotactic protein-1 (MCP-1),C-reactive protein (CRP),matrix metalloproteinase-2, plasminogen activator inhibitor-1(PAI-1),and activated nuclear factor kappa B (in mononuclear cells) in women with PCOS lean (body mass index, 18-25 kg/m²) and obese (body mass index 30-40 kg/m²) ,and in weight-matched controls (lean and obese) were measured.An analysis revealed higher IL-6, sICAM-1, CRP, PAI-1, systolic and diastolic blood pressures, triglycerides, fasting insulin, and homeostasis model assessment of insulin resistance index in women with PCOS compared with weight-matched controls, and the highest levels in the obese regardless of PCOS status. Fasting MCP-1 levels resulted significantly correlated with activated nuclear factor kappa B during hyperglycemia ,and with androstenedione. Therefore, this study concluded that both PCOS and obesity contribute to a proatherogenic state but, in women with PCOS, abdominal adiposity and hyperandrogenism may exacerbate the risk of atherosclerosis [15]. Obese females are at higher risk for metabolic syndrome due to severe hyperandrogenemia, which also leads to high blood pressure. The study of Tamimi et al.investigated , among patients with PCOS, the correlation of body mass index (BMI) with the clinical manifestations of PCOS and blood pressure. Sixty-two patients were divided into two BMI groups: nonobese (BMI less than 25 kg/m²) and obese (BMI more than 25 kg/m²). Patients' waist to hip ratio, acne, hirsutism, and systolic and diastolic blood pressures were also recorded as clinical manifestations in PCOS and compared between the two BMI groups. The mean age of the patients was 35.85 ± 5.03 years, BMI was 31.91 ± 6.40 kg/m². When the groups were compared according to BMI, a significant increase in systolic and diastolic blood pressures (p = 0.001 and 0.003, respectively) was seen in obese patients, but there was no significant rise in the waist-hip ratio and hirsutism score. In conclusion, it was observed a significant and progressive effect of BMI on clinical manifestations and blood pressure levels in patients with PCOS [16]. Another study evaluated the prevalence of central and general obesity, arterial hypertension, and alterations in cholesterol, triglycerids, glycemia and uric acid levels in patients with PCOS compared with women not showing this syndrome. The age of the patients with PCOS varied between 18 and 39 years old.The prevalence of general obesity (BMI ≥ 30) was of 50.9% in PCOS group and 18.2% in the control groups. The systolic hypertension (BP ≥ 140 mm Hg) was found in 9% against 7.3%.in controls. A diastolic hypertension (BP ≥ 90 mm Hg)was reported in 25.5% against 7.3%; while,were found hypercholesterolemia (≥ 220 mg/dL)in 30.9% against 10.9%, hypertriglyceridemia (≥ 160 mg/dL) in 30.9% against 16.4%, hyperglycaemia(≥115 mg/dL) in 5.5% against 3.6% and, hyperuricemia (≥ 6.5 mg/L) in 23.6% against 3.6%. Indeed, this report showed that patients with PCOS have the possibility to present obesity, hypercholesterolemia, hypertriglyceridemia, hyperuricemia and diastolic hypertension, 4.6, 3.7, 2.3, 8.2 and 4.4 times more than the controls. The comparison of the variable averages of both groups showed significant differences for BMI, WHI, systolic BP, cholesterol and uric acid. In addition, it was found a consistent association between PCOS and hyperuricemia , obesity, hypercholesterolemia, hypertriglyceridemia, and diastolic hypertension. No such thing for hyperglycaemia and systolic hypertension [17]. The prevalence of polycystic ovary syndrome (PCOS) is estimated to be nearly 10% among reproductive age women. PCOS may represent the largest underappreciated segment of the female population at risk of cardiovascular disease. Cardiac risk factors associated with PCOS have public health implications and should drive early screening and intervention measures. There are no consensus guidelines regarding screening for cardiovascular disease in patients with PCOS. Fasting lipid profiles and glucose examinations should be performed regularly. Carotid intimal medial thickness examinations should begin at age 30 years, and coronary calcium screening should begin at age 45 years.Treatment of the associated cardiovascular risk factors, including insulin resistance, hypertension, and dyslipidemia , should be incorporated into the routine PCOS patient wellness care program [18]. Polycystic ovary syndrome is an extremely prevalent disorder in which elevated blood markers of cardiovascular risk and altered endothelial function have been found. An Italian study was performed to determine if abnormal carotid intima-media thickness (IMT) and brachial flow-mediated dilation (FMD) in young women with PCOS may be explained by insulin resistance and elevated adipocytokines. It was found that BMI or waist-hip ratio did not correlate with IMT or FMD; insulin and QUICKI (a marker of insulin resistance) correlated positively and negatively with IMT (P <.01),while adiponectin correlated negatively with IMT (P <.05). Differently, leptin and resistin resulted not different compared with matched controls. The data suggested that young women with PCOS have evidence for altered endothelial function and that adverse endothelial parameters were correlated with insulin resistance and low adiponectin. The Authors have hypothesized that the type of fat distribution may influence these factors [19]. Another study considered fifty young women with PCOS (overweight or obese 24 and nonobese 26) and 25 age-matched healthy controls.Plasma thrombin-activatable fibrinolysis inhibitor, serum FSH, LH, DHEAS, total T, E 2, total cholesterol, high-density lipoprotein cholesterol, low-density lipoprotein cholesterol, triglyceride, insulin resistance, and carotid intima-media thickness were evaluated. The data allowed to show that plasma thrombin-activatable fibrinolysis inhibitor levels in the overweight or obese PCOS group were significantly higher than those in the nonobese PCOS and control groups. Carotid intima-media thickness did not significantly differ between the groups. Obesity and insulin resistance were positively associated with plasma thrombin-activatable fibrinolysis inhibitor levels, but there was no association between carotid intima-media thickness and thrombin-activatable fibrinolysis inhibitor. Therefore, in young overweight or obese women with PCOS, impaired fibrinolysis may be responsible for the increased risk of cardiovascular diseases (20). Young women with PCOS presented a plasma viscosity that resulted increased by obesity and IR. Therefore, clinical management of young overweight women with PCOS and IR should always include a serious reduction in body weight and the use of oral contraceptive treatment with cautious [21]. Hypoadiponectinemia is evident only in obese adolescents with PCOS and therefore does not seem to be involved in the pathogenesis of PCOS in this age group [22].

References

[1] Vague J. La différenciacion sexuelle, facteur determinant des formes de l'obésité. *Presse Med.* 1947;30:339-40.

[2] Avogaro P,Crepaldi G,Enzi G,Tiengo A.Associazione di iperlipidemia, diabete mellito e obesità di medio grado. *Acta Diabetol. Lat.* 1967;4:572-590.

[3] Haller H. Epidemiology and associated risk factors of hyperlipoproteinemia. *Z. Gesante Inn. Med.* 1977;32(8):124-8).

[4] Singer P. Diagnosis of primary hyperlipoproteinemias. *Z. Gesante Inn. Med.* 1977;32(9):129-33.

[5] Phillips GB. Sex hormones, risk factors and cardiovascular disease. *Am. J. Med.* 1978; 65: 7-11.

[6] Phillips GB. Relationship between serum sex hormones and glucose ,insulin, and lipid abnormalities in men with myocardial infarction. *Proc. Natl. Acad. Sci. U.S.A.* 1977;74: 1729-1733.

[7] Reaven GM. Role of insulin resistance in human disease. *Diabetes* 1988; 37: 1595-607.

[8] Dagdelen S,Yildrim T, Erbas T.Global confusion on the diagnostic criteria for metabolic syndrome:what is the point that guidelines can not agree? *Anadolu Kardivol Derg* 2008 ,8(2):149-53[Article in Turkish].

[9] Cussons AJ,Watts GF,Burke V,Shaw JE,Zimmet PZ,Stuckey BG. Cardiometabolic risk in polycystic ovary syndrome:a comparison of different approaches to defining the metabolic syndrome. *Hum. Reprod.* 2008;23.

[10] 2352-8 10. Hayden MR,Sowers JR,Tyagi SC..The central role of vascular extracellular matrix and basement membrane remodeling in metabolic syndrome and type 2 diabetes: the matrix preloaded. *Cardiovascular Diabetology* 2005;28; 4(1): 9.

[11] Cupisti S,Haberle L, Dittrich R, Oppelt PG, Reissman C, Kronawitter D, Beckmann MW, Mueller A. Smoking is associated with increased free testosterone and fasting insulin levels in women with polycystic ovary syndrome, resulting in aggravated insulin resistance. *Fertil. Steril.* 2009 [Epub ahead of print].

[12] Samy N,Hashim M,Sayed M, Said M.Clinical significance of inflammatory markers in polycystic ovary syndrome: their relationship to insulin resistance and body mass index. *Dis. Markers* 2009;26(4): 163-70.

[13] Verit FF. High sensitive serum C-reactive protein and its relationship with other cardiovascular risk factors in normoinsulinemic polycystic ovary patients without metabolic syndrome. *Arch. Gynecol. Obstet.* 2010;281(6):1009-14.

[14] Chen MJ,Chen HF,Chen SU,Ho HN,Yang YS, Yang WS.The relationship between follistatin and chronic low-grade inflammation in women with polycystic ovary syndrome. *Fertil. Steril.* 2009; 92(6):2041-4.

[15] Gonzales F,Rote NS, Minium J,Kirwan JP. Evidence of proatherogenic inflammation in polycystic ovary syndrome. *Metabolism* 2009 ;58(7):954-62.

[16] Tamimi W, Siddiqui IA ,Tamim H, Aleisa N,Adham M. Effect of body mass index on clinical manifestations in patients with polycystic ovary syndrome. *Int. J.Gynaecol. Obstet.* 2009;107(1):54-7.

[17] Quinonez Zarza C,Silva Ruiz R,Torres Juarez JM. Obesity, arterial hypertension, metabolic disorders, and polycystic ovary syndrome. Obesity, arterial hypertension,metabolic disorders,and polycystic ovary syndrome. *Ginecol. Obstet. Mex.* 2000; 68: 317: 22.

[18] Alexander CJ, Tangchitnob EP,Lepor NE. Polycystic ovary syndrome: a major unrecognized cardiovascular risk factor in women.*Rev.Cardiovasc.Med.* 2009;10(2): 83-90.

[19] Carmina E, Orio F,Palomba S,Longo RA, Cascella T,Colao A, Lombardi G,Rini GB, Lobo RA.Endothelial dysfunction in PCOS: role of obesity and adipose hormones. *Am. J. Med.* 2006; 119(4): 356.

[20] Adali E,Yildizhan R,Kurdoglu M, Bugdayci G,Kolusari A,Sahin HG.Increased plasma thrombin-activatable fibrinolysis inhibitor levels in young obese women with polycystic ovary syndrome. *Fertil. Steril.* 2009; [Epub ahead of print].

[21] Vervita V,Saltamavros AD,Adonakis G,Tsapanos V,Decavalas G,Georopoulos NA. Obesity and insulin resistance increase plasma viscosity in young women with polycystic ovary syndrome. *Gynecol. Endocrinol.* 2009; 25(10): 640-646.

[22] Pinhas-Hamiel O, Singer S,Pilpel N,Koren I,Boiko V,Hemi R,Pariente C, Kanetv H. Adiponectin levels in adolescent girls with polycystic ovary syndrome. *Clin. Endocrinol.* (Oxf.). 2009 ;71(6):823-7.

Insulin Resistance

Insulin resistance (IR) is not a new entity. In fact, it was first associated with diabetes in the 1930s by Harold Percival Himsworth who used the term " insulin insensitivity". IR affects between 10% to 25% of the general population.It was estimated that one in three Americans is insulin resistant, a condition that puts them at high risk for developing type2 diabetes and cardiovascular disease.Two common disorders,frequently associated with IR, are PCOS affecting 4% to 6% of reproductive-aged women, and type 2 diabetes mellitus which is observed in about 2% to 6% of similarly aged women.

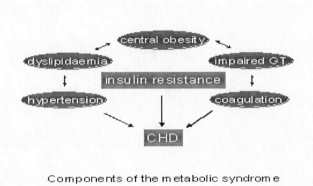

Components of the metabolic syndrome

Overall, about 50% to 70% of women with PCOS and 80% to 100% of patients with type 2 diabetes mellitus have variable degrees of Insulin resistance and its secondary hyperinsulinemia appear to underlie many of the endocrine features of PCOS in a large proportion of such patients.The risk of type 2 diabetes mellitus among PCOS patients is 5 to10-fold higher than normal. In turn, the risk of PCOS among reproductive-aged type 2 diabetes mellitus patients appears to be similarly increased [1]. People who are insulin resistant have high levels of circulating insulin because the pancreas continues to produce more and more insulin in an effort to lower rising blood glucose levels. Insulin resistance can be thought of as a set of metabolic dysfunctions associated with or contributing to a range of serious health problems.These disorders include type2 diabetes ,the metabolic syndrome, the obesity and the polycystic ovary syndrome. It is well known that, when the concentrations of blood glucose reaches a certain point, the pancreas is stimulated to release insulin in the blood.As the insulin reaches cells in muscle and fatty tissues, it attaches itself to insulin receptors on the surface of the cells. This interrelationship is the basis of the biochemical mechanism which leads to conversion of glucose to energy In the early stage of insulin resistance the pancreas steps up its production of insulin in order to control the increased levels of glucose in the blood. As a result, it is not unusual for patients to have high blood sugar and high blood insulin levels at the same time. If insulin resistance is not detected and treated, the islet of Langerhans may eventually shut down and decrease in number .

Insulin resistance (IR) increases during puberty in normal children but is also the first adverse metabolic event of obesity and the marker of the metabolic syndrome.

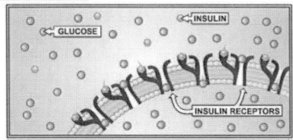

The insulin may fail to bind to the insulin receptors because of:
1) inherited gene mutation of insulin
2) abnormalities of the insulin receptor :
- type A when the receptor is missing from the cell surface or does not function properly;
- type B when the immune system produces autoantibodies to the insulin receptor

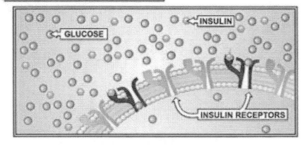

A study considered the effect of puberty on IR, in obese and normal-weight children. IR was estimated ,using the HOMA-IR index, in .424 obese children (207 pre-pubertal and 217 pubertal divided in Tanner stages 2-3, 4, and 5) Data were compared to those obtained in 123 healthy normal-weight children (40 pre-pubertal and 83 pubertal divided in Tanner stages 2-3, 4, and 5). In the obese children mean HOMA-IR increased progressively across Tanner stages, and was significantly higher in all groups (pre-pubertal and Tanner stages 2,3,4,and 5) of obese than in control children. HOMA-IR was significantly correlated with BMI.

$$\text{HOMA-IR} = \frac{(\text{Glucose in mg/dL} \times 0.05551) \times \text{insulin in } \mu IU/mL}{22.5}$$

$$\text{HOMA-}\beta\text{-cell} = \frac{20 \times \text{insulin in } \mu IU/mL}{(\text{Glucose in mg/dL} \times 0.05551) - 3.5}$$

Therefore, HOMA-IR in obese children increases at puberty more than in normal-weight children and does not return to pre-pubertal values at the end of puberty [2]. MS is clinically important since cardiovascular risk exponentially increases when a patient has more than one risk factor. A better understanding of the underlying pathophysiology might provide the basis for a more rational clinical approach to patients with MS. It remains to be determined whether PCOS and type 2 diabetes mellitus represent no more than different clinical manifestations of the same IR syndrome, with their phenotypic differences due to the presence or absence of a coincidental genetic defect at the level of the ovary or pancreas, respectively, or representing the result of etiologically different subtypes of IR syndromes [3] . Evidence shows that not all women with PCOS should be considered as being similar in term of cardiovascular risk profiles [4]. Insulin resistance, defined as a diminished effect of a given dose of insulin on glucose homeostasis, is a highly prevalent feature of women with PCOS. Insulin resistance in PCOS is closely associated with an increase in truncal-abdominal fat mass, elevated free fatty acid levels, increased androgens, particularly free testosterone through reduced SHBG levels, and anovulation. The causes for insulin resistance in PCOS are still unknown. Evidence suggests that an increase in truncal-abdominal fat mass and subsequently increased free fatty acid levels induce IR in women with PCOS. Increased effects of corticosteroids and a relative reduction in estrogen and progesterone seem to be involved in the aberrant body fat distribution. Conversely, there are also results supporting primary, genetic target cell defects as a cause of insulin resistance in PCOS.An explanation for these seemingly contradictory results could be that the group of women with PCOS is heterogeneous with respect to the primary event in carbohydrate /insulin disturbances.Also insulin secretion in PCOS is characterized by heterogeneity.At one end of the spectrum there is a large subgroup of mainly obese women with reduced insulin secretion, which appears to result from failure of the beta cells to compensate for insulin resistance in susceptible women, resulting in glucose intolerance and NIDDM.In the insulin-resistant patients with normal glucose tolerance, most of the hyperinsulinaemia is probably due to secondarily increased insulin secretion and decreased insulin degradation. However, a component of the increased first-phase insulin release is not due to measurable insulin resistance. Notably, this is also found in lean women with normal insulin sensitivity, and is not reversed after weight reduction, in contrast to the findings for insulin resistance.The implications of this enhanced insulin release are not fully clear, but it may tentatively be associated with carbohydrate craving and subsequently increased risks for development of obesity and insulin resistance. It may represent a primary disturbance of insulin secretion in PCOS or may be associated with the perturbed steroid balance in anovulation.The insulin-androgen connection in PCOS appears to be amplified by several different mechanisms, notably in both directions, the initiating event probably varying between individuals.Thus, insulin increases the biological availability of potent steroids, primarily testosterone, through the suppression of SHBG synthesis. Insulin is also involved as a progonadotrophin in ovarian steroidogenesis, with the possible net result of interfering with ovulation and/or increasing ovarian androgen production in states of hyperinsulinaemia. Conversely, testosterone may indirectly contribute to insulin resistance through facilitating free fatty acid release from abdominal fat, but perhaps also through direct muscular effects at higher serum levels. It seems likely that this constitution, presumably genetic, would provide evolutionary advantages in times of limited nutrition, given the energy-saving effects of insulin resistance.Hypothetically, hyperinsulinaemia primary could provide a stimulus to ensure intake of nourishment, but unlimited food supplies could in some cases initiate a vicious 'anabolic' circle, in which several of the proposed amplifying mechanisms between insulin and androgens , in both directions ,could take part [5].

The Relationships between IR and Obesity

In industrial societies, the prevalence of overweight, diabetes, dyslipidemia, and hypertension is steadily increasing. Since many of these apparently different conditions appear in the same patients, it has been suggested that they represent a true syndrome, and the term "metabolic syndrome" (MS) has been uniformly accepted. For researchers, the word "syndrome" implies a common pathophysiology for all observed abnormalities. It was studied the interaction between increased sympathetic activity and elevated blood pressure (BP), obesity, and the insulin resistance/diabetes components of MS, which is clinically important since cardiovascular risk exponentially increases when a patient has more than one risk factor.

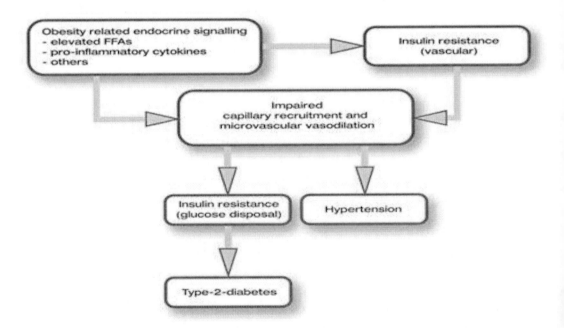

The worldwide epidemic of obesity may increase the frequency and the importance of the problems PCOS-related. Particularly , reproductive function is strongly dependent on body weight and metabolic status. Therefore, obesity may increase the risk of infertility and may impair pregnancy outcome [6,7,8,9]. A study compared the body fat distribution ,evaluated by dual X-ray absorbsiometry (DEXA),in PCOS women with age and body mass index (BDI) and investigated if the androgens and insulin resistance were associated with fat distribution. The results of this study showed that fat mass in trunk and arms were significantly higher in PCOS women than in the controls and there was a positive correlation between free testosterone and arms fat mass distribution also after controlling for age and BMI [10]. The evaluation of some metabolic risk markers as adiponectin, ghrelin, leptin and body composition in hirsute PCOS patients showed that adiponectin levels are significantly decreased in obese PCOS patients compared with weight-matched controls ($P<0.05$), that mean ghrelin was significantly lower in hirsute PCOS patients than in controls ($P<0.001$) and this remained significant after subdividing subjects according to waist circumference and BMI. In addition, testosterone correlates positively with adiponectin and negatively with ghrelin independent of BMI, WHR and total fat mass. Therefore, obese hirsute PCOS patients demonstrate significantly lower adiponectin levels than weight-matched controls suggesting a very high risk for the metabolic syndrome.Furthermore, ghrelin levels were decreased in hirsute PCOS patients and showed a significant, negative correlation with testosterone independent from body composition [11].Adipocytokines are produced by adipose tissue and have been thought to be related to insulin resistance and other health consequences. An Italian study measured leptin, adiponectin, and resistin simultaneously in women with polycystic ovary syndrome and age- and weight-matched controls. Fifty-two women with PCOS and 45 normal ovulatory women who were age- and weight-matched were studied. Blood was obtained for adipocytokines (leptin, adiponectin, and resistin) as well as hormonal parameters and markers of insulin resistance as assessed by the quantitative insulin-sensitivity check index. Body mass index was stratified into obese, overweight,and normal subgroups for comparisons between PCOS and controls. The results showed that adiponectin was lower ($P < 0.05$) and resistin was higher ($P < 0.05$) while leptin was similar to matched controls.Furthermore,a strong body mass relationship for leptin with no changes in resistin although adiponectin was lower in PCOS, was found.In controls, leptin and adiponectin and leptin and resistin correlated ($P < 0.05$) but not in PCOS. In controls, all adipocytokines correlated with markers of insulin resistance but not in PCOS. Therefore, when matched for BMI status, decreased adiponectin in PCOS represents the most marked change. This alteration may be the result of altered adipose tissue distribution and function in PCOS but no correlation with insulin resistance was found [12]. Current knowledges show that, in most obese patients, obesity is associated with a low-grade inflammation of white adipose tissue (WAT) resulting from chronic activation of the innate immune system and which can subsequently lead to insulin resistance, impaired glucose tolerance and even diabetes.

References

[1]   Kousta E, Tolis G, Franks S. Polycystic ovary syndrome-Revised diagnostic criteria and long-term health consequences. *Hormones (Athens)* 2005; 4(3): 133-47.

[2]   Pilia S, Casini MR, Foschini ML,Minerba L,Musiu MC,Marras V,Civolani P,Loche S. The effect of puberty on insulin resistance in obese children. *J. Endocrinol. Invest.* 2009; 32(5): 401-5.

[3]   Ovalle F,Azziz R. Insulin resistance, polycystic ovary syndrome, and type 2 diabetes mellitus. *Fertil. Steril.* 2002; 77(6): 1095-105.

[4] Jovanovic VP,Carmina E,Lobo RA. Not all women diagnosed with PCOS share the same cardiovascular risk profiles. *Fertil. Steril.* 2009.
[5] Holte J. Disturbances in insulin secretion and sensitivity in women with the polycystic ovary syndrome. *Baillieres Clin. Endocrinol. Metab.* 1996;10(2):221-47.
[6] Hirschberg AL.Polycystic ovary syndrome,obesity and reproductive implications. *Women Health (Lond)* 2009; 5(5): 529-40.
[7] Glueck CJ, Papanna R, Wang P,Goldenberg N,Sieve-Smith L. Incidence and treatment of metabolic syndrome in newly referred women with confirmed polycystic ovarian syndrome. Atherosclerosis, Obesity and Stroke) *Metabolism* 2003;52:908-915.
[8] Apridonidze T, Essah P,Iuorno M,Nestler JE. Prevalence and characteristics of metabolic syndrome in women with polycystic ovary syndrome. *Journal of Clinical Endocrinology and Metabolism* 2005;90:1929-1935).
[9] Essah PA,Nestler JE.The metabolic syndrome in polycystic ovary syndrome. *J. Endocrinol. Invest.* 2006;29(3):270-80.
[10] Yucel A, Noyan V,Sagsoz N. The association of serum androgens and insulin resistance with fat distribution in polycystic ovary syndrome. *Eur. J. Obstet. Gynecol. Reprod. Biol.* 2006; 126 (1):81-6.
[11] Glinborg D, Andersen M, Hagen C,Frystvk J, Hulstrom V, Flyvbjerg A, Hermann AP. Evaluation of metabolic risk markers in polycystic ovary syndrome (PCOAdiponectin, ghrelin, leptin and body composition in hirsute PCOS patients and control *Eur. J. Endocrinol.* 2006; 155(2): 337-45.
[12] Carmina E, Orio F,Palomba S,Cascella T,Longo RA,Calao AM,Lombardi G,Lobo RA Evidence for altered adipocyte function in polycystic ovary syndrome. *Eur. J. Endocrinol.* 2005; 152 (3): 389-94.

White Adipose Tissue (WAT)

White adipose tissue is one of two types of adipose tissue found in humans. It composes as much as 25% of the body weight in women. Upon release of insulin from the pancreas, the insulin receptors of the white adipose cells cause a dephosphorylation cascade that lead to the inactivation of hormone -sensitive lipase. Upon release of glucagons from the pancreas, glucagons receptors cause a phosphorylation cascade that inactivates hormone-sensitive lipase, causing the breakdown of the stored fat to fatty acid, which is exported into the blood and bound to albumin, and glycerol, which is exported into the blood freely. Fatty acid are taken up to muscle and cardiac tissue as a fuel source, and glycerol is taken up by the liver for gluconeogenenesis.

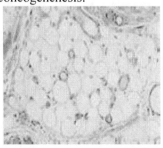

WAT serves tree functions: heat insulation, mechanical cushion, and most importantly, a source of energy. WAT acts as a thermal insulator , helping to maintain body temperature. The degree of insulation is dependent upon the thickness of the fat layer. As the major form of energy storage ,fat provides a buffer for energy imbalances when energy intake is not equal to energy output. It is an efficient way to store excess energy, because it is stored with very little water.

Consequently, more energy can be derived per gram of fat than per gram of carbohydrate protein. White adipose tissue is not as richly vascularized as brown adipose tissue, but each adipocyte in WAT is in contact with at least one capillary. Blood flow to adipose tissue varies depending upon body weight and nutritional state, with blood flow increasing during fasting [1]. In humans, adipose tissue is located beneath the skin (subcutaneous fat),around internal organs (visceral fat) and in the bone marrow (yellow bone marrow).

Adipose derived hormones

- Adiponectin
- Leptin
- Resistin
- Plasminogen activator inhibitor-1(PAI-1)

- TNF-α
- IL-6
- Angiotensin
- Estradiol

Furthermore, adipose tissue is the major peripheral source of aromatase contributing to the production of estradiol

---

Adipose tissue contains several cell types with the highest percentage of cells being adipocytes. Other cell types include: fibroblasts, macrophages and endothelial cells. White adipose tissue cells have receptors for insulin, growth hormones, norepinephrine and glucocorticoids. WAT has an endocrine function by secreting leptin and adiponectin and other molecules named adipokines including cytokines and chemokines., involved in inflammatory process. The release of adipokines by adipose tissue infiltrated macrophages lead to a chronic sub-inflammatory state [2]. .It has been more recently recognized as an active participant in numerous physiological and patho-physiological processes. In obesity, WAT is known to express and secrete a wide range of products named adipokines including adiponectin, leptin, resistin and others. In obesity, WAT is known to express and secrete a wide range of products named adipokines including adiponectin, leptin, resistin and visfatin, cytokines and chemokines such as tumor necrosis factor- alpha, interleukin-6 (IL-6) and monocyte chemoattractant protein-1 which may have local effects on WAT physiology but also systemic effects on other organs.

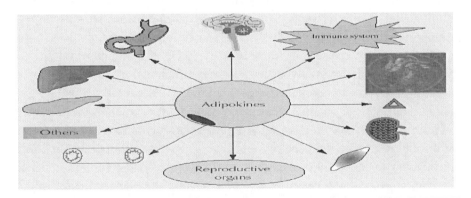

Recent data indicate that, in obese, WAT is infiltrated by macrophages which may be a major source of locally-produced pro-inflammatory cytokines (Antuna-Puente 2008) [3].

Interestingly, weight loss is associated with a reduction in the macrophage infiltration of WAT and an improvement of the inflammatory profile of gene expression. TNF-alpha is overproduced in adipose tissue of several rodent models of obesity and has an important role in the pathogenesis of insulin resistance in these species. However, its actual involvement in glucose metabolism disorders in humans, remains controversial. IL-6 production by human adipose tissue increases during obesity. It may induce hepatic CRP synthesis and may promote the onset of cardiovascular complications. Both TNF-alpha and IL-6 can alter insulin sensitivity by triggering different key steps in the insulin signaling pathway [4].In rodents, resistin can induce insulin resistance, while its implication in the control of insulin

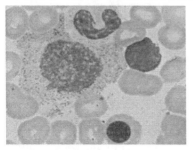

sensitivity is still a matter of debate in humans.Adiponectin is highly expressed in WAT, and circulating adiponectin levels are decreased in subjects with obesity related to insulin resistance, type 2 diabetes and coronary heart disease. Adiponectin inhibits liver neoglucogenesis and promotes fatty acid oxidation in skeletal muscle. In addition,adiponectin counteracts the pro-inflammatory effects of TNF-alpha on the arterial wall and probably protects against the development of atheriosclerosis. In obesity, the pro-inflammatory effects of cytokines through intracellular signaling pathways involve the NF-kappa B and JNK systems.Genetic or pharmacological manipulations of the inflammatory response effectors have been shown to modulate insulin sensitivity in different animal models. In humans, it has been suggested that the improved glucose tolerance observed in the presence of thiazolidinediones or statins is likely related to their anti-inflammatory properties.Thus, it can be considered that obesity corresponds to a sub-clinical inflammatory condition that promotes the production of pro-inflammatory factors involved in the pathogenesis of insulin resistance [5]. Metabolic syndrome is a major risk factor for cardiovascular and metabolic diseases playing a central role in the development of metabolic dysfunction and in its clinical consequences like visceral obesity. Adipose tissue is now considered to be an active endocrine organ that secretes various humoral factors (adipokines), and its shift to production of proinflammatory cytokines in obesity likely contributes to the low-level systemic inflammation that is seen in metabolic syndrome-associated chronic pathologies such as atherosclerosis. Recent studies have shown that obesity induces chronic local inflammation in adipose tissue, and that cells of the innate immune system, particularly macrophages, are crucially involved in adipose inflammation and systemic metabolic abnormalities. Moreover, it was recently revealed that T cells are key regulators of adipose inflammation, and that the adaptive immune system is also crucially important. In mouse models modulation of T cell function may improve not only adipose inflammation but also systemic insulin resistance induced by obesity. Thus clarification of the inflammatory processes ongoing in obese adipose tissue would seem essential for the understanding of metabolic syndrome and for developing novel therapeutic strategies to treat it [6].

The Relationships between IR and Dyslipidemia

Dyslipidemia is a feature of PCOS . It seems that mothers of women with PCOS have an elevated LDL levels and markers of insulin resistance as well as an increased prevalence of the metabolic syndrome. Particularly, it is possible to identify a subgroup of mothers with a history of irregular menses who have other features of PCOS: hyperandrogenemia, markers of insulin resistance and high levels of LDL[7,8,9]. Some studies suggested a role for androgens rather than insulin resistance in the pathogenesis of alteration in LDL levels.These considerations were based on the following observations:1) Flutemide blocking androgen action, induces an important decrease in total and LDL cholesterol in PCOS women independently from changes in body weight and insulin sensitivity [10,11]The improvement of insulin sensitivity with a thiazolidendione or with a hypocaloric diet alone or combined with metformin did not alter LDL levels in affected women [12]. Mothers of PCOS women seem to have elevated LDL levels consistent with an heritable trait. In addition, they have elevated androgen levels and markers of insulin resistance. Mothers with a history of irregular menses seem to be more severely affected.[13]. Another investigation consider the impact of fatness, insulin and gynaecological age on luteinizing hormone secretory dynamics in female adolescents.In this study LH sampling were obtained every 10 minutes/24 hours and at 20 minutes after a GnRH challenge. The results showed as the percent body fat ,and younger gynaecological age predict faster LH pulse frequency.Furthermore,fatness was negatively linked to LH-AUC (LH integrated concentration).Therefore, higher adiposity and younger gynaecological age predict rapid LH pulse frequency (LHPF).The post-menarcheal years represent a vulnerable window for an exaggerated LHPF with weight gain [14,15]. It is now recognised that by studying the immersed part of the iceberg, one can characterise a large number of people who, although not ill, are suffering from several metabolic disorders: high blood pressure, disturbed lipid and sugar metabolism, and a tendency to be overweight. This combination, without any obvious illness, is what the Scientific Community call Metabolic Syndrome. Many years ago it was recognised that a person's metabolic profile, which at that time was still poorly defined, can be very atherogenic .We know today that this is responsible for causing cardiovascular accidents such as myocardial infarction and angina pectoris, resulting in excess mortality. Recent studies have demonstrated that patients suffering from Metabolic Syndrome are 3 times more likely to experience a cardiovascular accident than persons not presenting the syndrome. In the face of this threat, we now consider it essential to go beyond the conventional risk factors and to identify the population concerned by MS . Finally,metabolic syndrome helps to identify individuals who are at high risk of developing diabetes and cardiovascular diseases (heart attack, stroke, peripheral arterial diseases).

Obesity

The prevalence of obesity is increasing in the world, affecting men,women and children. Hence, the global epidemic of overweight and obesity is rapidly becoming a major public health problem in many parts of the world. Particularly, between early 1960 and late 1980, the prevalence of obesity tripled in young black girls 6 to 11 years of age, while it doubled in white girls.Similarly,overweight and obesity in girls 12 to 17 years of age , increased with a statistically significant increase in black adolescents [16,17, 18]

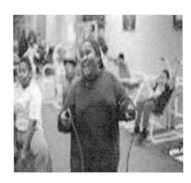

From available data, the worldwide prevalence of obesity has been found to range from less than 5% in rural China, Japan and some African countries to levels as high as 75% of the adult population in urban Samoa. Therefore,there is a different prevalence of obesity within different countries. Obesity levels also vary depending on ethnic origin. In the USA, particularly among women, there are large differences in the prevalence of obesity between populations of the different ethnic origins within the same country. In developed countries the levels of obesity are higher in the lower socio-economic groups; while, in developing countries this relationship is reversed. The transition from a rural to an urban lifestyle is associated with increased levels of obesity,which has been linked with dramatic changes in lifestyles. Epidemiological studies have showed the association with overweight and obesity of some findings : parental overweight, high weight gain during pregnancy, maternal smoking during pregnancy, high birth weight, high media consumption. Furthermore,a positive association was found between overweight/obesity and low socio-economic status (SES);while a negative association was found between these and sleep duration for 3 to 10 – years olds [19,20]. Paradoxically, coexisting with undernutrition in developing countries, the increasing prevalence of overweight and obesity is associated with many diet-related chronic diseases including diabetes mellitus, cardiovascular disease, stroke, hypertension and certain cancers. Several factors may lead to obesity: genetic, environmental, physiological, and unknown. Rare recessive causes of obesity are: the syndrome of Bardet –Biedl, the syndrome of Lawrence-Moon, the syndrome of Prader-Labhart-Willi ,as well as the syndromes related to trygliceride storage. It is not only the most common cause of insulin resistance but is a growing health concern in its own right. According to the National Institutes of Health (NIH),the percentage of Americans adults who meet the criteria for obesity rose from 25% to 33% between 1990 and 2000 with an increased of a third within the space of a decade.

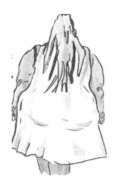

Obesity is an important risk factor for the development of type 2 diabetes, hypertension and coronary artery disease
Obesity is a leading preventable cause of death worldwide, with increasing prevalence in adults and children, and authorities view it as one of the most serious public health problems of the 21st century (Barness 2007)(21).

Insulin resistance, hyperleptinaemia and low plasma levels of adiponectin are also widely related to features of the MS. The functional capacity of the adipose tissue varies among subjects explaining the incomplete overlapping among the metabolic syndrome and obesity. Far turnover is determined by a complex equilibrium in which insulin is a main factor but not the only one. Chronically inadequate energy balance may be a key factor, stressing the system. In this situation, an adipose tissue functional failure occurs resulting in changes in systemic energy delivery, impaired glucose consumption and activation of self-regulatory mechanisms that extend their influence to the whole body homeostasis system. Lipid metabolism alterations in liver and peripheral tissues are addressed, with particular reference to adipose and muscle tissues, and the mechanisms by which some adipokines, as leptin and adiponectin, mediate the regulation of fatty acid oxidation in those tissues. The activation of the AMPK (AMP-dependent kinase) pathway, together with a subsequent increase in the fatty acid oxidation, appear to constitute the main mechanism of action of these hormones in the regulation of lipid metabolism. A decreased activation of AMPK appears to have a role in the development of features of the MS. In addition, the alteration of its signalling in the hypothalamus , which may function as a sensor of nutrient availability, integrating multiple nutritional and hormonal signals, may have a key role in the appearance of the MS [22] Worldwide, along with the increasing prevalence of obesity, the number of people with pre diabetes is increasing. The diagnostic criteria for prediabetes include impaired fasting glucose, impaired glucose tolerance, and metabolic syndrome. The presence of two or more of these three criteria makes a person at high risk for future diabetes. The treatment goal of prediabetes is to prevent future development of type 2 diabetes and diabetes-related cardiovascular complications. The treatment approach is twofold: glycemic control and control of cardiovascular risk factors, mainly hypertension and hyperlipidemia. Intensive lifestyle modification is the mainstay of treatment in low-risk patients. When lifestyle modification fails and in high-risk patients, medications such as metformin and others are recommended. For high-risk patients and those who progress despite intensive lifestyle modification, thiazolidinediones are also recommended. The goals for cardiovascular risk factor control are similar to those for patients with diabetes [23]. Systemic insulin resistance has been implicated as one possible factor that links visceral obesity to adverse metabolic consequences; however, the mechanism whereby adipose tissue causes alterations in insulin sensitivity remains unclear. Infection and inflammation are commonly associated with insulin resistance and visceral obesity is associated with a chronic, low-grade inflammatory state suggesting that inflammation may be a potential mechanism whereby obesity leads to insulin resistance. Moreover,adiposetissue is now recognized as an immune organ that secretes many immunomodulatory factors and seems to be a significant source of inflammatory signals known to cause insulin resistance. Therefore, proinflammatory cytokines and hormones released by adipose tissue can induce the chronic inflammatory profile associated with visceral obesity [24].Chronic inflammation may represent a triggering factor in the origin of the metabolic syndrome; stimuli such as overnutrition, physical inactivity, and aging would result in cytokine hypersecretion and eventually lead to insulin resistance and diabetes in genetically or metabolically predisposed subjects [25]. The metabolic syndrome,of course, could be driven by the epidemic of obesity. Obese patients (BMI>35) after blunt trauma are at increased risk compared to non-obese for organ dysfunction, prolonged hospital stay, infection, prolonged mechanical ventilation, and mortality

Classification of Obesity

Obesity is defined as the quantity of adipose tissue and not just as total body weight[26]. It is defined by body mass index (BMI) and further evaluated in terms of fat distribution via the waist hip ratio (WHR) and total cardiovascular risk factors. BMI is highly related to both percentage body fat and total body fat. A formula combining BMI, age and gender can be used to estimate a person's body fat percentage with an accuracy of 4% [27]. The most commonly used definitions, established by the World Health Organization (WHO) in 1997 and published in 2000,provide the values listed in the following table:

BMI	Classification
< 18.5	Underweight
18.5–24.9	Normal weight
25.0–29.9	Overweight
30.0–34.9	Class I obesity
35.0–39.9	Class II obesity
> 40.0	Class III obesity

The surgical Literature breaks down "class III" obesity into further categories:
- A BMI > 40 is severe obesity
- A BMI of 40.0–49.9 is morbid obesity
- A BMI of >50 is super obese

Different BMI classifications were adopted in some countries. Hence, Asian populations develop negative health consequences at a lower BMI than Caucasians, and some nations have redefined obesity. The Japan has defined obesity as any BMI greater than 25, while China uses a BMI greater than 28 [28].

Waist Circumference and Waist–Hip Ratio

The waist circumference (>102 cm in men and >88 cm in women) and the waist–hip ratio (circumference of the waist divided by circumference of the hips >0.9 for men and >0.85 for women) are both used as measures of central obesity. In those with a BMI under 35, intra-abdominal body fat is related to negative health outcomes independent of total body fat. Intra-abdominal or visceral fat has a particularly strong correlation with cardiovascular disease.. In a study of 15,000 people, waist circumference results also better correlated with metabolic syndrome than BMI.

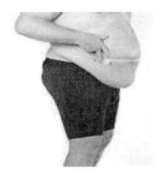

Fat distribution is also significant; in fact, insulin resistance is associated with "apple shaped figure", in which much of the excess weight is carried around the abdomen. Generally, the patient's waist-to-hip ratio(WHR) was used. A ratio greater than 0.8 in women is strongly correlated with IR (Kanazawa 2002)(28) .

Women with abdominal obesity have a cardiovascular risk similar to that of men..However,in people with a BMI over 35, measurement of waist circumference adds little to the predictive power of BMI. In any case,the majority of the individuals with this BMI have an abnormal waist circumferences. BMI values are age-independent and the same for both sexes.BMI may not correspond to the same degree of fatness in different populations;it is due, in part, to different body proportions [30]. The health risks associated with increasing BMI are continuous and the interpretation of BMI gradings in relation with risk may differ for different populations. In recent years, there was a growing debate on whether there are possible needs for developing different BMI cut-off points for different ethnic groups due to the increasing evidence that the associations between BMI, percentage of body fat, and body fat distribution differ across populations and therefore, the health risks increase below the cut-off point of 25 kg/m² that defines overweight in the current WHO classification.BMI cut-offs in Asian and Pacific populations contributed to the growing debates. Therefore, to shed some light on this debates, WHO convened the Expert Consultation on BMI in Asian populations (Singapore, 8-11 July, 2002) The WHO Expert Consultation concluded that the proportion of Asian people with a high risk of type 2 diabetes and cardiovascular disease is substantial at BMI's lower than the existing WHO cut-off point for overweight (= 25 kg/m²).However, the cut-off point for observed risk varies from 22 kg/m² (circumference of the waist divided by circumference of the hips >0.9 for men and >0.85 for women) to 25 kg/m² in different Asian populations and for high risk, it varies from 26 kg/m² to 31 kg/m² . The Consultation, therefore, recommended that the current WHO-BMI cut-off points should be retained as the international classification. But the cut-off points of 23, 27.5, 32.5 and 37.5 kg/m² are to be added as points for public health action. It was, therefore, recommended that countries should use all categories (i.e. 18.5, 23, 25, 27.5, 30, 32.5 kg/m² , and in many populations, 35, 37.5, and 40 kg/m²) for reporting purposes, with a view to facilitate international comparisons.

Body Fat Percentage

Body fat percentage is total body fat expressed as a percentage of total body weight. It is generally agreed that men with more than 25% body fat and women with more than 33% body fat are obese. Body fat percentage can be estimated from a person's BMI by the following formula:Body fat% = (1.2 BMI) + (0.23 age) − 5.4 − (10.8 gender) where gender is 0 if female and 1 if male This formula takes into account the fact that body fat percentage is 10 percentage points greater in women than in men for a given BMI. It recognizes that a person's percentage body fat increases as they age even if their weight remains constant. The results of this formula have an accuracy of 4%. There are many other methods used to determine body fat percentage. Hydrostatic weighing, one of the most accurate methods of body fat calculation, involves weighting a person underwater. Two other simpler and less accurate methods have been used historically but are now not recommended. The first is the skinfold test, in which a pinch of skin is precisely measured to determine the thickness of the subcutaneous fat layer. The other is bioelectrical impedance analysis which uses electrical resistance. Bioelectrical impedance has not been shown to provide an advantage over BMI. Body fat percentage measurement techniques mainly used for research include computed tomography (CT scan), magnetic resonance imaging (MRI), and dual energy X-ray absorptiometry (DEXA). These techniques provide very accurate measurements, but it can be difficult to obtain in the severely obese due to weight limits of most equipment and insufficient diameter of many CT or MRI scanners.

References

[1]   Greenwood MRC, Johnson PR.Genetic differences in adipose tissue metabolism and regulation. *Ann. N. Y. Acad. Sci.* 1993; 676: 253-269.

[2]   Fève B, Bastard JP, Vidal H. Relationship between obesity, inflammation and insulin resistance: new concepts. *C. R. Biol.* 2006;329(8):587-97.

[3]   Antuna-Puente B,Feve B,Fellahi S,Bastard JP. Adipokines : the missing link between insulin resistance and obesity. *Diabetes Metab.* 2008; 34(1): 2-11.

[4]   Fève B, Bastard JP. The role of interleukins in insulin resistance and type 2 diabetes mellitus. *Nat. Rev. Endocrinol.* 2009; 5(6): 305-11.

[5]   Bastard JP,Maachi M, Lagathu C,Kim M,Caron M,Vidal H,Capeau J.Feve B. Recent advances in the relationship between obesity, inflammation, and insulin resistance. *Eur. Cytokine Netw.* 2006; 17(1): 4-12.

[6]   Nishimura S, Manabe I, Nagai R. Adipose tissue inflammation in obesity and metabolic syndrome. *Discov. Med.* 2009; 8(41):55-60.

[7]   Dunaif A,Graf M,Mandeli J,Laumas V, Dobrjansky A. Characterization of groups of hyperandrogenic women with acanthosis nigricans, impaired glucose tolerance, and/or hyperinsulinemia. *J. Clin. Endocrinol. Metab.* 1987; 65(3):499-507.

[8] Legro RS, Kunselman AR,Dunaif A. ;111(8):607-13.Prevalence and predictors of dyslipidemia in women with polycystic ovary syndrome. *Am. J. Med.* 2001; 111(8):607-13.

[9] Graf MJ,Richards CJ,Brown V,Meissner L,Dunaif A. The independent effects of hyperandrogenaemia, hyperinsulinaemia, and obesity on lipid and lipoprotein profiles in women. *Clin. Endocrinol.* (Oxf.) 1990;33 (1):119-31.

[10] Diamanti-Kandarakis E,Mitrakou A, Raptis S,Tolis G,Duleba AJ. The effect of a pure antiandrogen receptor blocker, flutamide, on the lipid profile in the polycystic ovary syndrome. *J. Clin. Endocrinol. Metab.* 1998;83(8): 2699-2705.

[11] Gambineri A,Pelusi C, Genghini S, Morselli –Labate AM, Cacciari M, Pagotto U, Pasquali R Effect of flutamide and metformin administered alone or in combination in dieting obese women with polycystic ovary syndrome. *Clin. Endocrinol.* (Oxford) 2004; 60(2 :241-249.

[12] Legro RS, Azziz R,Ehrmann D,Fereshetian AG, O'Keefe M,Ghazzi M.N. Minimal response of circulating lipids in women with polycystic ovary syndrome to improvement in insulin sensitivity with troglitazone. *J. Clin. Endocrinol. Metab.* 2003; 88(11):5137-5144.

[13] Sam S,Legro RS,Essah PA, Apridonidze T,Dunaif A. Evidence for metabolic and reproductive phenotypes in mothers of women with polycystic ovary syndrome. *Proc. Natl. Acad. Sci.* 2006; 103(18): 7030-35.

[14] Kasa-Vubu JZ,Jain V,Welch K. Impact of fatness,insulin and gynaecological age on luteinizing hormone secretory dynamics in adolescent females. *Fertil. Steril.* 2009 [Epub ahead of print].

[15] Ovalle F,Azziz R.Insulin resistance, polycystic ovary syndrome, and type 2 diabetes mellitus. *Fertil. Steril.* 2002;77(6):1095-105.

[16] Kimm SY,Barton BA,Obarzanek E,McMahon RP,Sabry ZI, Waclawiw MA,Schreiber GB,Morrison JA,Similo S,Daniels SR.Racial divergence in adiposity during adolescence:The NHLBI Growth and Health Study. *Pediatrics* 2001;107(3): E34.

[17] Crawford PB,Story M,Wang MC,Ritchie LD,Sabry ZI.Ethnic issues in the epidemiology of childhood obesity. *Pediatr. Clin. North. Am.* 2001;48(4):855-878.

[18] Lee JM, Appugliese D,Kaciroti N,Corwyn RF, Bradley RH,Lumeng JC.Weight Status in young girls and the onset of puberty. *Pediatrics* 2007; 119(3):624-630.

[19] Maffeis C.Aetiology of overweight and obesity in children and adolescents. *Eur. J. Pediatr.* 2000; 159(Suppl.1):35-44.

[20] Reilly JJ,Armstrong J,Dorosty AR,Emmett PM,Ness A,Rogers I,Steer C,Sherriff A.Early life risk factors for obesity in childhood:cohort sudy. *Br. Med. J.* 2005; 330: 1357-1364.

[21] Barness LA,Opitz JM, Gilbert--Barness E. Obesity:genetic,molecular,and environmental aspects. *Am. J .Med. Genet.* 2007; 143(24): 3016-34.

[22] Sumarac –Dumanovic M,Jeremic D .Adipokines and lipids. *Med. Pregl.* 2009; Suppl.3: 47-53.

[23] Sharma MD, Garber AJ. What is the best treatment for prediabetes? *Curr. Diab. Rep.* 2009; 9 (5):335-41.

[24] Wisse BE.The inflammatory syndrome: the role of adipose tissue cytokines in metabolic disorders linked to obesity. *J. Am. Soc. Nephrol.* 2004;15(11):2792-800.

[25] Esposito K,Giugliano D. The metabolic syndrome and inflammation: association or causation? *Nutr. Metab. Cardiovasc. Dis.* 2004; 14(5):228-32.

[26] Janssen I,Katzmarzyk PT,Ross R. Waist circumference and not body mass index explains obesity-related health risk. *Am. J. Clin. Nutr.* 279(3):379-84.

[27] Gray DS,Fujioka K.Use of relative weight and Body Mass Index for the determination of adiposity. *J. Clin. Epidemiol.* 1991;44(6): 545-50.
[28] Kanazawa M,Yoshilke N,Osaka Y,Numba Y,Zimmet P, Inove S.Criteria and classification of obesity in Japan and Asia- Oceania. *Asia Pac. J. Clin. Nutr.* 2002; 11(Suppl.8): 732-737.
[29] Bei-Fan Z. Predictive values of body mass index and waist circumference for risk factors of related diseases in Chinese adults: study on optimal cut-off points of body mass index and waist circumference in Chinese adults. *Asia Pac. J. Clin. Nutr.* 2002; 11 (Suppl 8): 685-93.
[30] Yusuf S,Hawken S,Ounpuun S, Dans T, Avezum A,Lanas F,McQueen M,Budaj A,Varigos J,Lisheng L.Effects of potentially modifiable risk factors associated with myocardial infarction in 52 countries. *Lancet* 2004; 364: 937-52.

Overweight and obesity in Children and Adolescents

The prevalence and magnitude of childhood obesity are dramatically increasing in recent years. There is an epidemic of obesity affecting childhood and adolescents worldwide.In fact,childhood obesity has reached epidemic levels in 21st century with rising rates in both developed and developing countries.Rates of obesity in Canadian boys have increased from 11% in 1980s to over 30% in 1990s, while during this same time period, rates increased from 4 to 14% in Brazilian children. In the USA, the percentage of overweight children has doubled in the last 30 years, from 15% to 32%. Data from 79 developing countries and a number of industrialised countries suggest that about 22 million children under 5 years old are overweight worldwide (WHO 1998). .

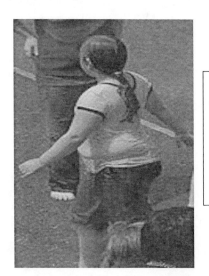

The healthy BMI range varies with the age and sex of the child. Obesity in children and adolescents is defined as a BMI greater than the 95th percentile and thus this definition has not been affected by the recent evaluations.

Recent reports indicated that 16% of American children, 2 to 19 years old, are overweight [1]. As with obesity in adults, many different factors contribute to the rising rates of childhood obesity. Changing diet and decreasing physical activity are believed to be the two most important factors in causing the recent increase of the obesity rate. Young adults are becoming more and more obese because of their poor nutritional habits. Metabolic consequences of obesity, including insulin resistance, type 2 diabetes mellitus, hyperlipidemia, hypertension, polycystic ovarian syndrome and non-alcoholic fatty liver infiltration, are rapidly emerging in the pediatric population.

Weight categories in Childhood and Adolescence

- Underweight : $< 5^{th}$ percentile
- Normal : 5th to $< 85^{th}$ percentile
- At risk of overweight : 85th to $< 95^{th}$ percentile
- Overweight : 95th percentile and above

Looking for effective strategies to identify and treat these obesity related comorbidities in children are crucial for the prevention of future cardiovascular disease and poor health outcomes [2].Considering that childhood obesity often persists into adulthood, and is associated with several health complications, it is important that obese children could be tested for hypertension, diabetes , hyperlipidemia, and fatty liver. A recent survey of the Center for Disease Control and Prevention found that 25% of obese adults were overweight as children. Furthermore, it seems that, if overweight begins before 8 years of age,obesity in adulthood is likely to be more severe.Treatments used in children are primarily lifestyle interventions and behavioral techniques. Medications are not FDA approved for their use in this age group. There are many things that teens can do to become less obese, such as a regular exercise and a right nutritional diet. Teens who are obese usually have an environment around them that shows them to be the way they are. Many factors contribute to a teen's weight. Results from Examination Survey showed that 17% of children ages 2-19 years old are overweight. Children between the ages of 6-11 have increased from 11 to 19% from 1988-94 to 2003-2004. Based on these data, overweight in children and adolescents was stable from the 1960s to 1980 whether, since 1994, overweight in youths has increased In 2003-2004, NHANES estimated that 66% of U.S. adults are either obese or overweight .Over the last 25 years there has been an increase in the prevalence of individuals who are either overweight or obese.A complex interaction of different factors may induce childhood overweight and obesity: genetic feature, lifestyle, environment,ethnic minority, familial low income. Among adults,it has been established a negative relationship between socioeconomic status (SES) and being overweight or obese; however, the relationship appears weaker and less consistent in children [3,4].A number of studies find that SES is negatively associated with children being overweight or obese.It likely appears that the relationship between SES and obesity varies by race/ethnicity, such that the negative relationship is only apparent among white adolescents and is not apparent among black or Mexican-American adolescents [5].In other words, Black and Latino children from families with higher socioeconomic status are no less likely to be overweight or obese than those in families with lower socioeconomic status. Despite the more pronounced impact of SES among White children, they are substantially less likely to be overweight or obese than Black, Latino, or Native American children, who are disproportionately affected by obesity [6,7].In 2003, a regional survey in the Aberdeen area, showed as American Indian boys ages 5-17 years old had a prevalence of overweight at 22 percent and children/girls at 18 percent for the same age group [8].

Adolescent Girls.Prevalence of Obesity by Race/Ethnicity (Aged 12–19 Years)		
	Survey Periods	
	NHANES III 1988–1994	NHANES 2003–2006
Non-Hispanic White	7.4%	14.5%
Non-Hispanic Black	13.2%	27.7%
Mexican American	9.2%	19.9%

Furthermore, the prevalence at which obesity has been increasing in children in the recent years has been even more pronounced and rapid among minority children: between 1986 and 1998, obesity prevalence among African Americans and Hispanics increased up to 120 percent, as compared to a 50 percent increase among non-Hispanic whites. Findings from studies suggest that the effects of race/ ethnicity and SES on the prevalence of childhood obesity cannot be individually determined because they are collinear.

Therefore, evidence is often inconsistent as a result of the difficulty of separating the overlapping factors [5]. Furthermore, the relationship among race/ ethnicity, SES, and childhood obesity may result from a number of underlying causes, including less healthy eating patterns, engaging in less physical activity, more sedentary behavior, and cultural attitudes about body weight. Clearly, these factors tend to co-occur and are likely to jointly contribute to differentials in increased risk of obesity in children [6,9].Obesity is a serious health concern for children and adolescents and disproportionately affects certain minority youth populations. NHANES found that African American and Mexican American adolescents ages 12-19 were more likely to be overweight than non-Hispanic White adolescents. In children 6-11 years old, 22 percent of Mexican American children were overweight, whereas 20 percent of African American children and 14 percent of non-Hispanic In addition to the children and teens who were overweight in 1999-2002, another 15 percent were at risk of becoming overweight. In a national survey on American Indian children 5-18 years old, 39 percent were found to be overweight or at risk for overweight [10] Data from National Health and Nutrition Examination Survey (NHANES) (1976–1980 and 2003–2006) show that the prevalence of obesity has increased: for children aged 2–5 years, prevalence increased from 5.0% to 12.4%; for those aged 6–11 years, prevalence increased from 6.5% to 17.0%; and for those aged 12–19 years,prevalence increased from 5.0% to 17.6%.

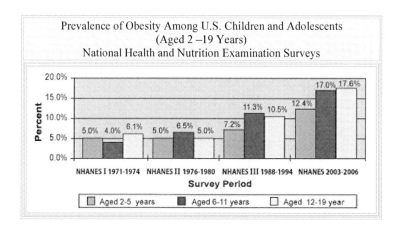

Obese children and adolescents are at risk for health problems during their youth and as adults. For example, during their youth, obese children and adolescents are more likely to have risk factors associated with cardiovascular disease ,high blood pressure, high cholesterol, and Type 2 diabetes, than are other children and adolescents. The prevalence of the metabolic syndrome is high among obese children and adolescents, and it increases with worsening obesity.Biomarkers of an increased risk of adverse cardiovascular outcomes are already present in these youngsters[3,11]. The constellation of elevated levels of abdominal adiposity, blood pressure, glucose, and triglycerides and lowered high-density lipoprotein-cholesterol has been termed the metabolic syndrome (Third Report of the National Cholesterol Education Program (NCEP). Expert Panel on Detection, Evaluation, and Treatment of High Blood Cholesterol in Adults -Adult Treatment Panel III-: Final Report. Bethesda, 2002). Given the current pediatric obesity epidemic, it is perhaps not surprising that recent reports suggest the emergence of the metabolic syndrome during childhood and adolescence[12,13,14].Data of the National Health and Nutrition Examination Survey (NHANES III 1988–1994) (U.S.) showed that the prevalence rate of the metabolic syndrome was 4% in 12–19 yr old adolescents .Currently, there is no agreement regarding the definition of the metabolic syndrome in children or adolescents. Several investigators have selected various criterion values to estimate the prevalence of the metabolic syndrome in children and adolescents, on the basis of absolute values of fasting plasma triglyceride levels, fasting plasma HDLcholesterol levels, and fasting plasma glucose levels, coupled with age and gender specific 90th percentile values for waist circumference and blood pressure [15, 16,17]. However, it is more informative to link the adult metabolic syndrome directly to childhood risk factors in the same individuals,and to establish criterion values according to age and gender that are associated with metabolic and cardiovascular health later in life.Significant tracking of obesity and blood pressure from childhood into adulthood has been observed, and the onset of obesity and hypertension often begins in childhood [18]. However, little is known about the accuracy of age and gender specific cut-off values for blood pressure in childhood in predicting hypertension and the metabolic syndrome later in life, because of the paucity of serial data collected for the same individuals over several decades. Lacking such serial data, earlier studies were not capable of ascertaining the age in childhood when values for risk factors diverge between subjects who develop hypertension or the metabolic syndrome in adulthood and those who do not. A study identifies the earliest age of divergence of blood pressure in childhood among adults with the metabolic syndrome and age and gender matched adults without the metabolic syndrome. The same study also establishes age and gender specific criterion values of childhood blood pressure for predicting hypertension and the metabolic syndrome later in life and validates the predictiveness of these childhood criterion values independent of the effects of age when the metabolic syndrome was first diagnosed and independent of childhood BMI. Based on current estimates,more than 2 million of U.S adolescents have the metabolic syndrome phenotype [1,19,20,21]. Obese children and adolescents are more likely to become obese as adults For example, one study found that approximately 80% of children who were overweight at aged 10–15 years were obese when adults at age 25 years. Another study found that 25% of obese adults were overweight as children[22,23]. In girls, abdominal fat distribution is associated with cardiovascular risk factors, independently of overall adiposity. International definition of abdominal obesity in children is required to standardize studies and to progress in the evaluation of childhood obesity and its consequences [24]. Obesity is associated with elevated blood pressure (BP) both in adults and children. Childhood obesity has become a severe health problem, especially during the last few decades. So far there has not been any large-scale study specifically focusing on the association between obesity and BP in early life. A study systematically examined the association between obesity and BP in preschool Chinese children. In 1996, measurements of weight, height, and BP values were collected in a nationwide, case-control study of 748 boys and 574 girls who ranged in age from 0.1 to 6.9 years in 8 cities in mainland China. The BP differences of the mean-matched pair were approximately 5 mm Hg for systolic blood pressure (SBP) and approximately 4 mm Hg for diastolic blood pressure (DBP) ; a higher value was noted in obese children.The BP value of 19.4% children in the obese group and 7.0% children in the nonobese group was higher than the 95th percentile value,which is defined as high BP by the Task Force on Blood Pressure Control in Children.Both SBP and DBP were significantly positively related to body mass index values for children in obese and nonobese groups .To be specific, an increase of 1 BMI unit was associated with, on average, an increase of 0.56 mm Hg and 0.54 mm Hg in SBP and DBP,respectively,for obese children.In nonobese children , the increase in SBP and DBP was 1.22 mm Hg and 1.20 mm Hg, respectively. An increase in the BMI is conclusively associated with elevated SBP and DBP in nonobese children. Furthermore, an increase in the BMI was associated with an increase in SBP and DBP in obese and nonobese children [25]. Some studies suggest that the presence of metabolic syndrome before adulthood may identify those at high risk for later cardiovascular morbidity, but there are few data examining the reliability of pediatric metabolic syndrome.To examine the short and long-term stability of pediatric metabolic syndrome a study was performed. Metabolic syndrome was defined as having at least three of the following: waist circumference,blood pressure,and fasting serum triglycerides in the 90th or higher percentile for age/sex; high-density lipoprotein-cholesterol 10th or lower percentile for age/sex; and fasting serum glucose of at least 100 mg/dl. Short-term metabolic syndrome stability was assessed in 220 obese youth ages 6-17 yr. Long-term metabolic syndrome stability was studied in 146 obese and nonobese children age 6-12 yr at baseline.The results showed as the diagnosis of metabolic syndrome was unstable in 31.6% of cases. At their short-term follow-up visit, incidence of metabolic syndrome among participants who did not have metabolic syndrome at baseline was 24%. In the long term, the diagnosis of metabolic syndrome was unstable in 45.5% of cases. Therefore, cut-off point based definitions for pediatric metabolic syndrome have substantial instability in the short and long term [25]. Popular media, health experts and researchers talk about a paediatric obesity epidemic with exponentially increasing rates of obesity and overweight. However, some recent reports suggest that prevalence may have plateaued. It was examined the trend in the prevalence of Australian childhood overweight and obesity since 1985. Specifically, the aim of this investigation was to determine whether there have been overall increases in average body mass index (BMI), differential patterns of change within age groups and increases in BMI within each weight-status category. Forty-one Australian studies of childhood weight status, performed between 1985 and 2008 were reviewed.The studies included data on 264.905Australians aged 2-18 years,with data being available on 70 758 children (27%). Children were classified as overweight or obese based on BMI using the criteria of Cole et al. [25] There has been a plateau, or only slight increase, in the percentage of boys and girls classified as overweight or obese, with almost no change over the last 10 years. In boys and girls, prevalence rates have settled around 21-25% for overweight and obesity together, and 5-6% for obesity alone. Similar trends were found for BMI scores. These patterns were fairly consistent across the age span. Within each weight-status category, average BMI has not increased.. Although levels of Australian paediatric overweight remain high, the prevalence of overweight and obesity seems to have flattened. Fasting plasma non-esterified fatty acid levels were lower in the obese versus normal-weight children (P=0.021). Both at baseline and postprandially, plasma adiponectin levels were lower in the obese versus normal-weight children (P<0.001). It was observed that levels of tumor necrosis factor-alpha were lower in the obese versus normal-weight children. Adiponectin was inversely associated with insulin in the obese children ,after adjustment for BMI and sex.At prepubertal age,obese children showed lower fasting and postprandial plasma adiponectin levels in comparison to normal-weight children, whereas non-esterified fatty acids and tumor necrosis factor-alpha(TNF alpha) were not yet increased. Therefore, adiponectin appears to be a good marker of early metabolic alterations associated with childhood obesity [26,27]. Considering the high prevalence and the increasing trends,obesity is now considered as a public health problem in numerous countries.Consequently, the main aim of the National Program of Nutrition and Health is to stop the increasing prevalence of childhood obesity. When a child is identified as having a real risk of obesity,simple preventive measures,adapted for each subject,could avoid a development toward massive obesity,wich may become difficult to reduce if managed too late [28].

References

[1] Ogden CL,Carroll MD,Flegal KM. High body mass in dex for age among US children and adolescents, 2003-2006. *Jama* 2008; 299(20): 1401-2405.

[2] Ode KL,Frohnert BI,NathanBM. Identification and treatment of metabolic complications in pediatric obesity. *Rev. Endocr. Metab. Disord.* 2009; 10(3):167-88.

[3] Strauss, R.S. and Knight, J. . Influence of the home environment on the development of obesity in children. *Pediatrics* 1999; 103 (6): 85.

[4] Hyattsville, MD.; Berkowitz, R.I. and Stunkard, A.J. Development of childhood obesity. In Wadden, and Stunkard (ed). Handbook of obesity treatment 2002; pp. 515-531.

[5] Troiano, R.P. and Flegal, K.M. (1998). Overweight children and adolescents: Description, epidemiology, and demographics. *Pediatrics* 1998;101 (3): 497-504.

[6] Crawford BP, Story M, Wang MC, Ritchie LD, Sabry ZI . Ethnic issues in the epidemiology of childhood obesity. *Pediatr. Clin. North Am.* 2001; 48 (4), 855-878.

[7]   Strauss RS, Pollack HA. Epidemic increase in childhood overweight, 1986-1998. *JAMA* 2001; 286 (22), 2845-2848.

[8]   Zephier E, Himes JH, Story M. Prevalence of overweight and obesity in American Indian school children and adolescents in the Aberdeen area: A population study. (1999) *International Journal of Obesity* 1999; 23, S28-S30.

[9]   Sobal, J. and Stunkard, A.J. Socioeconomic status and obesity: A review of the literature. *Psychological Bulletin* 1989; 105, 260-275.

[10]   Yvonne.J. Height, weight, and body mass index of American Indian school children, 1990-1991. *Journal of the American Dietetic Association* 1993; 93(10) 1136-1140.

[11]   Engelmann G., Lenhartz H., Grulich-Henn J., Davis T. M.E., Ee C. K., Invitti C., Gilardini L., Viberti G., Weiss R., Yeckel C. W., Caprio S. Obesity and the Metabolic Syndrome in Children and Adolescents. *N. Engl. J. Med.* 2004; 351:1146-1148.

[12]   Anderson PM, Butcher KE. Childhood obesity: trends and potential causes. *Future* Child. 2006;16:19–45.

[13]   Eisenmann JC. Secular trends in variables associated with the metabolic syndrome of North American children and adolescents. *Am. J. Hum. Biol.* 2003;15: 786–794.

[14]   Cook S,Weitzman M, Auinger P, Nguyen M, Dietz WH. Prevalence of a metabolic syndrome phenotype in adolescents. *Arch. Pediatr. Adolesc. Med.* 2003;137 :821 –827.

[15]   Cruz ML, Goran MI. The metabolic syndrome in children and adolescents. *Curr. Diabetes Rep.* 2004;4 :53 –62.

[16]   16.Weiss R, Dziura J, Burgert T. Obesity and metabolic syndrome in children and adolescents. N Engl J Med. 2004;350 :2362 –2374.

[17]   17.Berenson GS, Srinivasan SR, Bao W, Newman WP III, Tracy RE, Wattingney WA.Association between multiple cardiovascular risk factors and atherosclerosis in children and young adults. N Engl. J Med. 1998;338 :1650 –1656.

[18]   Duncan GE, Li SM, Zhou XH. Prevalence and trends of a metabolic syndrome phenotype among u.s. Adolescents, 1999-2000. *Diabetes Care.* 2004;27:2438–2443.

[19]   Ogden CL, Flegal KM, Carroll MD, Johnson CL. Prevalence and trends in overweight among U.S. children and adolescents, 1999–2000. *JAMA* 2002;288:1728–1732.

[20]   Hedley AA, Ogden CL, Johnson CL, Carroll MD, Curtin LR, Flegal KM. Prevalence of overweight and obesity among US children, adolescents, and adults, 1999–2002. *JAMA* 2004; 291:2847–2850.

[21]   American Academy of Pediatrics. Prevention of pediatric overweight and obesity. *Pediatrics* 2003; 112(2):424-30.

[22]   Botton L,Heude B,Kettaneh A,Borys JM,Lommez A,Bresson JL,Ducimetiere P,Charles MA; FLVS Study Group. Cardiovascular risk factor levels and their relationships with overweight and fat distribution in children: the Fleurbaix Laventie Ville Santé II study. *Metabolism* 2000;56(5): 614-22.

[23]   He Q,Ding ZY,Fong DY, Karlberg J.Blood pressure is associated with body mass index in both normal and obese children. *Hypertension* 2000; 36(2): 165-70..

[24]   Gustafson JK,Yanoff LB,Easter BD,Brady SM,Keil MF,Roberts MD,Sebring NG,Han JC, Yanovski SZ, Hubbard VS,Yanovski JA.The stability of Metabolic Syndrome in Children and Adolescents .*Clin. Endocrinol. Metab.* 2009 94(12):4828-34.

[25]   Cole TJ,Bellizzi MC,Flegal KM,Dietz WH. Establishing a standard definition for child overweight and obesity worldwide:international survey. *BMJ*, 2000; 320:(7244): 1240-3

[26] Olds TS,Tomkinson GR,Ferrar KE,Maher CA. Trends in the prevalence of childhood overweight and obesity in Australia between 1985 and 2008. *Int. J. Obes. (Lond)*2010;34(1):57-66.

[27] Gil-Campos M,Ramirez Tortosa MC,Aquilera CM,Canete R,Gil A. Fasting and postprandial adiponectin alterations anticipate NEFA and TNF-alpha changes in prepubertal obese children. *Nutr. Metab. Cardiovasc. Dis.* 2009; [Epub ahead of print].

[28] Thibault H,Rolland-Cachera MF.Prevention strategies of childhood obesity. *Arch. Pediatr.* 2003;10(12): 1100-8.

Genetic Factors

Animal studies showed some genetic causes of obesity : recessive, dominant or polygenic. Up to now,a specific genetic cause of obesity has yet to be detected in humans, in absence of other concurrent genetic syndromes . However, twin and familial studies suggested a genetic component of obesity that can be modulated by environmental factors in which food intake and the degree of physical activity are of great importance. Other factors may be an alterated adipose tissue metabolism, hormonal changes such as hyperinsulinemia and defects regarding the control satiety by the hypothalamus. In fact, some subjects show an evident eating disorder. Some depressed or stressed subjects may eat large meals as reaction to their psychological state. In any case, an excessive weight gain generally remains resulting a lifelong obesity [1]. Elevated free fatty acids (FFAs) seem to be involved in insulin resistance of polycystic ovary syndrome (PCOS). It was investigated the role of fatty acid transporter CD36, hormone-sensitive lipase (HSL) and adipose triglyceride lipase (ATGL) in regulation of lipolysis,in insulin-resistant women with PCOS . CD36, HSL and ATGL proteins were analyzed in omental adipose tissue from 10 women with PCOS and 10 healthy women. Women with PCOS had higher fasting and 2 h insulin levels, a higher homeostasis model insulin resistance index and a lower fasting glucose-to-insulin ratio than controls. CD36 protein levels in the PCOS women were higher (268% with respect to control levels) and HSL protein levels were lower (43% with respect to control levels). However, ATGL protein levels were not different in the two groups. Fasting serum insulin levels showed a positive correlation with CD36 levels and a negative correlation with HSL levels . Furthermore, a positive correlation was found between serum testosterone levels and CD36 protein levels but the correlation did not reach significance after controlling for HOMA-IR.After adjusting insulin resistance index of HOMA-IR , only CD36 differed between PCOS and control . Therefore, it was suggested that, in insulin-resistant women with PCOS, changes in CD36 and HSL expression may result in altered FFA uptake [2]. Currently, a study investigated serum adiponectin concentrations in adolescent girls with and without polycystic ovary syndrome with the aim to assess possible correlations of adiponectin levels with insulin and androgen levels. Forty four adolescent girls were grouped as follows: 14 were overweight with PCOS; 16 were lean with PCOS; and 14 were lean without PCOS. Blood samples were collected from all girls between 8 and 11 am, after an overnight fast. Serum levels of adiponectin, leptin, insulin,Müllerian inhibiting substance (MIS), luteinizing hormone (LH), follicle-stimulating hormone (FSH), testosterone (T),17-alpha-hydroxy progesterone (DHEAS), androstendione, and 17-oestradiol were measured. The results of this study showed that adiponectin concentrations were significantly decreased in obese adolescents with PCOS (10.5 ± 5.5 mug/ml) compared with lean girls with or without PCOS (16.9 ± 8.64 and 18.0 ± 7.4 mcg/ml, respectively). Leptin levels were significantly elevated in obese adolescents with PCOS compared with levels in normal weight adolescents with PCOS, and compared with normal weight controls. Insulin levels were markedly higher in obese adolescents with PCOS compared with normal weight adolescents (12.3 ± 12.2 vs. 4.5 ± 2.9, p<0.05), and compared with normal weight PCOS adolescents (7.4 ± 4.9), however this difference was not statistically significant. Insulin levels did not differ between normal weight adolescents with PCOS and normal controls. Adiponectin concentrations correlated inversely with BMI, leptin and insulin. Therefore, hypoadiponectinemia is evident only in obese adolescents with PCOS and does not seem to be involved in the pathogenesis of PCOS, in this age group [3]. Adipocytokines are produced by adipose tissue and have been thought to be related to insulin resistance and other health consequences. A study simultaneously considered leptin, adiponectin, and resistin in women with polycystic ovary syndrome (PCOS) and age- and weight-matched controls. Fifty-two women with PCOS and 45 normal ovulatory women who were age- and weight-matched were studied. Body mass index (BMI) was stratified into obese, overweight, and normal subgroups for comparisons between PCOS and controls. The results of this investigation showed as adiponectin was lower (P < 0.05) and resistin was higher (P < 0.05) while leptin was similar to matched controls. Breakdown of the groups into subgroups showed a strong body mass relationship for leptin with no changes in resistin although adiponectin was lower in PCOS, even controlling for BMI. In controls, leptin and adiponectin and leptin and resistin correlated but not in PCOS. In conclusion .it seems that when matched for BMI status, decreased adiponectin in PCOS represent the most marked change. This alteration may be the result of altered adipose tissue distribution and function in PCOS but no correlation with insulin resistance was found [4].Another study compared serum levels of resistin and adiponectin in women with polycystic ovary syndrome (PCOS) and normal controls. Seventy-six patients (36 obese, 40 non-obese) with PCOS and 42 healthy subjects were included in the study. Serum levels of resistin, adiponectin, follicle-stimulating hormone, luteinising hormone, dehydroepiandrosterone sulfate (DHEA-S), 17 hydroxyprogesterone, free testosterone, androstenedione,glucose,insulin and lipid parameters were measured. Insulin resistance and carbohydrate metabolism were evaluated by using the homeostasis model (HOMA) and the area under the insulin curve (AUCI). This study confirmed that plasma resistin levels, HOMA -IR and AUCI were significantly higher and adiponectin level was lower in women with PCOS than those in healthy women. Plasma resistin levels were similar among obese and non-obese women with PCOS. No correlation was observed between resistin, body mass index (BMI), HOMA-IR, AUCI, insulin, lipid parameters and serum androgen levels. In obese PCOS patients, adiponectin levels were lower than in the lean PCOS patients. A negative correlation was observed among adiponectin, HOMA-IR, AUCI, BMI, testosterone, DHEAS, total-cholesterol, LDL-cholesterol and lipoprotein levels.Therefore, these results suggest that the serum adiponectin level may be involved in the pathogenesis of PCOS ; while, resistin levels are independently associated with insulin resistance and BMI, in PCOS patients [5]. Polycystic ovary syndrome is associated with an increased incidence of insulin resistance (IR), obesity, and type 2 diabetes. Resistin, an adipocytokine, may represent a link between obesity, and these metabolic disorders. There is also evidence that inflammation is a hyperresistinemic state in humans, and cytokine induction of resistin may contribute to insulin resistance in endotoxemia, obesity, and other inflammatory states. In contrast, adiponectin, increases insulin sensitivity, improves glucose tolerance, inhibits inflammatory pathways, while adenovirus-expressed adiponectin reduces atherosclerotic lesions in a mouse model of atherosclerosis. It was investigated , in women with PCOS, whether there is a relationship between adiponectin and resistin and the indices of IR, and whether serum levels of these adipocytokines are altered by glucose-induced hyperinsulinaemia. In 19 women with PCOS (BMI 29.3 ± 7.7 kg/m²) serum levels of resistin and adiponectin were measured at 0, 60, and 120 min during 75 g oral glucose tolerance test (OGTT) and correlated with the indices of IR, such as HOMA-IR, QUICKI, and the insulin resistance index, calculated from glucose and insulin levels obtained during OGTT. There was no change in resistin concentrations but there was an increase in adiponectin from 11.32 ± 4.64 microg/ml at baseline to 14.78 ± 7.41 microg/ml, at 120 min of OGTT (P < 0.01). The magnitude of the overall rise in adiponectin was greater from 60 to 120 min. Neither resistin, nor adiponectin correlated with the indices of IR, lipids, or other hormonal parameters of the PCOS. There was, however, a significant negative correlation between serum resistin and adiponectin (P = 0.001). In conclusion, it was observed a strong negative correlation between serum adiponectin and resistin, despite the lack of direct correlation with the indices of IR. Given the opposite effects of resistin and adiponectin on the inflammatory process, may be hypothesized that relative proportion of adiponectin-to-resistin potentially influence cardiometabolic risk in women with the PCOS, independently of IR parameters.In any case, this observed increase in adiponectin during OGTT requires further studies [6]. It has been suggested that changes in adiponectin levels may contribute to improved insulin sensitivity in insulin resistant individuals both after weight loss and after treatment with thiazolidinedione compounds. If this is correct, then changes in total circulating adiponectin and/or distribution of its multimeric complexes should coincide with improvements in insulin sensitivity after both interventions. To address this issue, fasting adiponectin concentrations and distribution of adiponectin complexes were measured in plasma samples in 24 insulin-resistant, nondiabetic subjects before and after 3-4 months of treatment with either rosiglitazone or caloric restriction. The degree of insulin resistance in each group of 12 subjects was equal at baseline and improved to a similar extent (approximately 30%) after each therapy. Whereas total adiponectin levels increased by nearly threefold and the relative amount of several higher molecular weight adiponectin complexes increased significantly in the rosiglitazone treatment group; while, there were no discernible changes in adiponectin levels or in the distribution between high or low molecular weight complexes in the weight loss group. These data indicate that, although changes in total adiponectin and several specific adiponectin complexes paralleled improvements in insulin resistance in thiazolidinedione-treated subjects, neither circulating adiponectin concentrations nor multimeric complexes changed in association with enhanced insulin sensitivity after moderate weight loss in 12 insulin-resistant, obese individuals were detected. [7]. In the adiponectin gene polymorphisms, single-nucleotide polymorphism (SNP)-45 and SNP276 have reported to be associated with obesity, type 2 diabetes, and other features of metabolic syndrome. Recent studies suggest that altered adipocytokine gene expression is closely associated with insulin resistance and that single nucleotide polymorphisms (SNPs)modulate the expression and/or function of these genes, thereby affecting insulin sensitivity . With that in mind, it was investigated whether SNPs at position -420 of the resistin gene (RETN) and/or -11377 of the adiponectin gene (ADIPOQ) modulate the susceptibility to PCOS. The evaluation of the genotypes of 117 women with PCOS and 380 healthy fertile controls measuring the index of insulin resistance and hormonal profiles showed that the RETN-420G/G homozygous variant genotype occurred significantly more frequently among the PCOS group than among the control group (15.4% vs. 8.4%, p = 0.035). PCOS women with the RETN-420G/G genotype also showed significantly higher BMIs and greater insulin resistance than those with RETN-420 C/C or C/G genotypes. The ADIPOQ SNP at -11377 showed no association with PCOS. It was concluded that the RETN G/G at -420 genotype is associated with PCOS in Japanese women [8]. Furthermore, it was investigated whether these adiponectin SNP affect obesity-related parameters during caloric restriction in obese subjects. Thirty- two obese Japanese women were treated by meal replacement with a low calorie diet for 8 weeks and asked to maintain their habitual lifestyle. Obesity-related parameters were measured before and after the treatment period. Four SNP were determined (T45G, I164T, G276T, and C-11377G) using a fluorescent allele-specific DNA primer assay system and FRET probe assay system.These findings indicate that each SNP in the adiponectin gene might modify the change in obesity-related parameters during meal replacement with a low calorie diet [9].It has been known that women with polycystic ovary syndrome benefit from metformin therapy. A randomized, placebo-controlled,double-blind study of obese (body mass index >30 kg/m2),oligo/amenorrhoeic women with PCOS compared Metformin (850 mg) twice daily with placebo, over 6 months. All received the same advice from a dietitian. A total of 143 subjects was randomized [metformin (MET) = 69; placebo(PL) = 74]. Both groups showed significant improvements in menstrual frequency [median increase (MET = 1, $P < 0.001$; PL = 1, $P < 0.001$)] and weight loss [mean (kg) (MET = 2.84; $P < 0.001$ and PL = 1.46; $P = 0.011$)]. Only the percentage weight loss correlated with an improvement in menses ($P = 0.047$). There were no significant changes in insulin sensitivity or lipid profiles in either groups. Those who received metformin achieved a significant reduction in waist circumference and free androgen index. Therefore ,Metformin does not improve weight loss or menstrual frequency in obese patients with PCOS. Weight loss alone through lifestyle changes improves menstrual frequency [10].

References

[1] Jeor ST. The role of weight management in the health of women. *J. Amer. Dietetic Assoc.* 1993; 93:1007-1012.

[2] Seow KM,Tsai YL, Hwang JL,Hsu WY,Ho LT,Juan CC. Omental adipose tissue overexpression of fatty acid transporter CD36 and decreased expression of hormone-sensitive lipase in insulin-resistant women with polycystic ovary syndrome. *Hum. Reprod.* 2009 ; 24(8):1982-8.

[3] Pinhas-Hamiel O,Singer S, Pilpel N,Koren I,Boiko V,Hemi R,Pariente C,Kanety H. Adiponectin levels in adolescent girls with polycystic ovary syndrome. *Clin. Endocrinol.* (Oxf) 2009 71(6):823-7.

[4] Carmina E,Orio F,Palomba S, Cascella T,Longo RA, Colao AM, Lombardi G, Lobo RA. Evidence for altered adipocyte function in polycystic ovary syndrome. *Eur. J. Endocrinol.* 2005; 152(3): 389-94.

[5] Yilmaz M,Bukan N,Demirci H,Ozturk C, Kan E,Avvaz G,Arslan M.Serum resistin and adiponectin levels in women with polycystic ovary syndrome. *Gynecol. Endocrinol.* 2009; 25(4): 246-52.

[6] Lewandowski KC, Szosland K, O'Callaghan C,Tan BK,Randeva HS,Lewinski A. Adiponectin and resistin serum levels in women with polycystic ovary syndrome during oral glucose tolerance test: a significant reciprocal correlation between adiponectin and resistin independent of insulin resistance indices. *Mol. Genet. Metab.* 2005; 85(1): 61-9.

[7] Abbasi F,Chang SA,Chu JW,Ciaraldi TP,Lamendola C,McLaughlin T,Reaven GM,Reaven PD. Improvements in insulin resistance with weight loss, in contrast to rosiglitazone, are not associated with changes in plasma adiponectin or adiponectin multimeric complexes. *Am. J. Physiol. Regul. Integr. Comp. Physiol.* 2006 ; 290 (1):139-44.

[8] Baba T,Endo T,Sata F,Nagasawa K,Honnma H,Kitajima Y,Hayashi T,Manase K,Kanaya M,Moriwaka O,Kamiya H,Yamada H,Minakami H,Kishi R,Saito T. The contributions of resistin and adiponectin gene single nucleotide polymorphisms to the genetic risk for polycystic ovary syndrome in a Japanese population. *Gynecol. Endocrinol.* 2009; 25(8):498-503.

[9] Tsuzaki K,kotani K,Nagai N,Saiga K,Sano Y,Hamada T,Moritani T,Yoshimura M,Egawa K,Horikawa C,Kitagawa Y,Kiso Y,Sakane N. Adiponectin gene single-nucleotide polymorphisms and treatment response to obesity. *J. Endocrinol. Invest.* 2009 May;32(5):395-400.

[10] Tang T,Glanville J,Hayden CJ,White D,Barth JH,Balen AH. Combined lifestyle modification and metformin in obese patients with polycystic ovary syndrome. A randomized, placebo-controlled, double-blind multicentre study. *Hun. Reprod.* 2006; 21(1): 80-9.

Effects of Adiposity on Health

Excessive body weight is associated with various diseases, particularly cardiovascular diseases, type 2 diabetes mellitus, obstructive sleep apnea, some types of cancer, and osteoarthritis.Obesity has been found to reduce life expectancy; in fact, it is one of the leading preventable causes of death worldwide [1,2].

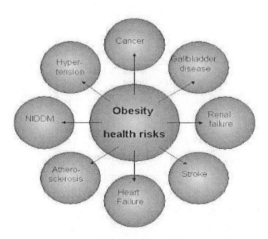

Large-scale American and European studies have found that mortality risk is lowest at a BMI of 22.5–25 kg/m2 in nonsmokers and at 24–27 kg/m2 in current smokers, with risk increasing along with changes in either direction. Obesity increases the risk of death in current and former smokers as well as in those who have never smoked [3].A BMI above 32 has been associated with a doubled mortality rate among women over a 16-year period. In fact, it is estimated, to reduce life expectancy,an average of six to seven years   leading to an excess of 111,909 to

365,000 death per year in the US. In particular, a BMI of 30–35 reduces life expectancy by 2 to 4 years while severe obesity (BMI > 40) reduces life expectancy by 20 years for men and five years for women [4]. Obesity increases the risk of many physical and mental conditions. These comorbidities are predominantly reflected in the metabolic syndrome being it a combination of medical disorders which includes diabetes mellitus type 2,high blood pressure, high blood cholesterol, and high triglyceride levels [5,6]. Complications are either directly caused by obesity or indirectly related through mechanisms sharing a common cause such as a poor diet or a sedentary lifestyle. The strength of the link between obesity and specific conditions varies. One of the strongest is the link with type 2 diabetes.Excess body fat underlies 64% of the cases of diabetes in men and 77% of the cases in women [7].Health consequences can be categorized by the effects of increased fat mass (obstructive sleep apnea, osteoarthritis, psychological disorders and others) or by the increased number of fat cells (diabetes, cancer, cardiovascular disease, non-alcoholic fatty liver disease) [5,7]. Increases in body fat alter the body's response to insulin,potentially leading to insulin resistance. Increased fat also creates a proinflammatory state, increasing the risk of thrombosis.The consequences of the metabolic syndrome envolve several organs and tissues and can be summarized as follow.

- Cardiovascular: ischemic hearth disease,angina,myocardial infarction,congestive hearth
- Heart failure, hypertension,deep vein thrombosis, pulmonary embolism.
- Brain diseases: stroke,migraine,idiopatic intracranial hypertension
- Endocrinological: diabetes mellitus,infertility, pregnancy complications(birth defects,
- and Reproductive intrauterine fetal death)
- Pulmonary diseases: obstructive sleep apnoea, ipoventilation syndrome, asthma
- Gatrointestinal : gastroesophageal reflux, fatty liver disease,cholelitiasis
- Urologic : urinary incontinence,chronic renal failure
- Dermatological : acanthosis nigricans,lymphedema,intertrigo
- Reumatological: gout, osteoarthritis,low back pain
- Psychiatric: depression
- Neoplastic: breast,ovary,cervical,.endometrial cancer, esophageal, colorectal, liver, stomac and pancreatic cancer, kidney and prostate cancer, multiple mieloma, non-Hodgkin lymphoma.

Although the negative health consequences of obesity in the general population are well supported by the available evidence,health outcomes in certain subgroups seem to be improved at an increased BMI, a phenomenon known as the obesity survival paradox [8,9].The paradox was first described in 1999 in overweight and obese people undergoing hemodialysis, and has subsequently been found in those with heart failure, and peripheral artery disease (PAD). In people with heart failure, those with a BMI between 30.0–34.9 had lower mortality than those with a normal weight. This has been attributed to the fact that people often lose weight as they become progressively more ill [10]. Similar findings have been made in other types of heart disease. People with class I obesity and heart disease do not have greater rates of further heart problems than people of normal weight who also have heart disease. In people with greater degrees of obesity, however, risk of further events is increased [11,12]. Even after cardiac bypass surgery, no increase in mortality is seen in the overweight and obese [13].One study found that the improved survival could be explained by the more aggressive treatment that obese people receive after a cardiac event. In any case, it is found that if one takes into account chronic obstructive pulmonary disease (COPD) in those with PAD the benefit of obesity no longer exists [14].

Causes

At an individual level, a combination of excessive caloric intake, lack of physical activity, and genetic susceptibility is thought to explain most cases of obesity, with a limited number of cases due solely to genetics, medical reasons, or psychiatric illness [15]. In contrast ,at a social level, increasing rates of obesity are felt to be due to an easily accessible and palatable diet, increased reliance on cars, and mechanized manufacturing [16,17,18]. A 2006 review identified ten other possible contributors to the recent increase of obesity: (1) insufficient sleep, (2) endocrine disruptors (environmental causes), (3) decreased variability in ambient temperature, (4) decreased rates of smoking, because smoking suppresses appetite, (5) increased use of medications that can cause weight gain (antipsychotics), (6) proportional increases in ethnic and age groups that tend to be heavier, (7) pregnancy at a later age (which may cause susceptibility to obesity in children), (8) epigenetic risk factors passed on generationally, (9) natural selection for higher BMI, and (10) assortative mating leading to increased concentration of obesity risk factors [19].However, there is not conclusive evidence for these mechanisms[1,2].

Ectopic Accumulation of Lipids in Peripheral Tissues

Ectopic accumulation of lipids in peripheral tissues, such as pancreatic beta cells, liver, heart and skeletal muscle leads to lipotoxicity,a process that contributes substantially to the pathophysiology of insulin resistance, type 2 diabetes, steatotic liver disease, kidney disease and heart failure. Accumulation of lipid metabolites within non-adipose tissues can induce chronic inflammation by promoting macrophage infiltration and activation. Oxidized and glycated lipoproteins, free fatty acids, free cholesterol, triacylglycerols, diacylglycerols and ceramides have long been known to induce cellular dysfunction through their pro-inflammatory and proapoptotic properties. Emerging evidence suggests that macrophage activation by lipid metabolites and further modulation by lipid signaling represents a common pathogenic mechanism underlying lipotoxicity in atherosclerosis, obesity-associated insulin resistance and inflammatory diseases related to metabolic syndrome such as liver steatosis and chronic kidney disease [20].The latest discoveries support the role of lipids in modulating the macrophage phenotype in different metabolic diseases. Lipid derivatives induce their action , through modulation of macrophage function, and promote plaque instability in the arterial wall, impair insulin responsiveness, and contribute to inflammatory liver, muscle and kidney disease. Current data suggest the primary role of triglycerides that have a storage function. The toxicity might be induced mainly from long- chain nonesterified fatty acid (NEFA) and their products such as ceramides and diacylglycerols. The results of this fat accumulation are the chronic dysfunction and injury [21]. Current evidence has demonstrated that hypothalamic sensing of circulating lipids and modulation of hypothalamic endogenous fatty acid and lipid metabolism are two important mechanisms modulating energy homeostasis at the whole body level.Key enzymes, such as AMP-activated protein kinase(AMPK) and fatty acid synthase (FAS), as well as intermediate metabolites, such as malonyl-CoA and long chain fatty acids-CoA (LCFAs-CoA), play a major role in this neuronal network,integrating peripheral signals with classical neuropeptide- based mechanisms [22]. However, one key question may be if impairment of lipid metabolism and accumulation of specific lipid species in the hypothalamus, leading to lipotoxicity, may have deleterious effects on hypothalamic neurons [22].

Social Consequences of Obesity

Obesity has a great number of negative health, social and economic consequences. Mortality and morbidity rates are higher among overweight and obese individuals than lean people. Increased BMI is linked with a greater risk of CHD, hypertension, hyperlipidaemia , NIDDM and certain cancers. Furthermore, obesity has been identified in 1997 by the American Heart Association as a major independent risk factor for CHD. Modest weight reduction can significantly reduce the risk of these serious health conditions. In addition to the physical consequences on health, obesity creates a massive social burden.Often over shadowed by the health and social consequences of obesity is the economic cost to society and to the individual.In several developed countries obesity has been estimated to account for 2-7% of the total health care costs (WHO TRS 894). In addition to the direct costs of obesity are costs in terms of the individuals ,including ill health and reduced quality of life,and society in terms of loss of productivity due to sick-leave and premature pensions. Prevention is clearly more cost effective than treatment, both in terms of economic and personal costs. Health care providers and policy makers need to appreciate the importance of obesity and its prevention, and develop effective polices and programmes to prevent obesity.

References

[1] Mokdad AH,Marks JS,Stroup DF,Gerberding JL.Actual causes of death in the United States. *Jama* 2000; 291(10): 1238-45.

[2] Allison DB,Fontaine KR,Manson JE,Stevens J,Vanitallie TB. Annual deaths attributable to obesity in the United States. *Jama* 1999;282(16): 1530-8.

[3] Pischont T,Boeingh H,Hoffmann K et al. General and abdominal adiposity and risk death in Europe. *N. Engl. J. Med.* 2008; 359 (20):2105-20.

[4] Peters A,Barendregt JJ,Willekens F,Mackenbach JP,AlMamun A,Bonneux L.Obesity in adulthood and its consequences for the life expectancy. *Ann. Intern. Med.* 2003; 138(1): 24-32.

[5] Haslam DW, James WP . "Obesity". *Lancet* 2005;366 (9492):1197–209.

[6] Grundy SM . "Obesity, metabolic syndrome, and cardiovascular disease". *J. Clin. Endocrinol. Metab.* 2004; 89 (6): 2595.

[7] Bray GA "Medical consequences of obesity". *J. Clin. Endocrinol. Metab.* 2004;.89 (6): 2583–9.

[8] Yosipovitch G, DeVore A, Dawn A "Obesity and the skin: skin physiology and skin manifestations of obesity". *J. Am. Acad. Dermatol.* 2007; 56 (6): 901–16.

[9] Schmidt DS, Salahudeen AK . "Obesity-survival paradox-still a controversy?". *Semin. Dial.* 2007; 20 (6): 486–92.

[10] Habbu A, Lakkis NM, Dokainish H. "The obesity paradox: Fact or fiction?". *Am. J. Cardiol.* 2006; 98 (7): 944–8.

[11] Romero-Corral A, Montori VM, Somers VK, et al. . "Association of bodyweight with total mortality and with cardiovascular events in coronary artery disease: A systematic review of cohort studies". *Lancet* 2006; 368 (9536): 666–78.

[12] Oreopoulos A, Padwal R, Kalantar-Zadeh K, Fonarow GC, Norris CM, McAlister FA . "Body mass index and mortality in heart failure: A meta-analysis". *Am. Heart J.* 2008;156 (1): 13–22.

[13] Oreopoulos A, Padwal R, Norris CM, Mullen JC, Pretorius V, Kalantar-Zadeh K . "Effect of obesity on short- and long-term mortality postcoronary revascularization: A meta-analysis". *Obesity* (Silver Spring) 2008;16 (2): 442–50.

[14] Diercks DB, Roe MT, Mulgund J et al. . "The obesity paradox in non-ST-segment elevation acute coronary syndromes: Results from the Can Rapid risk stratification of Unstable angina patients Suppress ADverse outcomes with Early implementation of the American College of Cardiology/American Heart Association Guidelines Quality Improvement Initiative". *Am. Heart J.* 152 (1): 140–8.

[15] Bleich S, Cutler D, Murray C, Adams A . "Why is the developed world obese?". *Annu. Rev. Public Health* 2008; 29: 273–95.

[16] Drewnowski A, Specter SE . "Poverty and obesity: the role of energy density and energy costs". *Am. J. Clin. Nutr.* 2004; 79 (1): 6–16.

[17] Nestle M, Jacobson MF . "Halting the obesity epidemic: A public health policy approach". *Public Health Rep.* 2000; 115 (1): 12–24.

[18] James WP "The fundamental drivers of the obesity epidemic". *Obes. Rev.* 2008; 9 Suppl 1: 6–13.

[19] Keith SW, Redden DT, Katzmarzyk PT, et al. "Putative contributors to the secular increase in obesity: Exploring the roads less traveled". *Int. J. Obes.* (Lond)2006; 30 (11): 1585–94.

[20] Weinberg JM. Lipotoxicity. *Kidney Int.* 2006;70 (9):1560-6.

[21] Prieur X,Roszer T,Ricote M. Lipotoxicity in macrophages: Evidence from diseases associated with the metabolic syndrome. *Biochim. Biophys. Acta* 2010; 1801(3):327-37.

[22] Martinez de Morentin PB,Varela L,Ferna J,Noqueiras R,Diequez C,Lopez M. Hypothalamic lipotoxicity and the metabolic syndrome. *Hum. Reprod.* 2005;21(1): 80-9.

Obstructive Sleep Apnoea

Sleep apnoea is a sleep disorder characterized by pauses in breathing during sleep. The individual with sleep apnea is rarely aware of having difficulty breathing, even upon awakening. Sleep apnea is recognized as a problem by others witnessing the individual during episodes or is suspected because of its effects on the body. Persons who sleep alone without a long-term human partner may not be told about their sleep disorder symptoms. Symptoms may be present for years without identification, during which time the sufferer may become conditioned to the daytime sleepiness and fatigue associated with significant levels of sleep disturbance. There are three distinct forms of sleep apnea: central, obstructive , and complex constituting 0.4%, 84% and 15% of cases, respectively [1,2]. Breathing is interrupted by the lack of respiratory effort in central sleep apnea and by a physical block to airflow despite respiratory effort in obstructive sleep apnea; while, in complex or "mixed" sleep apnea, there is a transition from central to obstructive features during the events themselves. In obstructive sleep apnea, the muscles of the soft palate around the base of the tongue and the uvula relax, obstructing the airway. The airway obstruction causes the level of oxygen in the blood to fall, increases the stress on the heart, elevates blood pressure, and prevents the patient from entering the REM sleep,the restful and restorative stage of sleep. In other words, sleep apnea causes deprivation of quality sleep.These episodes, each lasting long enough that one or more breaths are missed, repeatedly occur throughout the sleep.Obstructive sleep apnea is a chronic condition and its symptoms,occurring in 4% and 2% of middle-aged men and women respectively, include loud snoring and/or abnormal pattern of snoring with pauses and gasps. Other symptoms include excessive daytime sleepiness, memory changes, depression, and irritability. Estimates of disease prevalence are in the range of 3% to 7%, with certain subgroups of the population bearing higher risk. Factors that increase vulnerability for the disorder include age, male sex, obesity, family history,menopause, craniofacial abnormalities,and certain health behaviors such as cigarette smoking and alcohol use. OSA is being increasingly recognized as an important cause of medical morbidity and mortality. The health consequences of obstructive sleep apnea are numerous. If left untreated, it leads to excessive daytime sleepiness, cognitive dysfunction, impaired work performance, and decrements in health-related quality of life.

Relationship between OSA, Obesity and Diabetes

During the day there is a sufficient muscle tone to keep the airway open allowing for normal breathing. As already mentioned, snoring is a common finding in people with this syndrome. Although not everyone who snores is experiencing difficulty breathing, snoring in combination with other conditions such as overweight and obesity has been found to be highly predictive of OSA risk [3]. Excess body weight is a common clinical finding and it is present in more than 60% of the patients referred for a diagnostic sleep evaluation [2]. There are multiple metabolic pathways involved in the interaction between OSA,obesity, and metabolic derangements. Over the last 10 to 15 years, there have been dramatic increases in the number of overweight and obese adults in the United States [4] . Obesity, particularly visceral obesity, is an important factor in the assessment of adverse metabolic outcome in OSA. The study of Coughlin and colleagues showed that the prevalence of metabolic syndrome is about 40% greater in patients with OSA. Studies from around the world have consistently identified body weight as the strongest risk factor for obstructive sleep apnea[5]. In the Wisconsin Sleep Cohort study, a one standard deviation difference in body mass index was associated with a 4-fold increase in disease prevalence [6]. Chronic intermittent hypoxia and sleep fragmentation with sleep loss in OSA are likely key triggers that initiate or contribute to the sustenance of inflammation as a prominent phenomenon, but their complex interplay remains to be elucidated [7]. Increased obesity in subjects reporting short sleep duration leads to speculation that, during recent decades, decreased sleeping time in the general population may have contributed to the increasing prevalence of obesity. Recently, it has been suggested that obstructive sleep apnea (OSA), an increasingly prevalent condition, may contribute to the development of MS and diabetes [8,9,10,11]. Despite substantial evidence from clinical and population studies, it seems that the link between OSA and metabolic abnormalities might be independent; however, the issue still remains controversial [5]. In healthy subjects, experimental sleep restriction can cause insulin resistance (IR) and can increase evening cortisol and sympathetic activation. In the general population, obstructive sleep apnoea is associated with glucose intolerance and its severity is also associated with the degree of IR. However, OSA at baseline does not seem to significantly predict the development of diabetes. Prevalence of the metabolic syndrome is higher in patients with OSA than in obese subjects without OSA. Treatment with continuous positive airway pressure seems to improve glucose metabolism both in diabetic and nondiabetic OSA but, mainly, in nonobese subjects. The relative role of obesity and OSA in the pathogenesis of metabolic alterations is still unclear and it is intensively studied in clinical and experimental models. In the intermittent hypoxia model in rodents, strong interactions are likely to occur between haemodynamic alterations, systemic inflammation and metabolic changes, modulated by genetic background. Molecular and cellular mechanisms are currently being investigated [12]. The severity of OSA was a highly significant predictor of the fasting concentrations of glucose and insulin as well as the 2-h glucose concentration and HOMA index. The Homeostasis Assessment Model (HOMA IR) can also be used to estimate insulin resistance using the formula: fasting insulin (mU/ml) X fasting plasma glucose (mmol/l) / 22.5 [13,14]. The IDF consensus statement on sleep apnoea and type 2 diabetes wants to raise awareness of the association between the two conditions, which have significant implications on public health and on the lives of individuals [15,16,17].

Relationship between OSA and cardiovascular disease

Sleep-disordered breathing is associated with an increased risk of cardiovascular disease, stroke, high blood pressure, arrhythmias, diabetes, and sleep deprived driving accidents [18,19,20,21]. OSA has been increasingly implicated in the initiation and progression of cardiovascular diseases [22,23]. It seems that SA increases risks for cardiovascular disease independently of individuals' demographic characteristics or risk markers (smoking, alcohol, obesity,diabetes, dyslipidemia) [24]. The mechanism explaining the association between OSA and CVD is not entirely known .However, oxidative stress, intrathoracic pressure changes, sympathetic activation, such as coagulation factors ,platelet activation and increased inflammation mediators might have a role in the patogenesis of CVD.Particularly, both obesity and OSA are associated with vascular endothelial inflammation and increased risk for cardiovascular diseases [25]. Furthermore, stroke is also associated with obstructive sleep apnea [26]. In 2008, some researchers revealed that people with OSA show tissue loss in brain regions that help store memory, thus linking OSA with memory loss. Using magnetic resonance imaging (MRI), it was discovered that sleep apnea patients' mammillary bodies were nearly 20 percent smaller, particularly on the left side. One of the key investigators hypothesized that repeated drops in oxygen lead to the brain injury [27].

Pathogenesis

Despite substantial evidence from clinical and population studies, it seems that the link between OSA and metabolic abnormalities might be independent; however, the issue still remains controversial [5]. In healthy subjects, experimental sleep restriction caused insulin resistance (IR) and increased evening cortisol and sympathetic activation. In the general population, obstructive sleep apnoea is associated with glucose intolerance and its severity is also associated with the degree of IR. However, OSA at baseline does not seem to significantly predict the development of diabetes. Prevalence of the metabolic syndrome is higher in patients with OSA than in obese subjects without OSA. Treatment with continuous positive airway pressure seems to improve glucose metabolism both in diabetic and nondiabetic OSA but mainly in nonobese subjects. The relative role of obesity and OSA in the pathogenesis of metabolic alterations is still unclear and is intensively studied in clinical and experimental models. In the intermittent hypoxia model in rodents, strong interactions are likely to occur between haemodynamic alterations, systemic inflammation and metabolic changes, modulated by genetic background. Molecular and cellular mechanisms are currently being investigated [12]. The severity of OSA was a highly significant predictor of the fasting concentrations of glucose and insulin as well as the 2-h glucose concentration and HOMA index.[13,14].There is evidence that adipocyte-fatty acid binding protein (A-FABP) may be involved in the development of cardiometabolic dysfunction. Some researchers hypothesise that A-FABP is upregulated in OSA. Serum adipocyte-fatty acid binding protein levels correlated with obstructive sleep apnoea and insulin resistance, independently of obesity, and were significantly higher in severe obstructive sleep apnoea. Therefore,adipocyte-fatty acid binding protein may play a role in obstructive sleep apnoea and metabolic dysfunction [28]. Excessive daytime sleepiness (EDS), obesity and insulin resistance (IR) frequently occur in patients with obstructive sleep apnoea syndrome(OSAS). A study showed that in these patients, EDS is a marker of IR, independent of obesity.In fact, despite the fact that age, BMI and apnoea–hypopnoea index (AHI) were similar, patients with EDS had higher plasma levels of glucose (p<0.05) and insulin (p<0.01), as well as evidence of IR (p<0.01) compared with patients without EDS or healthy controls. Therefore,EDS in OSAS is associated with IR, independently of obesity. Hence, EDS may be a useful clinical marker to identify patients with OSAS at risk of metabolic syndrome [29]. Another study suggested that, independently from adiposity, sleep-disordered breathing (SDB) is associated with impairments in insulin sensitivity, glucose effectiveness, and pancreatic β-cell function. Collectively, these defects may increase the risk of glucose intolerance and type 2 diabetes mellitus in SDB [8].A growing body of evidence supports an association between obstructive sleep apnoea and cardiovascular disease. Pathophysiologic mechanisms that are present in patients with OSA , including sympathetic activation, endothelial dysfunction, oxidative stress, systemic inflammation, hypercoagulability, hyperleptinemia, and insulin resistance , may influence the development and progression of cardiac and vascular pathologies. OSA is widely prevalent in patients with obesity, diabetes, and hypertension. The understanding of the relative importance and interactions of these cardiovascular disease mechanisms and risk factors in patients with OSA may have direct implications for the development of targeted preventive and therapeutic strategies. The National Cholesterol Education Program (NCEP) Adult Treatment Panel III (2001) proposed a clinically practical approach that establishes the diagnosis of metabolic syndrome when an individual has three of these five characteristics: increased waist circumference, high blood pressure, increased fasting glucose, increased triglycerides, and decreased high-density lipoprotein (HDL) cholesterol. Other important features of the metabolic syndrome include microalbuminuria, hypercoagulability, increased inflammation, endothelial dysfunction, poor cardiorespiratory fitness, and sympathetic activation [1] The clustering of cardiovascular disease mechanisms in the metabolic syndrome and OSA are remarkably similar. Patients with OSA have abnormalities in each of the "core" components of the metabolic syndrome : high blood pressure, high fasting glucose, increased waist circumference, low HDL cholesterol, and high triglycerides , as well as in many of its other features, including sympathetic activation, endothelial dysfunction, systemic inflammation, hypercoagulability, and insulin resistance. It has even been suggested that the metabolic syndrome should encompass OSA ("Syndrome Z"). However, there is little information about the extent to which the cardinal features of the metabolic syndrome are simultaneously present in patients with OSA [30] The prevalence of metabolic syndrome (by NCEP) was evaluated about 40% greater in patients with OSA [5]. The obesity epidemic and its impact on the prevalence of both metabolic syndrome and OSA make these data especially relevant and timely. The association of OSAS with insulin resistance and diabetes type 2 has been confirmed. Effective treatment of OSA with continuous positive airway pressure (CPAP) decreases blood pressure and may increase insulin sensitivity [31,32]. Reductions in blood pressure lower cardiovascular risk. Therapies that increase insulin sensitivity also improve cardiovascular risk factors and surrogate endpoints, and outcomes trials are currently underway. As such, effective OSA therapy, via these mechanisms alone, might be expected to reduce cardiovascular morbidity and mortality. Some investigators conducted a prospective cohort study of the effects of OSA therapy on cardiovascular morbidity and mortality. They studied 54 patients who had 70% coronary artery stenosis during elective coronary angiography (86% underwent revascularisation) and subsequently had a polysomnogram that confirmed OSA. Patients were offered therapy and then followed up for an average of 7 years for a composite endpoint of cardiovascular death, acute coronary syndrome, coronary revascularisation, or hospitalisation for heart failure. Patients who accepted OSA therapy experienced only one third of the risk for the composite endpoint compared to those who refused OSA therapy. It is clear that OSA and the metabolic syndrome share a similar pathophysiologic milieu that would be expected to increase the risk of cardiovascular disease. In patients with established coronary artery disease, treatment of OSA may confer long-term cardiovascular benefits [11].Several studies highlight the need for rigorous experimental approaches to understand the pathophysiology and implications of OSA. Identification of the mechanisms by which CPAP acts to mitigate cardiovascular risk would also be of great interest. Both of these studies highlight the need for rigorous experimental approaches to understanding the pathophysiology and implications of OSA. Given the obesity epidemic at hand, the prevalences of both metabolic syndrome and OSA are rising. The implications of these trends for cardiovascular disease are enormous. Levels of adiponectin in the blood are decreased under conditions of obesity, insulin resistance, and type 2 diabetes. It was found that plasma level of adiponectin is decreased in OSAS patients compared with that in obese control subjects without OSAS. The level of adiponectin is associated with the severity of OSAS as indicated by apnea-hypopnea index (AHI), rather than obesity indexed as body mass index. The lower adiponectin level is also associated with increased levels of hsCRP and IL-6 [33]. At the inflammatory point of view, the levels of TNF-α, IL-6, hsCRP, adhesion molecules, and monocyte chemoattractant protein-1 were markedly and significantly elevated in patients with sleep apnea than those in normal control subjects. IL-6 and hsCRP levels were independently associated with OSAS severity as indicated by the AHI. In addition, hsCRP level is associated with visceral adipose tissue and is significantly associated with the components of insulin resistance syndrome. These data support the belief that inflammatory processes and metabolic syndrome are activated in atherosclerotic lesions in patients with OSAS. C-reactive protein and other inflammatory cytokines accelerate the progression of atherosclerosis in patients with OSAS. In addition, increase in circulating levels of adenosine and urinary uric acid in patients with obstructive sleep apnea are implicated with increased production of reactive oxygen species. Activation of redox-sensitive gene expression is suggested by the increase in some protein products of these genes, including vascular endothelial growth factor, erythropoietin, endothelin-1, inflammatory cytokines, and adhesion molecules. These results implicate the participation of redox-sensitive transcription factors as hypoxia-inducible factor-1, activator protein-1 and nuclear factor-kB. Importantly, the elevated levels of atherogenic inflammatory mediators were improved by the OSAS-specific treatment such as nasal continuous positive airway pressure. Thus, OSAS plays a crucial role in metabolic syndrome and systemic inflammatory disorders [34].

Familial and Genetic Predisposition

Familial aggregation of obstructive sleep apnea was first recognized in the 1970s by Strohl and coworkers in a family with several affected individuals Since then, several large-scale studies have confirmed a role for inheritance and familial factors in the genesis of obstructive sleep apnea [35].First-degree relatives of those with the disorder are more likely to be at risk compared with first-degree relatives of those without the disorder. Familial susceptibility to obstructive sleep apnea increases directly with the number of affected relatives [36]. Segregation analyses of the Cleveland Family Study show that, independently from BMI, up to 35% of the variance in disease severity (AHI) can be attributed to genetic factors with possible racial differences in the mode of inheritance [37] Genome-wide association scans have identified susceptibility loci for obstructive sleep apnea and show that linkage patterns for the disorder may differ between whites and African Americans [38,39]. However, someone has been argued that confounding factors, such as obesity, hamper definitive conclusions on genetic underpinnings for obstructive sleep apnea and that additional studies are needed to further define whether the disorder truly has a genetic component [40].

Diagnosis

Obstructive sleep apnea typically affects middle-age, overweight men, and may affect women in later years. OSA can be aggravated by alcohol, sleeping pills and tranquilizers taken at bedtime. It can range from very mild to very severe. Hypopneas in adults are defined as a 50% reduction in air flow for more than ten seconds, followed by a 4% desaturation.

AHI	Rating
<5	Normal
5-15	Mild
15-30	Moderate
>30	Severe

Apnoea/Hypopnoea Index

Apnoea/Hypopnoea Index (AHI) The Apnea-Hypopnea Index (AHI) is expressed as the number of apneas and hypopneas per hour of sleep. Clinically significant levels of sleep apnea are defined as five or more episodes per hour of any type of apnea. The severity is often established using the apnoea/hypopnoea index (AHI), which is the number of apnoeas plus the number of hypopnoeas per hour of sleep . An AHI of less than 10 is not likely to be associated with clinical problems. The ultimate investigation is the polysomnography of sleep apnea which shows pauses in breathing that are followed by drops in blood oxygen and increases in blood carbon dioxide. In adults, a pause must last 10 seconds to be scored as an apnea. However, young children normally breath at a much faster rate and may have the pause many seconds shorter than adults,apnea may be also considered . Currently, the diagnosis of OSA is based on the following evaluations:

- Electro-encephalography (EEG) - brain wave monitoring
- Electromyography (EMG) - muscle tone monitoring
- Recording thoracic-abdominal movements - chest and abdomen movements
- Recording oro-nasal airflow - mouth and nose airflow
- Pulse oximetry - heart rate and blood oxygen level monitoring
- Electrocardiography (ECG) - heart monitoring
- Sound and video recording

Treatment

General measures in treating obstructive sleep apnea include losing excessive weight, avoiding alcohol and sedatives, sleeping on one side, and medications to relieve nasal congestion.CPAP is an effective treatment for sleep apnea inducing continuous positive airway pressure. A mask is worn over the nose during sleep while compressed air is gently forced through the nose to keep the airway open. Different patients need different mask sizes and different pressure levels for optimal treatment results. Another type of treatment for obstructive sleep apnea is the ENT surgery. An operation called UPPP, consent to remove the excess of soft tissue from the back of the throat to relieve obstruction

Conclusion

Sleep apnoea deeply affects metabolic pathways. Chronic intermittent hypoxia and sleep fragmentation with sleep loss in OSA are likely key triggers that initiate or contribute to the sustenance of inflammation as a prominent phenomenon, but their complex interplay remains to be elucidated [7] Recent research demonstrates the likelihood of a relationship between type 2 diabetes and obstructive sleep apnoea, the most common form of sleep disordered breathing. However, obesity, particularly visceral obesity, may be an important factor in the assessment of adverse metabolic outcome in OSA. Sleep-disordered breathing is associated with an increased risk of cardiovascular disease, stroke, high blood pressure, arrhythmias, diabetes, and sleep deprived driving accidents [18,19,20,21]. There are multiple mechanistic pathways involved in the interaction between OSA, obesity, and metabolic derangements [21,22,41]. Early recognition and appropriate therapy can ameliorate the neurobehavioral consequences and may also have favorable effects on cardiovascular health [41].

References

[1]   Teramoto, S, Ohga, E, Ouchi, Y Obstructive sleep apnoea. *Lancet* 1999;354,1213-1214.

[2]   Strohl KP, Redline S. Recognition of obstructive sleep apnea. *Am. J. Respir. Crit. Care Med.* 1996;154:279–289.

[3]   Morris LG, Kleinberger A, Lee KC, Liberatore LA, Burschtin O "Rapid risk stratification for obstructive sleep apnea, based on snoring severity and body mass index". Otolaryngology. *Head and Neck Surgery* 2008;139 (5): 615–8.

[4]   Flegal KM, Carroll MD, Ogden CL, Johnson CL. Prevalence and trends in obesity among US adults, 1999–2000. *JAMA* 2002;288:1723–1727.

[5]   Coughlin, SR, Mawdsley, L, Mugarza, JA, et al Obstructive sleep apnoea is independently associated with an increased prevalence of metabolic syndrome. *Eur. Heart J.* 2004;25,735-741.

[6]   Young T, Palta M, Dempsey J, Skatrud J, Weber S, Badr S. The occurrence of sleep-disordered breathing among middle-aged adults. *N. Engl. J. Med.* 1993;328:1230–1235.

[7]   Esra Tasali , Mary S. M. Obstructive Sleep Apnea and Metabolic Syndrome.Alterations in Glucose Metabolism and Inflammation. *The Proceedings of the American Thoracic Society* 2008; 5:207-217.

[8]   Punjabi NM, Polotsky VY. Disorders of glucose metabolism in sleep apnea. *J. Appl. Physiol.* 2005;99:1998–2007.

[9]   Lévy P, Bonsignore M. R ,Eckel J.. Sleep, sleep disordered breathing and metabolic consequences. *Eur. Respir. J.* 2009; 34:243-260.

[10]   Peppard PE, Young T, Palta M, Skatrud J. Prospective study of the association between sleep-disordered breathing and hypertension. *N. Engl. J. Med.* 2000;342:1378–1384.

[11]   Peker Y, Carlson J,Hedner J. Increased incidence of coronary artery disease in sleep apnoea: a long-term follow-up. *Eur. Respir. J.* 2006;28:596–602.

[12]   Lévy P. Obstructive sleep apnoea (OSA) is associated with insulin resistance and metabolic syndrome. *Eur. Respir. J.* 2009; 34(1):243-60.

[13] Matthews DR, Hosker JP, Rudenski AS, Naylor BA, Treacher DF, Turner RC. Homeostasis assessment model: Insulin resistance and beta cell function from fasting plasma glucose and insulin concentrations in man. *Diabetologia* 1985;28:412-9.

[14] 14. Tasali E, Van Cauter E, Hoffman L,Ehrmann DA.Impact of Obstructive Sleep Apnea on Insulin Resistance and Glucose Tolerance in Women with Polycystic Ovary Syndrome. J. Clin. Endocr. Metab. 2008;93(10): 3878-3884.

[15] Meslier N, Gagnadoux F, Giraud P, Person C, Ouksel H, Urban T, Racineux JL: Impaired glucose-insulin metabolism in males with obstructive sleep apnea syndrome. *Eur. Respir. J.* 2003; 22(1): 156-160.

[16] West SD, Nicoll DJ, Stradling JR: Prevalence of obstructive sleep apnea in men with type 2 diabetes. *Thorax* 2006; 61(11): 945-950.

[17] Resnick HE, Redline S, Shahar E, Gilpin A, Newman A, Walter R, Ewy GA, Howard BV, Punjabi NM: Diabetes and sleep disturbances: findings from the Sleep Heart Health Study. *Diabetes Care* 2003; 26(3): 702-709.

[18] Yan-fang S, Yu-ping W "Sleep-disordered breathing: impact on functional outcome of ischemic stroke patients". *Sleep Medicine* 2009;10 (7): 717–9.

[19] Bixler EO, Vgontzas AN, Lin HM, et al. "Blood pressure associated with sleep-disordered breathing in a population sample of children". *Hypertension* 2008;52 (5): 841–6.

[20] Leung RS "Sleep-disordered breathing: autonomic mechanisms and arrhythmias". *Progress in Cardiovascular Diseases* 2009; 51 (4): 324–38.

[21] Yaggi HK, Concato J, Kernan WN, Lichtman JH, Brass LM, Mohsenin V "Obstructive sleep apnea as a risk factor for stroke and death". *The New England Journal of Medicine* 2005;353 (19): 2034–41.

[22] Bradley TD, Floras JS "Sleep apnea and heart failure: Part II: central sleep apnea". *Circulation* 2003;107 (13): 1822–6.

[23] Shamsuzzaman AS,Gersh BJ,Somers VK.Obstructive sleep apnea: implications for cardiac and vascular disease. *JAMA* 2003;290(14): 1906-14.

[24] Jean- Louis G, Zizi F, Clark LT, Brown CD, Mc Farlane SI. Obstructive sleep apnea and cardiovascular disease:role of the metabolic syndrome and its components. *J. Clin. Sleep Med.* 2008;4(3): 261-72.

[25] Lederer JS, Adams T,Padeletti M, Colombo PC,Factor PH, Le Jemtel TH. Vascular inflammation in obesity and sleep apnea. *Circulation* 2010;[Epub ahead of print].

[26] Grigg-Damberger M . "Why a polysomnogram should become part of the diagnostic evaluation of stroke and transient ischemic attack". *Journal of Clinical Neurophysiology* 2006; 23 (1): 21–38.

[27] Kumar R, Birrer BV, Macey PM, et al. "Reduced mammillary body volume in patients with obstructive sleep apnea". *Neuroscience Letters* 2008;438 (3): 330–4.

[28] Lam C.L.,Xu A, Lam SL,Lam B,Lam CM,Lui MS, Lam, A. XuK, Lam, B. Lam, J. C.M. Lam, Lui M. Serum adipocyte-fatty acid binding protein level is elevated in severe OSA and correlates with insulin resistance. *Eur. Respir. J.* 2009; 33:346-351.

[29] Barceló A, Barbé F , de la Peña M , Martinez P , J B Soriano J B , J Piérola J , A G N Agustí A G N. Insulin resistance and daytime sleepiness in patients with sleep apnoea.*Thorax* 2008;63:946-950.

[30] Teramoto, S, Kume, H, Matsuse, T, et al The risk of future cardiovascular diseases in the patients with OSAS is dependently or independently associated with obstructive sleep apnoea. *Eur. Respir. J.* 2001;17,573-574.

[31] Harsch, IA, Schahin, SP, Radespiel-Troger, M, et al Continuous positive airway pressure treatment rapidly improves insulin sensitivity in patients with obstructive sleep apnea syndrome. *Am. J. Respir. Crit. Care Med.* 2004;169,156-162.

[32] Wolk R, Shamsuzzaman ASM, Somers VK. Obesity, sleep apnea, and hypertension. *Hypertension.* 2003;42:1067-1674.

[33] Teramoto, S, Yamamoto, H, Yamaguchi, Y, et al A significant association of plasma adiponectin level with apnea-hypopnea index rather than BMI in patients with obstructive sleep apnea syndrome [abstract]. *Am. J. Respir. Crit. Care Med.* 2004;169,430.

[34] Teramoto, S, Kume, H, Yamamoto, H, et al Effects of oxygen administration on the circulating vascular endothelial growth factor (VEGF) levels in patients with obstructive sleep apnea syndrome. *Intern. Med.* 2003;42,681-685.

[35] Redline S, Tishler PV. The genetics of sleep apnea. *Sleep Med. Rev.* 2000;4:583–602.

[36] Redline S, Tishler PV, Tosteson TD, Williamson J, Kump K, Browner I, Ferrette V, Krejci P. The familial aggregation of obstructive sleep apnea. *Am. J. Respir. Crit. Care Med.* 1995;151:682–687.

[37] Buxbaum SG, Elston RC, Tishler PV, Redline S. Genetics of the apnea hypopnea index in Caucasians and African Americans: I. Segregation analysis. *Genet. Epidemiol.* 2002;22:243–253.

[38] Palmer LJ, Buxbaum SG, Larkin EK, Patel SR, Elston RC, Tishler PV, Redline S. Whole genome scan for obstructive sleep apnea and obesity in African-American families. *Am. J. Respir. Crit. Care Med.* 2004;169:1314–1321.

[39] Palmer LJ, Buxbaum SG, Larkin E, Patel SR,Elston RC, Tishler PV, Redline S. A whole-genome scan for obstructive sleep apnea and obesity. *Am. J. Hum. Genet.* 2003;72:340–350.

[40] Pack AI, Gislason T, Hakonarson H. Linkage to apnea-hypopnea index across the life-span: is this a viable strategy? *Am. J. Respir. Crit. Care Med.* 2004;170:1260–1261.

[41] Marin JM, Carrizo SJ, Vicente E, Agusti AG. Long-term cardiovascular outcomes in men with obstructive sleep apnoea-hypopnoea with or without treatment with continuous positive airway pressure: an observational study. *Lancet* 2005;365:1046–1053.

Hypertension and Cardiovascular Effects

Cardiovascular disease affects approximately 60% of the adult population over the age of 65 and represents the number one cause of death in the United States. Coronary atherosclerosis is responsible for the vast majority of the cardiovascular events, and a number of cardiovascular risk factors have been identified. Several studies have demonstrated that Metabolic Syndrome (MS) patients are three times more likely to experience a vascular event than persons not presenting the syndrome [1].Women with PCOS also have an increased prevalence of several established cardiovascular risk factors such as diabetes, hypertension, and dyslipidemia.

Metabolic Syndrome (Cardiometabolic Risk)

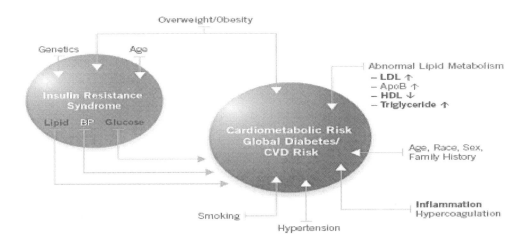

These factors contribute to the increased risk of endothelial dysfunction, increased carotid artery intima media thickness, and coronary artery calcification noted in women with PCOS compared with controls. Although, truncal obesity is very prevalent in PCOS, the markers of atherosclerosis have been shown to be independent of body weight in young, asymptomatic subjects [2]. Metabolic syndrome is a cluster of risk factors that also confer an increased risk of cardiovascular disease. Women with PCOS have also been shown to have a significantly higher prevalence of metabolic syndrome compared with age-matched controls.Few longitudinal studies confirm increased cardiovascular morbidity and/or mortality; however, evidence is accumulating that PCOS-postmenopausal women have an increased risk of cerebrovascular and cardiovascular events [3]. Therefore,the early presence of traditional and other cardiovascular risk factors underscores the need to screen and aggressively counsel and treat these women to prevent future symptomatic cardiovascular disease [4].Obese females are at higher risk for metabolic syndrome due to severe hyperandrogenemia, which also leads to high blood pressure. A study was performed with the aim to determine, among 62 patients (29-43 years) with PCOS, the correlation of body mass index with the clinical manifestations of PCOS and blood pressure. These patients were divided into two BMI groups: nonobese (BMI less than 25 kg/m^2) and obese (BMI more than 25 kg/m^2). Patients' waist to hip ratio, acne, hirsutism, systolic and diastolic blood pressures were also recorded as clinical manifestations in PCOS and compared between the two BMI groups. When the groups were compared according to BMI, a significant increase in systolic and diastolic blood pressures was seen in obese patients, but there was no significant rise in the waist-hip ratio and hirsutism score. Therefore,it seems that BMI may exert a significant and progressive effect on clinical manifestations and blood pressure levels in patients with PCOS [5]. The women with PCOS had significantly higher serum fasting insulin, CRP, protein carbonyl levels, HOMA-R, LH levels, and LH/FSH ratios than healthy women. However, TAOS (total antioxidant status) was significantly lower in women with PCOS. TAOS was negatively correlated with fasting insulin,HOMA-R,CRP, and protein carbonyls. Fasting insulin was positively correlated with protein carbonyls.High density lipoprotein(HDL) was inversely associated with fasting insulin, HOMA-R, and protein carbonyls. Therefore,it is hypothesized that increased oxidative stress and decreased antioxidant capacity may contribute to the increased risk of cardiovascular disease in women with PCOS, in addition to known risk factors such as insulin resistance, hypertension, central obesity, and dyslipidemia An adverse lipid profile has also been observed in PCOS-affected women, suggesting that these individuals may be at increased risk for coronary heart disease at a young age [6]. Although a positive relationship between insulin and blood pressure has been demonstrated in many populations, it is possible that this association does not exist in PCOS.[7,8] In fact, women with PCOS do not appear to be more hypertensive than control subjects, matched for body composition, even if they have significant insulin resistance [9,10,11]. Total plasma renin levels, however, were found to be higher in normotensive women with PCOS than in healthy women, independent of the degree of insulin resistance [12].Additionally, in a retrospective long-term study of postmenopausal women with a history of PCOS, Dahlgren et al. have found a significant higher rate of hypertension (39%) compared to controls (11%)[13].In any case, an effect of obesity or a longer-term impact of blood pressure could be not apparent in a younger healthier population. Women with PCOS would be expected to be at high risk for dyslipidaemia due to elevated androgen levels, body fat distribution and hyperinsulinaemic insulin resistance. Several studies have shown that women with PCOS exhibit an abnormal lipoprotein profile characterized by raised concentrations of plasma triglycerides, marginally elevated low-density lipoprotein (LDL) cholesterol, and reduced high-density lipoprotein (HDL) cholesterol. Recently, two studies have shown that women with PCOS have an atherogenic lipoprotein profile characterized not only by the above mentioned abnormalities but also by raised concentrations and proportions of atherogenic small, dense LDL- relative to body mass index (BMI)-matched controls [14].Furthermore, an increased hepatic lipase activity has been documented. These metabolic disturbances appear to be related more closely to adiposity/insulin metabolism than to circulating androgen levels[15].Indeed, it was supposed that suppressing androgen levels does not alter lipid profile in PCOS In contrast, Diamanti-Kandarakis et al.have observed for the first time that treatment with a pure androgen receptor blocker, flutamide, improves the lipid profile and that this effect may be due to direct inhibition of androgenic actions [16].It is also found that PCOS women have increased circulating levels of plasminogen activator inhibitor, PAI-1 [11]. Elevated PAI-1 activity levels are linked both to the insulin resistance state and to increased risk of thrombotic vascular events being an independent risk factor for atherosclerosis [17,18]. In PCOS, these levels decreased with improvement in insulin sensitivity mediated by weight loss or insulin-sensitizing agents [19,20,21]. Lately, Diamanti-Kandarakis et al. showed elevated endothelin-1 (ET-1) levels in women with PCOS, independently of the presence of obesity .In addition, they suggested that high ET-1, a potent vasoconstrictor peptide, may represent an early sign of abnormal vascular reactivity. In fact, a positive correlation between plasma ET-1 levels and testosterone levels was reported [22]. Considering that 6 months of metformin therapy may induce a reduction of ET-1 concentrations , it is licit to believe that increased insulin sensitivity may offer benefit by protecting and/or restoring the endothelial barrier. A study evaluated subclinical atherosclerosis among women with PCOS and age-matched control subjects. A total of 125 white PCOS cases and 142 controls, aged ≥30 years were evaluated.

During follow-up (1996 to 1999),these women underwent B-mode ultrasonography of the carotid arteries for the evaluation of carotid intima-media wall thickness (IMT) and the prevalence of plaque. A significant difference was observed in the distribution of carotid plaque among PCOS cases compared with controls: 7.2% (9 of 125) of PCOS cases had a plaque index of ≥ 3 compared with 0.7% (1 of 142) of similarly aged controls . Overall and in the group aged 30 to 44 years, no difference was noted in mean carotid IMT between PCOS cases and controls. Among women aged ≥ 45 years, PCOS cases had significantly greater mean IMT than did control women This difference remained significant after adjustment for age and BMI. These results suggest that lifelong exposure to an adverse cardiovascular risk profile in women with PCOS may lead to premature atherosclerosis,and the PCOS-IMT association is explained in part by weight and fat distribution and associated risk factors. There may be an independent effect of PCOS unexplained by the above variables that is related to the hormonal dysregulation of this condition[23].C Reactive Protein has been implicated as a vascular disease risk factor and, in PCOS patient its elevation is associated with increased carotid intima-media wall thickness.A recent study reported that body mass index seems to reduce the association of PCOS and CRP with IMT and was also associated with IMT. In any case,PCOS remains associated with IMT independent of insulin or visceral fat.and CRP does not appreciably seems to mediate the effect of PCOS on IMT. The effects of BMI on the PCOS-IMT relationship was not completely determined by hyperinsulinemia or visceral fat,and might be mediated by other aspects of PCOS-related adiposity [24]. A study focused on the subclinical atherosclerosis and on the question whether the IMT may be linked to low-grade inflammation, assessed by CRP in young women with PCOS. The conclusions of this research suggested that intima-media thickness (IMT) did not correlate with CRP but exhibited a significant correlation with total testosterone. In fact, CRP was significantly higher in PCOS than in control-women but no differences were found in IMT mean between PCOS and control women [25]. Therefore, PCOS itself seems not associated with structural arterial injury, and carotid IMT seems not linked to low-grade inflammation; while, hyperandrogenism could be associated with subclinical atherosclerosis and cardiovascular risk in young women with PCOS . Since, markers of inflammation (IL-6,CPR) are supposed to predict type 2 diabetes in combination with obesity features, may be interesting to know if insulin resistance may induce arterial injury. Current researches showed that the existence of insulin resistance alone may not be an adequate factor for deterioration of endothelial function and carotid IMT in young, nonobese patients with PCOS. However, other factors such as duration of IR,older age,obesity and inflammation markers may play an important role in this process [26]. Today,is again controversial whether the increased risk of CHD and T2DM is associated with endocrine abnormalities occurring as a consequence of PCOS or whether it is related to obesity or metabolic changes frequently seen in women with PCOS. A study indicated that most of these metabolic changes are related to increased levels of homocysteine and C-reactive protein;although, BMI seems to be the major factor determining CHD and D2DM in women with PCOS [27]. An interesting study performed at Keogh Institute for Medical Research of Nedlands(Australia) reported that the prevalence of Metabolic Syndrome was significantly higher among PCOS women when obese (BMI > 30kg/m²) and higher but not significantly in overweight(BMI= 25-30 kg/m²)[28].Briefly, an approximate 4-fold increase in the prevalence of Metabolic Syndrome in women with PCOS compared with the general population, consistent with the proposed major role of insulin and obesity in the syndrome, implies greater risk of cardiometabolic disease in women with PCOS [29]. Young, obese women with PCOS have a high prevalence of early asymptomatic coronary atherosclerosis, compared with obese controls. This increased risk is independent of traditional CV risk factors and novel markers of inflammation. These findings underscore the need to aggressively counsel and treat these women to prevent symptomatic CHD. It is well known as women with polycystic ovary syndrome could have associated risk for cardiovascular disease. The aim of a study was to investigate the relationship between age and metabolic factors on cardiovascular risk in obese women with PCOS. Obese patients with PCOS were divided into an adolescent group and an adult group. Basal values of glucose, insulin, lipid and fibrinolytic parameters were evaluated in all patients and matched controls. Significantly different concentrations between the groups with PCOS were obtained for glucose, total cholesterol,and triglycerides, LDL-cholesterol and Apo-B. Elevated concentrations of insulin, both insulin sensitivity indexes-G:I ratio and HOMA model and PAI-1 were obtained in the adolescent group with PCOS compared to controls, with further increase in the adult group with PCOS [30]. It seems that the youngest obese population with PCOS represents a cohort with potential cardiovascular disease in adulthood .Another study evaluated CHD risk factors in 488 adult premenopausal women with PCOS compared with 351 healthy free-living population control .The Authors reported that PCOS women had lower high-density lipoprotein cholesterol, higher systolic blood pressure , insulin,HOMA-IR, and HOMA insulin secretion than healthy women. In addition, when they considered only the PCOS women and the control women with BMI less than 25 kg/m², they found in the first group higher insulin, glucose and HOMA-IR than in the second group.In conclusion,this study lead to establish that the increased risk of CHD and the high HOMA-IR in PCOS women cannot be exclusively attributed to centripetal obesity [31].In recent years,it has become clear that endothelial dysfunction plays a role in the pathogenesis of atherosclerosis and might also increase the risk for insulin resistance and T2DM. From this point of view , it is essential to go beyond the conventional risk factors and to identify the individuals who are at high risk of developing diabetes and cardiovascular diseases (heart attack, stroke, peripheral arterial diseases). Epidemiological studies show a strong cross-sectional and longitudinal link between blood pressure (BP) elevation and obesity. This association starts in young adults, with a minimal BP elevation (borderline hypertension) and these subjects are 2.2 times more likely to be obese than normotensive subjects [32].Cholesterol, triglycerides, insulin, and insulin/ glucose ratio are significantly elevated and high-density lipoproteins (HDL) are significantly lower in borderline hypertension. Furthermore, in the entire population, both body weight and systolic BP strongly correlate with plasma insulin and dyslipidemia. This correlation seems to be linear and extended into the normotensive and nonobese range,suggesting that a physiological relationship between these variables may exist. Most of the older literature found increased catecholamine in young patients with hypertension and tachycardia (hyperkinetic hypertension). In a study,both groups ,hyperkinetic and normokinetic hypertensives, were overweight, but plasma norepinephrine was elevated only in the hyperkinetic subgroup [33]. A relationship between a faster heart rate, which is a reliable index of sympathetic tone,and insulin resistance has also been reported in nonstressed sleeping individuals [34].In another study where obese subjects free of MS and hypertension were used as the control group, obese hypertensives without MS or nonhypertensive obese patients with MS had increased MSNA (Muscle Sympathetic Nerve Activity). MSNA was even more increased in patients having both hypertension and MS[35].In subjects with prehypertension, a stress-induced increase in sympathetic tone was associated with insulin resistance[36].Clearly,MS also occurs in normotensive individuals;hence, other mechanisms than enhanced sympathetic tone have also been investigated Recent literature data have shown that all the components of the metabolic syndrome are associated with increased levels of CRP. It is showed that high levels of CRP are associated with increased risk for incident cardiovascular events, especially in women with the metabolic syndrome[37].The potential interrelationships between CRP, metabolic syndrome, and cardiovascular events were examined in participants to the Women's Health Study, which enrolled 15,745 women not using hormone-replacement therapy .At baseline, 14,719 not having diabetes, were considered for all components of the metabolic syndrome .All participants were apparently healthy women aged 45 and older with no prior history of cardiovascular disease or cancer..C-reactive protein level correlated with each of the ATP III criteria as well as with cardiovascular risk (CRP levels, ≥3.0 mg/L was defined as high).The lack of fasting glucose and waist measurement, 2 of the 5 criteria that define the metabolic syndrome, is a major limitation of the study. However,the use of a BMI >26.7 kg/m^2 leads to 24.4% of the women having the metabolic syndrome, similar to the 23.4% prevalence in women in NHANES study [38,39].Insulin resistance is considered to be a risk factor for coronary heart disease as it is associated with impaired glucose tolerance and type 2 DM, abdominal obesity and adverse lipid profiles , all features of the so-called 'metabolic syndrome X' [40,41,42,43]. Retrospective studies suggest that there is an evident association between PCOS and cardiovascular disease [44].A study considered 102 pre- and postmenopausal women undergoing cardiac catheterization for the investigation of chest pain. Arterial lesions were seen in 52 women and these women were more likely to report hirsutism, diabetes mellitus, hypertension and previous coronary artery disease.[44,45]. Another investigation evaluated a pelvic ultrasound scan for polycystic ovary morphology on 143 women undergoing cardiac catheterization.The authors reported no significant difference in the prevalence of polycystic ovaries in women with coronary artery lesions and normal arteries. However, women with PCOS had more affected segments. These studies suggest that there may be some association between PCOS and coronary artery disease risk. Furthermore, the carotid artery intima-media thickness was significantly increased in women with PCOS but there was no significant difference in the number of women with atherosclerotic plaques [46]. Haemodynamic changes have also been reported in women with PCOS.Prelevic et al. reported lower cardiac flow velocity and higher resting forearm flow during reactive hyperaemia and lower incremental forearm flow in PCOS than in age-matched control women [47].In a subsequent study, Lees et al reported a constrictor response to transdermal glyceryl trinitrate, a potent vasodilator which acts through the endothelial nitric oxide system on uterine artery [48]. Furthermore, it was reported a paradoxical constrictor response to 5% carbon dioxide,acting as a cerebrovasodilator, in the internal carotid artery in women with

PCOS compared with women with normal ovaries [49]. Recently, it has been showed a positive correlation between abnormal endothelial function and testosterone levels in hyperandrogenic insulin-resistant women with PCOS, an association which was stronger than that of insulin sensitivity. All of these findings probably represent an abnormality in endothelial function in women with PCOS and are indicative of widespread changes in cardiovascular function in these women. Finally,despite the strong association between PCOS and cardiovascular risk factors, a long-term follow-up study of 786 women diagnosed with PCOS reported no excess of coronary heart disease mortality or morbidity among middle-aged women with a history of PCOS, despite increased prevalence of several cardiovascular risk factors. However, mortality and morbidity from diabetes and risk of nonfatal cerebrovascular disease were higher among women with PCOS [50].The reason for the discrepancy between prevalence of cardiovascular risk factors and expected prevalence of cardiovascular disease is unknown.It is interesting to note the prevalence of a positive family history of type 2 DM among women with PCOS compared with controls in this study. In addition, it has been suggested that protective mechanisms may be operative in PCOS such as prolonged exposure to unopposed oestrogen or elevated levels of vascular endothelial growth factor (VEGF). Indeed, increased serum VGEF concentrations have been reported in women with polycystic ovaries and PCOS [51].

Atherosclerosis

In recent years, it has become clear that endothelial dysfunction plays a role in the pathogenesis of atherosclerosis and might also increase the risk for insulin resistance and T2DM. Several PCOS women present abdominal adiposity with a level of peripheral insulin resistance (IR), similar to that present in women with type 2 diabetes, in association with an increased incidence of impaired glucose tolerance.Several cardiovascular risk factors are often related to metabolic alterations,such as dyslipidemia, hypertension, endothelial dysfunction and low grade chronic inflammation that are present even at early age in PCOS women. Pathogenetic mechanisms of these impairments are not yet completely clarified ,but IR appears to play a critical role, such as the key factor linking obesity, hypertension, glucose intolerance,lipid abnormalities and coronary artery disease [52]. Evidence supports the presence of insulin resistance as the fundamental pathophysiologic disturbance responsible for the cluster of metabolic and cardiovascular disorders, collectively known as the metabolic syndrome.All of the processes involved in atherogenesis can be exacerbated by the insulin resistance and/or the metabolic syndrome. Hypertriglyceridemia is a strong predictor of coronary heart disease. Evidence that inflammation is another component of MS raises the possibility that this is an additional process that links metabolic syndrome to cardiovascular disease risk. Population studies strongly suggest the existence of a relationship between the metabolic abnormalities associated with Metabolic Syndrome and the development of diabetes and cardiovascular disease [53,54,55].

Endothelial dysfunction

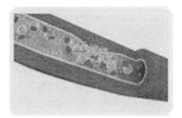

Endothelial dysfunction and increased arterial stiffness occur early in the pathogenesis of diabetic vasculopathy. They are both independent predictors of cardiovascular risk.The metabolic syndrome and type 2 diabetes mellitus are both becoming more prevalent, and both increase the risk of cardiovascular disease.Many patients are not receiving appropriate treatment for the type of dyslipidemia that commonly occurs in these disorders of high serum triglyceride levels, low serum high-density lipoprotein cholesterol (HDL-C) levels, and a preponderance of small, dense, low-density lipoprotein cholesterol (LDL-C) levels. There is also an inverse relationship between serum levels of HDL-C and triglycerides in diabetic patients, with low serum HDL-C levels possibly representing an independent risk factor for cardiovascular disease. Small, dense, LDL-C particles are also highly atherogenic as they are more likely to form oxidized LDL and are less readily cleared. Insulin resistance, which is central to the metabolic syndrome and type 2 diabetes mellitus, leads to high levels of very low-density lipoprotein(VLDL), which contain a high concentration of triglycerides, resulting in high serum triglyceride levels and low serum HDL-C levels [54,55]. Endothelial dysfunction primarily reflects decreased availability of nitric oxide,a critical endothelium-derived vasoactive factor with vasodilatory and anti-atherosclerotic properties.The pathogenesis of endothelial dysfunction in type 2 diabetes is multifactorial with principal contributors being oxidative stress, dyslipidaemia and hyperglycaemia. Elevated blood glucose levels drive production of reactive oxidant species (ROS) via multiple pathways, resulting in uncoupling of mitochondrial oxidative phosphorylation and endothelial NO synthase (eNOS) activity, reducing NO availability and generating further ROS. Hyperglycaemia also contributes to accelerated arterial stiffening by increasing formation of advanced glycation end-products (AGEs), which alter vessel wall structure and function. Diabetic dyslipidaemia is characterised by accumulation of triglyceride-rich lipoproteins, small dense low-density lipoprotein (LDL) particles, reduced high-density lipoprotein (HDL)-cholesterol and increased postprandial free fatty acid flux. These lipid abnormalities contribute to increasing oxidative stress and may directly inhibit eNOS activity [56,57,58]. Atherosclerosis, once largely regarded as a disorder of lipid accumulation,is now generally viewed as an inflammatory disease. Modified LDL is a major cause of endothelial injury in patients with type 2 diabetes and results from such factors as oxidation and glycation. Post-insult endothelial changes include increased leukocyte adhesion and migration into the arterial wall, increased permeability to lipoproteins and other plasma constituents, a switch from anticoagulant to procoagulant activity, and formation of cytokines, growth factors, and vasoactive molecules. As the inflammation continues,circulating monocytes and T lymphocytes migrate into the subendothelial space,and macrophages ingest oxidized LDL and are transformed into foam cells.The resulting fatty streak is augmented by migrating/ proliferating smooth muscle cells and adherent/aggregating platelets to form an intermediate atherosclerotic lesion. Activation of T lymphocytes and macrophages also leads to the release of hydrolytic enzymes, cytokines, chemokines, and growth factors, which induce further damage.Eventually,a fibrous cap, which represents a healing response, will form over the mixture of leukocytes, lipid, and debris to wall off the lesion from the lumen. The core of such an advanced lesion may become necrotic. Subsequent thinning and rupture of the fibrous cap appears to be caused by the continued influx and activation of macrophages. Their release of metalloproteinases and other proteolytic enzymes causes degradation of the matrix, followed by possible hemorrhage, thrombus formation, and arterial occlusion [59,60]. Endothelial dysfunction may be assessed by the ultrasonographic measurement of flow-mediated vasodilatation of the brachial artery and plethysmography measure of forearm blood flow responses to vasoactive agents. Arterial stiffness may be assessed by measures of pulse wave velocity, arterial compliance and wave reflection [57, 58]. Although lipid-regulating agents such as HMG-CoA reductase inhibitors and fibrates are used to treat diabetic dyslipidaemia, their impact on vascular function is less clear [60].Endothelial dysfunction is an important component of the metabolic or insulin resistance syndrome and this is demonstrated by inadequate vasodilation and/or paradoxical vasoconstriction in coronary and peripheral arteries in response to stimuli that release nitric oxide (NO).Endothelial dysfunction contributes to impaired insulin action, by altering the transcapillary passage of insulin to target tissues. Reduced expansion of the capillary, with attenuation of micro circulatory blood flow to metabolically active tissues, contributes to the impairment of insulin-stimulated glucose and lipid metabolism.This establishes a reverberating negative feedback cycle in which progressive endothelial dysfunction and disturbances in glucose and lipid metabolism develop secondarily to the insulin resistance [57].Positive interventions aimed to improve vascular function tend to obtain anti-inflammatory, anti-oxidative and direct effects on the arterial wall [52,53].Other treatments, such as renin-angiotensin-aldosterone system antagonists,insulin sensitisers and lifestyle-based interventions have shown beneficial effects on vascular function in type 2 diabetes. Combination therapy may potentially increase therapeutic efficacy and permit use of lower doses,thereby reducing the risk of adverse drug effects and interactions.The nonlipid parameters include elevated homocysteine and fibrinogen,and decreased endothelial-derived nitric oxide production. Among the new investigational agents there are the inhibitors of squalene synthetase, acylCoA: cholesterol acyltransferase, cholesteryl ester transfer protein, monocyte-macrophages and LDL cholesterol oxidation. Other applications may include thyromimetic therapy, cholesterol vaccination, somatic gene therapy, and recombinant proteins, in particular, apolipoproteins A-I and E. In the meantime before lipid-lowering therapy, dietary and lifestyle modification should be the first therapeutic intervention in the management of dyslipidaemia . Adherence to these recommendations is essential to lower the risk of atherosclerotic vascular disease, especially CHD. Clinical experience supports the concept that therapies which improve insulin resistance and endothelial dysfunction reduce cardiovascular morbidity and mortality.

Heart Failure

Heart failure (HF) is a condition in which a problem with the structure or function of the heart impairs its ability to supply sufficient blood flow to meet the body's needs.Common causes of heart failure include myocardial infarction and other forms of ischemic heart disease, hypertension, valvular heart disease and cardiomyopathy [61].Heart failure is often undiagnosed due to a lack of a universally agreed definition and challenges in definitive diagnosis. Treatment commonly consists of lifestyle measures and medications, and sometimes devices or even surgery. Heart failure is a common, costly, disabling and deadly condition. In developing countries, around 2% of adults suffer from heart failure but, in those over the age of 65 this increases to 6–10% [62, 63,64,65]. Heart failure is associated with significantly reduced physical and mental health, resulting in a markedly decreased quality of life [66].With the exception of heart failure caused by reversible conditions, the condition usually worsens with time.Although some patients survive many years, progressive disease is associated with an overall annual mortality rate of 10%[67].A 19 year study evaluating 13.000 healthy adults in the United States (the National Health and Nutrition Examination Survey (NHANES I) found the following causes ranked by Population Attributable Risk score [68]:

- Ischaemic Heart Disease 62%
- Cigarette Smoking 16%
- Hypertension (high blood pressure)10%
- Obesity 8%
- Diabetes 3%
- Valvular heart disease 2% (much higher in older populations)

An Italian registry of over 6200 patients with heart failure showed the following underlying causes [69].

- • Ischaemic Heart Disease 40%
- • Dilated Cardiomyopathy 32%
- • Valvular Heart Disease 12%
- • Hypertension 11%
- • Other 5%

Heart failure is caused by any condition which reduces the efficiency of the myocardium through damage or overloading. As such, it can be caused by an array of conditions as myocardial infarction , hypertension and amyloidosis in which proteins are deposited in the heart muscle, causing it to stiffen.Three concepts have emerged recently as possibly essential to understanding important aspects of cardiovascular disease (CVD):phenotype, metabolic syndrome and preserved ejection fraction.A study,reported at the 2006 Heart Failure Society of America Conference, among elderly patients with heart failure and preserved ejection fraction, affirmed that the metabolic syndrome is more often found in those with hypertension than those without hypertension.However, the study found no difference in cardiovascular structure and phenotype between these 2 groups [70]. Obesity, such a common problem in the United States, has been associated with myocardial infarction and coronary artery disease, but it has not been associated with heart failure[69]. In heart failure with normal or preserved ejection fraction, extracardiac factors such as anemia, renal dysfunction, and obesity play a major role. Since metabolic syndrome is also an extracardiac factor, it makes sense to try and associate it with diastolic heart failure. Subjects with metabolic syndrome have been reported to have higher left ventricular (LV) mass and more concentric LV hypertrophy, as indicated by higher relative wall thickness. This cardiovascular phenotype is often thought to characterize patients with heart failure in the setting of a preserved ejection fraction. . Hypertension is also commonly associated with heart failure with preserved ejection fraction. It was investigated the presence of the metabolic syndrome in a cohort of subjects with heart failure with preserved ejection fraction who were sorted according to the presence or absence of hypertension and stratified by the presence or absence of the metabolic syndrome.Among the patients with preserved ejection fraction, no significant differences were found between those with and without metabolic syndrome [70,71].Up to 25% of the adult population of the United States is thought to suffer from Metabolic Syndrome.Almost 58-73 million American men and women are at risk from the condition , which substantially increases the chances of damaging the cardiovascular system. Metabolic Syndrome has also been linked to an increased risk of developing Pre-and Type 2 Diabetes. Evidence showed that subjects suffering from Metabolic Syndrome were at significantly greater risk of dying from a heart attack than those without the condition. The study, conducted over a 15-year period, concluded that men with Metabolic Syndrome were from 2.9 to 4.2 times more likely to die of a heart attack [71].Growing scientific evidence demonstrates additional risk factors. A study by Philadelphia's Thomas Jefferson University found that men with Metabolic Syndrome had a 78% greater risk of having a stroke than those free of the condition. Women had a 50% greater risk. Stroke is the third leading cause of death in the United States. Recommendations for reducing heart disease risk are the same as those for reducing Insulin Resistance and the symptoms of Metabolic Syndrome: balancing glucose and insulin levels in the blood stream, losing weight, regulating cholesterol and triglyceride levels and lowering blood pressure to normal levels to prevent damage to the cardiovascular system. Previous research has estimated that these factors can cause up to a seven-fold increase in risk for heart attack for women with PCOS, compared to those without it. Plus, PCOS sufferers are also at greater risk of developing Gestational Diabetes during pregnancy, as well as liver, breast and colon cancer. In a study by the Royal Free and University Medical School in London,there was no significant difference in age or in total cholesterol, HDL or LDL cholesterol among the groups taking part. However,the comparison between PCOS women and women with normal ovaries, reveals that those with PCOS had significantly highest blood pressure and insulin levels,as well as more weight.than the other group Obesity is a major underlying cause of PCOS. As weight increases, stressors build up on the entire cardiovascular system, having to work harder to distribute an adequate amount of freshly oxygenated blood throughout the body. In addition to the increase in triglycerides and LDL cholesterol , there is a lowering of HDL cholesterol, which, in combination, increases the risk of stroke and heart attack.To lose weight and eat a balanced nutritional diet which includes low cholesterol food and a regular exercise are mandatory for these women. Before people develop the Type 2 Diabetes, most initially have a condition called Pre-Diabetes, which is characterized by blood glucose levels that are higher than normal, though not enough to trigger a diagnosis of Type II. It is crucial to address Pre-Diabetes because a growing body of scientific research suggests long term damage to the cardiovascular system may be occurring among people with this condition.Exercise has to be on a regular basis, choosing the preferred method whether it's walking, swimming, cycling, aerobics etc. and set aside a minimum of 30 minutes most days of the week to do it. Unfortunately, most Americans who are diagnosed with a form of Diabetes have Type 2 Diabetes. Obesity may be the result. More than 400,000 Americans die each year from smoking-related diseases, according to the Centers for Disease Control and Prevention. Cigarette smokers are four times more likely to have heart attacks and develop cardiovascular diseases than non-smokers. Men have a slightly higher risk than women. On average, lifetime smokers have a 50% chance of dying from a smoking-related disease. But quitting can quickly begin to nullify the risks .One year after quitting, the risk of heart disease drops by 50%, according to the World Health Organization (WHO). Within 15 years, a former smoker's risk of dying from heart disease approaches that of a lifetime non-smoker [72].

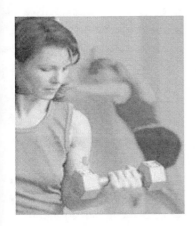

Although Type 2 Diabetes can be managed over a long life, almost 80% of diabetics eventually die from some form of heart or blood vessel diseases. A balanced, nutritional diet, that drastically lowers carbohydrate intake and ideally includes low cholesterol food, combined with regular exercise, are key factors that will help to lose weight and improve health of the heart.

Management of Hypertension

Increased pressure on the inner walls of blood vessels make the vessels less flexible over time and more vulnerable to the build-up of fatty deposits in a process known as atherosclerosis, a key risk factor in heart disease. Hypertension also forces the heart to work harder to pump adequate blood throughout the body.The underlying causes tend to be the same for everyone damage to the cardiovascular system,with a common key factor: insulin resistance-connected obesity. This condition can, in turn, lead to MS and to Prediabetes or Type 2 Diabetes, all major risk factors in heart-related disorders. All subjects with systolic pressure between 120 and 139 and/or diastolic pressure between 80 and 89 are included in the category of pre-hypertension.

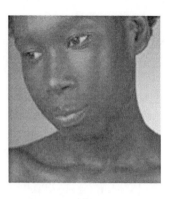

Life-threatening complications of the cardiovascular system can develop over a period of years when hypertension exists. Important differences are reported among the different etnic groups. In 1999, 78,574 African-Americans died from heart disease, the leading cause of death for all racial and ethnic groups. African-Americans were 30% more likely to die of heart disease than whites when differences in age distributions were taken into account. Diabetes, high blood pressure, high cholesterol, lack of exercise and smoking all put black women at high risk for heart disease.Heart disease risk and death rates are high among Mexican Americans partly because of increased rates of obesity and diabetes. Overall, Asian/Pacific Islander and Native Hawaiian women have much lower rates of heart disease than women of other minorities but it is still the leading cause of death within their own grouping. Heart disease risk and death rates are higher among Native Hawaiians and some Asian Americans ,especially Indians, partly because of higher rates of obesity, diabetes and high blood pressure. Heart disease is the leading cause of death for American Indians and Alaska Natives.Both sexes are at risk from factors such as insulin resistance leading to obesity, high cholesterol levels, smoking and high blood pressure, as well as diabetes, lack of exercise and genetic predisposition. In one study, married men who received support from their spouses were shown to be at less risk from heart disease.Therefore, considerably more men than women die of heart attacks each year in the U.S., with the average lifespan of an American white male about 5 years less than a woman's. Among African-Americans, the gap is seven years.The best ways to achieve the reduction in risk are: a balanced, nutritional diet, including low cholesterol food, regular exercise and weight loss in overweight individuals.Childhood obesity has tripled in the last 15 years in the U.S. Physically active parents who encourage nutritionally balanced meals at the dinner table can instill lifelong good habits in their children. In conclusion, parents can promote their children's heart health.

References

[1] Tziomalos K,Athyros VG,Karagiannis M,Mikhaillsis DP. Endothelial dysfunction in metabolic syndrome: Prevalence, pathogenesis and management. *Nutr. Metab. Cardiovasc. Dis.* 2009; [Epub ahead of print].

[2] Shroff R, Kerchner A, Maifeld M, Van Beek EJ, Jagasia D, Dokras A. Young obese women with polycystic ovary syndrome have evidence of early coronary atherosclerosis. *J. Clin. Endocrinol. Metab.* 2007 ;92(12):4609-14.

[3] Rizzo M,Berneis K,Spinas G,Rini GB, Carmina E. Long-term consequences of polycystic ovary syndrome on cardiovascular risk. *Fertil. Steril.* 2009:91(4):1563-7.

[4] Dokras A.Cardiovascular disease risk factors in polycystic ovary syndrome. *Semin. Reprod. Med.* 2008 ;26(1):39-44.

[5] Siddiqui IA, Tamimi W,Tamin H,Aleisa N,Adham M.A study on clinical and sonographic features in obese and nonobese patients with polycystic ovary syndrome. *Arch. Gynecol. Obstet.* 2009 [Epub ahead of print].

[6] Fenkci V, Fenkci S, Yilmazer M, Serteser M.Decreased total antioxidant status and increased oxidative stress in women with polycystic ovary syndrome may contribute to the risk of cardiovascular disease. *Fertil. Steril.* 2003 ; 80(1):123-7.

[7] Bonora E, Zavaroni I, Alpi O, Pezzarossa A, Bruschi F, Dall'Aglio E, Guerra L, Coscelli C, Butturini U. Relationship between blood pressure and plasma insulin in non-obese and obese non-diabetic subjects. *Diabetologia.* 1987 Sep;30(9):719-23.

[8] Zavaroni I, Bonora E, Pagliara M, Dall'Aglio E, Luchetti L, Buonanno G, Bonati PA, Bergonzani M, Gnudi L, Passeri M, et al. Risk factors for coronary artery disease in healthy persons with hyperinsulinemia and normal glucose tolerance. *N. Engl. J. Med.* 1989 Mar 16;320(11):702-6.

[9] Pollare et al., 1990) Pollare T, Lithell H, Berne C. Insulin resistance is a characteristic feature of primary hypertension independent of obesity. *Metabolism.* 1990 Feb;39(2):167-74.

[10] Zimmerman BJ, Anderson DC, Granger DN. Neuropeptides promote neutrophil adherence to endothelial cell monolayers. *Am. J. Physiol.* 1992 Nov;263(5 Pt 1):G678-82.

[11] Sampson M, Kong C, Patel A, Unwin R, Jacobs HS. Ambulatory blood pressure profiles and plasminogen activator inhibitor (PAI-1) activity in lean women with and without the polycystic ovary syndrome. *Clin. Endocrinol.* (Oxf). 1996 Nov;45(5):623-9.

[12] Hacihanefioglu B. Polycystic ovary syndrome nomenclature: chaos? *Fertil. Steril.* 2000 Jun;73(6):1261-2.

[13] Dahlgren E, Janson PO, Johansson S, Lapidus L, Odén A.Polycystic ovary syndrome and risk for myocardial infarction. Evaluated from a risk factor model based on a prospective population study of women. *Acta Obstet. Gynecol. Scand.* 1992 Dec;71(8):599-604.

[14] Dejager S, Pichard C, Giral P, Bruckert E, Federspield MC, Beucler I, Turpin G.Smaller LDL particle size in women with polycystic ovary syndrome compared to controls. *Clin. Endocrinol.* (Oxf). 2001 Apr;54(4):455-62.

[15] Pirwany et al., 2001 Pirwany IR, Fleming R, Sattar N, Greer IA, Wallace AM.Circulating leptin concentrations and ovarian function in polycystic ovary syndrome. *Eur. J. Endocrinol.* 2001 Sep;145(3):289-94.

[16] Diamanti-Kandarakis E, Mitrakou A, Raptis S, Tolis G, Duleba AJ.The effect of a pure antiandrogen receptor blocker, flutamide, on the lipid profile in the polycystic ovary syndrome. *J. Clin. Endocrinol. Metab.* 1998 Aug;83(8):2699-705.

[17] Dawson S, Henney A. The status of PAI-1 as a risk factor for arterial and thrombotic disease: a review. *Atherosclerosis.* 1992 Aug;95(2-3):105-17. Review.

[18] Hamsten A, de Faire U, Walldius G, Dahlén G, Szamosi A, Landou C, Blombäck M, Wiman B.Plasminogen activator inhibitor in plasma: risk factor for recurrent myocardial infarction. *Lancet.* 1987 Jul 4;2(8549):3-9.

[19] Andersen RE, Wadden TA, Bartlett SJ, Vogt RA, Weinstock RS. . Relation of weight loss to changes in serum lipids and lipoproteins in obese women. *Am. J. Clin. Nutr.* 1995 Aug;62(2):350-7.

[20] Ehrmann DA, Schneider DJ, Sobel BE, Cavaghan MK, Imperial J, Rosenfield RL, Polonsky KS.Troglitazone improves defects in insulin action, insulin secretion, ovarian steroidogenesis, and fibrinolysis in women with polycystic ovary syndrome. *J. Clin. Endocrinol. Metab.* 1997;82 (7): 2108-16.

[21] Velázquez E, Acosta A, Mendoza SG. Menstrual cyclicity after metformin therapy in polycystic ovary syndrome. *Obstet. Gynecol.* 1997 Sep;90(3):392-5.

[22] Diamanti-Kandarakis E, Spina G, Kouli C, Migdalis I. Increased endothelin-1 levels in women with polycystic ovary syndrome and the beneficial effect of metformin therapy. *J. Clin. Endocrinol. Metab.* 2001 Oct;86(10):4666-73.

[23] Talbott EO, Guzick DS, Sutton-Tyrrell K, McHugh-Pemu KP, Zborowski JV, Remsberg KE, Kuller LH. Evidence for association between polycystic ovary syndrome and premature carotid atherosclerosis in middle-aged women. *Arterioscler. Thromb Vasc. Biol.* 2000 ;20(11): 2414-21.

[24] Talbott EO,Zborowski JV,Boudreaux MY,McHugh-Pernu,KP, Sutton-Tyrrell K,Guzick DS. The relationship between C/reactive protein and carotid intima-media thickness in middle-aged women with polycystic ovary syndrome. *J. Clin. Endocrinol. Metab.* 2004;89(12); 6061-7.

[25] Costa LO,Dos Santos MP,Oliveira M,Viana A. Low-grade inflammation is not accompanied by structural arterial injury in polycystic ovary syndrome. *Diabetes Res. Clin. Pract.* 2008; 81(2): 179-83.

[26] Arikan S,Akay H,Bahceci M,Tuzcu A, Gokalp D. The evaluation of endothelial function with flow-mediated dilatation and carotid intima media thickness in young nonobese polycystic ovary syndrome patients; existence of insulin resistance alone may not represent an adequate condition for deterioration of endothelial function. *Fertil. Steril.* 2009;91(2):450-5.

[27] Guzelmeric K,Alkan N,Pirimoglu M,Unal O,Turan C. Chronic inflammation and elevated homocisteine levels are associated with increased body mass index in women with polycystic ovary syndrome. *Gynecol. Endocrinol.* 2007;23(9): 505-10.

[28] Cussons AJ,Watts GF,Burke V,Shaw JE,Zimmet PZ,Stuckey BG. Cardiometabolic risk in polycystic ovary syndrome:a comparison of different approaches to defining the metabolic syndrome. *Hum. Reprod.* 2008;23(10):2352-8.

[29] Elting MW, Korsen TJ, Schoemaker J.Obesity, rather than menstrual cycle pattern or follicle cohort size, determines hyperinsulinaemia, dyslipidaemia and hypertension in ageing women with polycystic ovary syndrome. *Clin. Endocrinol.* (Oxf). 2001 ;55(6):767-76.

[30] Macut D, Micić D, Cvijović G, Sumarac M, Kendereski A, Zorić S, Pejković D. Cardiovascular risk in adolescent and young adult obese females with polycystic ovary syndrome (PCOS). *J. Pediatr. Endocrinol. Metab.* 2001;14 Suppl 5:1353-59.

[31] Glueck CJ,Morrison JA,Goldenberg N,Wang P. Coronary heart disease risk factors in adult premenopausal white women with polycystic ovary syndrome compared with a healthy female population. *Metabolism* 2009;58 (5): 714-21.

[32] Julius S, Jamerson K, Mejia A, et al. The association of borderline hypertension with target organ changes and higher coronary risk. Tecumseh Blood Pressure Study. *JAMA.* 1990;264:354-358.

[33] Julius S, Krause L, Schork NJ, et al. Hyperkinetic borderline hypertension in Tecumseh, Michigan. *J. Hypertens.* 1991;9:77-84.

[34] Facchini FS, Stoohs RA, Reaven GM. Enhanced sympathetic nervous system activity: the link between insulin resistance, hyperinsulinemia, and heart rate. *Am. J. Hypertens.* 1996;9:1013-1017.

[35] Huggett RJ, Burns J, Mackintosh AF, Mary DA. Sympathetic neural activation in nondiabetic metabolic syndrome and its further augmentation by hypertension. *Hypertension.* 2004;44:847-852.

[36] Fossum E, Høieggen A, Reims HM, et al. High screening blood pressure is related to sympathetic nervous system activity and insulin resistance in healthy young men. *Blood Pressure.* 2004;13:89-94.

[37] Expert Panel on Detection, Evaluation, and Treatment of High Blood Cholesterol in Adults. Executive summary of the third report of the National Cholesterol Education Program (NCEP) Expert Panel on Detection, Evaluation, and Treatment of High Blood Cholesterol in Adults (Adult Treatment Panel III). *JAMA* 2001;285:2486-2497.

[38] Ridker PM, Buring JE, Cook NR, Rifai N. C-reactive protein, the metabolic syndrome, and risk of incident cardiovascular events: an 8-year follow-up of 14 719 initially healthy American women. *Circulation* 2003;107:391-397.

[39] Ford ES, Giles WH, Dietz WH. Prevalence of the metabolic syndrome among US adults: findings from the third National Health and Nutrition Examination Survey. *JAMA* 2002;287:356-359. \

[40] Orio F,Vuolo L,Lombardi G,Colao A.Metabolic and cardiovascular consequences of polycystic ovary syndrome. *Minerva Ginecol.* 2008; 60(1):39-51.

[41] Reaven GM. Insulin resistance, the insulin resistance syndrome, and cardiovascular disease. *Panminerva* 2005; 47(4): 201-10.).

[42] Petrie JR, Cleland SJ, Small M. The metabolic syndrome: overeating, inactivity, poor compliance or 'dud' advice? *Diabet Med.* 1998 Nov;15 Suppl 3:S29-31. Review.

[43] Ferrannini E, Buzzigoli G, Bonadonna R, Giorico MA, Oleggini M, Graziadei L, Pedrinelli R, Brandi L, Bevilacqua S.Insulin resistance in essential hypertension. *N. Engl. J. Med.* 1987 Aug 6;317(6):350-7.

[44] Orchard TJ, Becker DJ, Bates M, Kuller LH, Drash AL.Plasma insulin and lipoproteinconcentrations: an atherogenic association? *Am. J. Epidemiol.* 1983 Sep;118(3):326-37.

[45] Birdsall HH, Green DM, Trial J, Youker KA, Burns AR, MacKay CR, LaRosa GJ, Hawkins HK, Smith CW, Michael LH, Entman ML, Rossen RD.Complement C5a, TGF-beta 1, and MCP-1, in sequence, induce migration of monocytes into ischemic canine myocardium within the first one to five hours after reperfusion. *Circulation.* 1997 Feb 4;95(3):684-92.

[46] Guzick DS, Talbott EO, Sutton-Tyrrell K, Herzog HC, Kuller LH, Wolfson SK Jr.Carotid atherosclerosis in women with polycystic ovary syndrome: initial results from a case-control study. *Am. J. Obstet. Gynecol.* 1996 Apr;174(4):1224-9; discussion 1229-32.

[47] Prelevic GM, Beljic T, Balint-Peric L, Ginsburg J.Cardiac flow velocity in women with the polycystic ovary syndrome.Clin Endocrinol (Oxf). 1995 Dec;43(6):677-81.

[48] Lees KR.Multifactorial approach to stroke investigation and prevention. *Lancet.* 1998 Sep 19;352(9132):923-4.

[49] Lakhani K, Constantinovici N, Purcell WM, Fernando R, Hardiman P.Internal carotid-artery response to 5% carbon dioxide in women with polycystic ovaries. *Lancet.* 2000 Sep 30;356(9236):1166-7.

[50] Pierpoint T, McKeigue PM, Isaacs AJ, Wild SH, Jacobs HS.Mortality of women with polycystic ovary syndrome at long-term follow-up. *J. Clin. Epidemiol.* 1998 Jul;51(7):581-6.

[51] Agrawal R, Sladkevicius P, Engmann L, Conway GS, Payne NN, Bekis J, Tan SL, Campbell S, Jacobs HS.Serum vascular endothelial growth factor concentrations and ovarian stromal blood flow are increased in women with polycystic ovaries. *Hum. Reprod.* 1998 Mar;13(3):651-5.

[52] Theuma P, Fonseca V: Inflammation and emerging risk factors in diabetes mellitus and atherosclerosis. *Curr. Diab. Rep.* 2003; 3:248–254.

[53] Dandona P, Aljada A, Bandyopadhyay A: Inflammation: the link between insulin resistance, obesity and diabetes. *Trends Immunol.* 2004; 25:4–7.

[54] Nesto RW. Beyond low-density lipoprotein: addressing the atherogenic lipid triad in type 2 diabetes mellitus and the metabolic syndrome. *Am. J. Cardiovasc. Drugs* 2005;5(6): 379-87.

[55] Woodman RJ,Chew GT,Watts GF. Mechanisms, significance and treatment of vascular dysfunction in type 2 diabetes mellitus: focus on lipid-regulating therapy. *Drugs* 2005;65(1):31-74.

[56] Ross R. Atherosclerosis: An Inflammatory Disease. *N. Engl. J. Med.* 1999;340:115-126.

[57] Cerosino E, DeFronzo RA.Insulin resistance and endothelial dysfunction: the road map to cardiovascular diseases. *Diabetes Metab. Res. Rev.* 2006; 22(6): 423-36.

[58] Chong PH, Bachenheimer BS. Current, new and future treatments in dyslipidaemia and atherosclerosis. *Drugs* 2000; 60(1): 55-93.

[59] Willerson JT, Ridker PM: Inflammation as a cardiovascular risk factor. *Circulation* 2004 109 (Suppl. 1):II2–II10, 2004.

[60] Dilaveris P,Giannopoulos G, Riga M,Synetos A,Stefanadis C.Beneficial effects of statins on endothelial dysfunction and vascular stiffness. *Curr. Vasc. Pharmacol.* 2007; 5(3):227-37.

[61] McMurray JJ, Pfeffer MA (2005). "Heart failure". *Lancet* 2005; 365 (9474): 1877–89.

[62] Dickstein K, Cohen-Solal A, Filippatos G, et al. ESC Guidelines for the diagnosis and treatment of acute and chronic heart failure 2008: the Task Force for the Diagnosis and Treatment of Acute and Chronic Heart Failure 2008 of the European Society of Cardiology. Developed in collaboration with the Heart Failure Association of the ESC (HFA) and endorsed by the European Society of Intensive Care Medicine (ESICM) *Eur. Heart J.* 2008; 29 (19): 2388–442.

[63] Stewart S, Jenkins A, Buchan S, McGuire A, Capewell S, McMurray JJ . "The current cost of heart failure to the National Health Service in the UK". *Eur. J. Heart Fail.* 2002; 4 (3): 361–71.

[64] Rosamond W, Flegal K, Furie K, et al. "Heart disease and stroke statistics--2008 update: a report from the American Heart Association Statistics Committee and Stroke Statistics Subcommittee". *Circulation* 2008; 117 (4): 25–146.

[65] Juenger J, Schellberg D, Kraemer S, et al. . "Health related quality of life in patients with congestive heart failure: comparison with other chronic diseases and relation to functional variables". *Heart* 2002; 87 (3): 235–41.

[66] Hobbs FD, Kenkre JE, Roalfe AK, Davis RC, Hare R, Davies MK "Impact of heart failure and left ventricular systolic dysfunction on quality of life: a cross-sectional study comparing common chronic cardiac and medical disorders and a representative adult population". *Eur. Heart J.* 2002; 23 (23): 1867–76.

[67] Neubauer S "The failing heart :an engine out of fuel". *N. Engl. J. Med.* 2007; 356 (11): 1140–51.

[68] He J; Ogden LG; Bazzano LA; Vupputuri S, et al. "Risk factors for congestive heart failure in US men and women: NHANES I epidemiologic follow-up study.". *Arch. Intern. Med.* 2001;161 (7): 996–1002.

[69] Baldasseroni S; Opasich C; Gorini M; Lucci D, et al. (2002). "Left bundle-branch block is associated with increased 1-year sudden and total mortality rate in 5517 outpatients with congestive heart failure: a report from the Italian network on congestive heart failure.". *American Heart Journal* 143 (3): 398–405.

[70] Vindhya RKC, Wajahat R, Titova I, et al. The metabolic syndrome in patients with heart failure with normal ejection fraction. *J. Cardiac. Fail.* 2006; 12(6 suppl):S20.

[71] The Task Force for the Diagnosis and Treatment of Chronic Heart Failure of the European Society of Cardiology. Guidelines for the diagnosis and treatment of chronic heart failure: executive summary (update 2005). *Eur. Heart J.* 2005;26:1115-1140.

[72] Mc Laughlin T,Allison G,Abbasi F,Lamendola C,Reaven G.Prevalence of insulin resistance and associated cardiovascular risk factors among normal weight, overweight,and obese individuals. *Metabolism* 2004; 53(4):495-9.

Nonalcoholic Fatty Liver Disease

Metabolic syndrome (MS) is one of the most prevalent diseases in the developed countries and is closely associated with the incidence of cardiovascular as well as other diseases. Predominant sign is the abdominal type of obesity with increased visceral fat mass and the associated insulin resistance. Glucose metabolism disorder, dyslipidemia and arterial hypertension are other important attributes. Metabolic syndrome is also closely associated with the liver steatosis, mostly benign and reversible liver disease.

Fatty liver disease: histological features

Nonalcoholic fatty liver disease and its subset nonalcoholic steatohepatitis represent the liver manifestations of insulin resistance. Nonalcoholic fatty liver disease (NAFLD) is now considered to be the most common liver disease in the United States and involves a spectrum of progressive histopathologic changes. Common risk factors associated with NAFLD include obesity, diabetes, and hyperlipidemia.Although most patients with NAFLD have simple hepatic steatosis, a significant number develop nonalcoholic steatohepatitis, which may progress to fibrosis, cirrhosis, or end-stage liver disease.

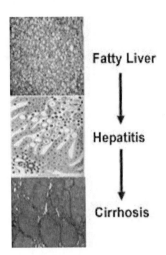

Nevertheless, uncomplicated steatosis may, under certain conditions, progress to inflammation and the disease may, through the stage of NASH (nonalcoholic steatohepatitis) and liver fibrosis, result in liver cirrhosis and hepatocellular carcinoma.

There is increasing evidence that NAFLD is a common feature in patients with the cardiometabolic syndrome, a constellation of metabolic, cardiovascular, renal, and inflammatory abnormalities in which insulin resistance is thought to play a key role in end-organ pathogenesis. NAFLD is usually diagnosed after abnormal liver chemistry results found during routine laboratory testing. No therapy has been proven effective for treating NAFLD/ nonalcoholic steatohepatitis. Expert opinion emphasizes the importance of exercise, weight loss in obese and overweight individuals, treatment of hyperlipidemia, and glucose control. Anglo-Saxon literature uses the term NAFLD (non-alcoholic fatty liver disease) to refer to these various stages of the liver disease (uncomplicated liver steatosis, steatohepatitis, fibrosis and cirrhosis). Non-alcoholic fatty liver disease (NAFLD) is the most common liver disorder in Western industrialized countries, affecting 20-40% of the general population. Patients enrolled in the Dallas Heart Study were found to have a 33% prevalence of nonalcoholic fatty liver disease and children dying of accidental deaths in San Diego were found to have a 13% prevalence of non alcoholic fatty liver disease.Because about 10% of people with nonalcoholic fatty liver disease are at risk for progressive fibrosis, the burden of this disease is now quite substantial [2].Nonalcoholic fatty liver disease (NAFLD) has been consistently associated with obesity and insulin resistance. Nonalcoholic steatohepatitis (NASH) is a histological entity within NAFLD that can progress to cirrhosis.The exact prevalence of NASH in severe obesity is unknown. It is unclear whether differences in insulin sensitivity exist among subjects with NASH and simple fatty liver.A study evaluated the prevalence and correlates of NASH and liver fibrosis in a racially diverse cohort of severely obese subjects. Ninety-seven subjects were enrolled.Liver biopsies, indirect markers of insulin resistance,metabolic parameters, and liver function tests were obtained. Thirty-six percent of subjects had NASH and 25% had fibrosis. No cirrhosis was diagnosed on histology. Markers of hyperglycemia, insulin resistance, and the metabolic syndrome but not body mass index were associated with the presence of NASH and fibrosis. Elevated transaminase levels correlated strongly with NASH and fibrosis but 46% subjects with NASH had normal transaminases. Subjects with NASH had more severe insulin resistance when compared to those with simple fatty liver.A signal detection model incorporating AST and the presence of diabetes predicted the presence of NASH while another incorporating

ALT and HbA1C predicted the presence of fibrosis. NAFLD is associated with the metabolic syndrome rather than excess adipose tissue in severe obesity. Insulin resistance is higher in subjects with NASH versus those with simple fatty liver [3]. Large population-based surveys in China, Japan, and Korea indicate that the prevalence of NAFLD is now 12% to 24% in population subgroups, depending on age, gender, ethnicity, and location.There is strong evidence that the prevalence of NAFLD has increased recently in parallel with regional trends in obesity, type 2 diabetes, and metabolic syndrome; and that further increases are likely. The relationship between NAFLD, central obesity, diabetes, and metabolic syndrome is clearly evident in retrospective and prospective Asian studies, but the strength of association with these metabolic risk factors is only appreciated when regional definitions of anthropometry are used [4].While, simple steatosis is not dangerous for the patient, NASH is the sign of developing cirrhosis . Etiopathogenesis of NASH features have identical characteristics of those of insulin resistance and metabolic syndrome [5]. Even though liver biopsy remains the gold standard in the diagnosis, new diagnostic approaches are emerging that could be useful in distinguishing simple steatosis from NASH [6]. Draft proposals were presented and discussed at Asia-Pacific Digestive Week at Cebu,Philippines, in late November 2006, and are published separately as an Executive Summary. The present document reviews the APWP-NAFLD proposals for definition, assessment, and management of NAFLD in the Asia-Pacific region. Based particularly on large community-based studies using ultrasonography, case-control series and prospective longitudinal studies, the prevalence of NAFLD in Asia is between 12% and 24%, depending on age, gender, locality and ethnicity. Further, the prevalence in China and Japan has nearly doubled in the last 10-15 years. A detailed analysis of these data shows that NAFLD risk factors for Asians resemble those in the West for age at presentation, prevalence of type 2 diabetes mellitus (T2DM) and hyperlipidemia. The apparent differences in prevalence of central obesity and overall obesity are related to the criteria used to define waist circumference and body mass index (BMI), respectively. The strongest associations are with components of the metabolic syndrome, particularly the combined presence of central obesity and insulin resistance. Non-alcoholic fatty liver disease likely represents the hepatic manifestation of metabolic syndrome. Not surprisingly therefore, Asians with NAFLD are at high risk of developing diabetes and cardiovascular disease. Conversely,metabolic syndrome may precede the diagnosis of NAFLD. The increasing prevalence of obesity, coupled with T2DM, dyslipidemia, hypertension and ultimately metabolic syndrome puts more than half the world's population at risk of developing NAFLD/non-alcoholic steato- hepatitis/cirrhosis in the coming decades. Public health initiatives are clearly imperative to halt or reverse the global pandemic diabetes, the underlying basis of NAFLD and metabolic syndrome. In addition, a perspective of NAFLD beyond its hepatic consequences is now warranted; this needs to be considered in relation to management guidelines for affected individuals [7].Nonalcoholic fatty liver disease is commonly associated with type 2 diabetes mellitus but its prevalence is not well studied. It was conducted a prospective study of prevalence and risk factors of NAFLD in patients with type 2 diabetes.Two hundred four type 2 DM patients attending an out-patient diabetic clinic underwent abdominal sonography. Ninety of 127 patients with fatty infiltration on ultrasound consented for liver biopsy, clinical and biochemical workup.Eighty seven percent had NAFLD on histology with 62.6% steatohepatitis and 37.3% fibrosis. Age, duration of diabetes mellitus, degree of glycemic control, body mass index, waist circumference, family history of diabetes mellitus, did not predict the presence or severity of NAFLD or fibrosis. Serum alanine aminostranferase (ALT) and alkaline phosphatase levels, though within normal limits, were significantly higher in patients with steatohepatitis. Prevalence of NASH increased with increase in the components of metabolic syndrome.Serum AST/ALT ratio were also significantly higher in patients with severe fibrosis. All patients with severe fibrosis had metabolic syndrome. Prevalence of NAFLD and NASH in this cohort of type 2 DM patients is high and increases with multiple components of metabolic syndrome. NASH and advanced fibrosis can occur in diabetic patients without any symptom,sign or routine laboratory test abnormalities. [8].Another study investigated the prevalence of NAFLD in those patients attending the routine health checkup and the relationship between NAFLD and metabolic syndrome. The prevalence of NAFLD among these subjects was determined and the presence of risk factors for metabolic disease in each individual was analysed. A relationship between NAFLD and metabolic syndrome was then established. Of the 1003 people 225 (22.6%) had NAFLD with higher prevalence among males 164/565 (29%) than among females 61/438 (13.9%). In the NAFLD group normal body mass index (BMI) was present in only 49/225 (20%) of the subjects while 119/225 (52.8%) were overweight and 56/225 (24.8%) were obese. Though liver enzymes were normal the mean AST among cases was 37.41 ± 14.50 and 33.93 ± 14.15 among controls and the mean ALT was 38.74 ± 17.96 among cases and 31.62 ± 13.49 among controls. Prevalence of metabolic syndrome was 106/225 (47%) among cases and 179/778 (23%) among controls.Therefore,a diagnosis of fatty liver on ultrasound in an asymptomatic person should alert us of metabolic syndrome and its progression to cardiovascular disease. NAFLD may be considered as the hepatic component of metabolic syndrome. [9]. Particularly, it seems that the elevation of serum aminotransferase activity increases the risk of carotid atherosclerosis in these patients. Carotid ultrasonography was used to measure maximal intima-media thickness (IMT) of the common carotid artery (CCA) and IMT (mean) > 1.0 mm was defined as the presence of carotid atherosclerosis.NAFLD patients with ALT elevation had increased risk of carotid atherosclerosis than those with normal ALT by Fisher's exact test ($P < 0.05$). In addition,higher serum ALT levels showed every 10 IU/L increment, greater risk of carotid atherosclerosis. In conclusion,serum ALT levels are positively associated with the risk of carotid atherosclerosis in patients with NAFLD, suggesting that serum ALT levels could serve as a surrogate marker of cardiovascular risk in this special clinical setting [10]. It was also affirmed that obesity and non-alcoholic fatty liver disease produce a low grade systemic inflammatory response syndrome (SIRS) with compromised hepatic blood flow,which impairs with body mass index. It was hypothesized that obesity further aggravates liver dysfunction by reduced hepatic perfusion following resuscitated hemorrhagic shock (HEM) [11]. The long-term prognosis of NAFLD in children remains uncertain.A clinical study focused on the long-term outcomes and survival of children with NAFLD.This retrospective longitudinal hospital-based cohort study evaluated sixty-six children with NAFLD who were followed up for up to 20 years with a total of 409.6 person-years of follow-up. The metabolic syndrome was present in 19(29%)children at the time of NAFLD diagnosis with 55(83%) presenting with at least one feature of the metabolic syndrome including obesity, hypertension, dyslipidaemia and/or hyperglycaemia.

Four children with baseline normal fasting glucose developed type 2 diabetes 4-11 years after NAFLD diagnosis. A total of 13 liver biopsies were obtained from five patients over a mean of 41.4 months showing progression of fibrosis stage in four children. During follow-up, two children died and two underwent liver transplantation for decompensated cirrhosis.

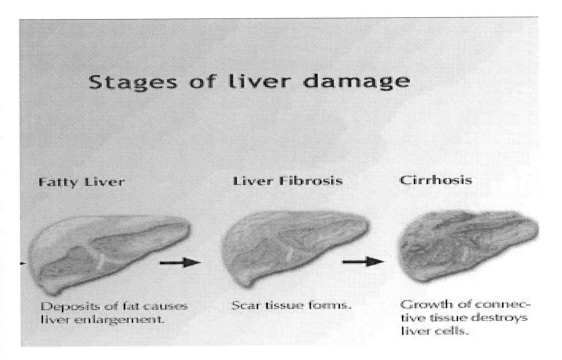

The observed survival free of liver transplantation was significantly shorter in the NAFLD cohort as compared to the expected survival in the general United States population of the same age and sex, with a standardised mortality ratio of 13.6. NAFLD recurred in the allograft in the two cases transplanted, with one patient progressing to cirrhosis and requiring re-transplantation.Children with NAFLD may develop end-stage liver disease with the consequent need for liver transplantation. NAFLD in children seen in a tertiary care centre may be associated with a significantly shorter survival as compared to the general population [12].It was investigated the metabolic profile of women with polycystic ovary syndrome and non-alcoholic fatty liver disease with the aim to determine whether circulating androgens differ in PCOS women with NAFLD compared to PCOS subjects without NAFLD.The results of this study showed that PCOS subjects with NAFLD demonstrate greater insulin resistance but have similar circulating androgen levels. Therefore,in this pilot study, insulin resistance was the most prominent feature characterising NAFLD complicating PCOS. Total testosterone, FAI, DHEAS and 17-hydroxy progesterone levels were similar between patients with PCOS and without NAFLD [13]. Experimental data also suggest that MCP-1 may be important in the regulation of hepatic insulin resistance and may represent a link between inflammation and metabolic diseases. Therefore,dietary cholesterol upregulation of hepatic MCP-1 may help to understand the role of circulating MCP-1 in conditions where liver derangements are clinically important and in the association of liver steatosis with the metabolic syndrome [14]. Incremental progress in understanding NAFLD and nonalcoholic steatohepatitis promises to lead to new therapeutic options for this disease.In the last 15 years evidence has been accumulating, suggesting that hepatic steatosis may be the starting point for a progressive liver disease. Non alcoholic steatosis is now considered a metabolic pathway to advanced liver disease, cirrhosis and hepato cellular carcinoma.Liver disease of other etiology may interact with NAFLD, although the underlying mechanisms have not been fully elucidated. Type 2 diabetes mellitus, obesity and dyslipidemia are the principal factors associated with NAFLD, which is now considered the hepatic expression of metabolic syndrome. Several studies have dealt with the relationship of NAFLD and MS, the risk of liver disease associated with the classical features of MS, the importance of insulin resistance as the common key factor of different diseases. There is still need to clarify the mechanisms responsible for liver disease progression from fatty liver, to steatohepatitis and to cirrhosis, and the reasons why only a few NAFLD cases progress to terminal liver failure while the majority will have a cardiovascular outcome. The epidemics of obesity and diabetes of Western countries is expected to produce a significant increase of metabolic liver disease in the next years. Prevention and intervention programs based on lifestyle are therefore mandatory to reduce the burden of metabolic liver disease [15].

References

[1]   Abdeen MB, Chowdhury NA,Hayden MR,Ibdah JA. Nonalcoholic steatohepatitis and the cardiometabolic syndrome. *J. Cardiometab. Syndr*. 2006;1(1):36-40.

[2]   Neuschwander -Tetri BA.Fatty liver and the metabolic syndrome. *Curr. Opin. Gastroenterol.* 2007;23(2):193-8.

[3]   Gholam PM, Flancbaum L,Machan JT,Charney DA,Kotler DP.Nonalcoholic fatty liver disease in severely obese subjects. *Am. J. Gastroenterol.* 2007;102(2):399-408.

[4]   Fan JG, Saibara T.Chitturi S,Kim BI, Sung JJ,Chutaputti A;Asia –Pacific Working Party for NAFLD.What are the risk factors and settings for non-alcoholic fatty liver disease in Asia-Pacific? *J. Gastroenterol. Hepatol.* 2007; 22(6):794-800.

[5]   Hulek P,Dresslerova I.Metabolic syndrome and the liver (NAFLD/ NASH) *Vnitr. Lek.* 2009;55(7-8):646-9.

[6]   Chitturi S,Farrell GC,Hashimoto E,Saibara T,Lau GK, Sollano JD,Asia-Pacific Working Party on NAFLD.Non-alcoholic fatty liver disease in the Asia-Pacific region: definitions and overview of proposed guidelines. *J. Gastroenterol. Hepatol.* 2007; 22(6):778-87.

[7]   Fan JG,Saibara T.Chitturi S,Kim BI, Sung JJ,Chutaputti A;Asia –Pacific Working Party for NAFLD.What are the risk factors and settings for non-alcoholic fatty liver disease in Asia-Pacific? *J. Gastroenterol. Hepatol.* 2007; 22(6):794-800.

[8]   Prashanth M,Ganesh HK,Vima MV, John M,Bandgar T,Joshi SR,Shah SR,Rathi PM, Joshi AS,Thakkar H,Menon PS,Shah NS. Prevalence of nonalcoholic fatty liver disease in patients with type 2 diabetes mellitus. *J. Assoc. Physicians India* 2009;57: 205-10.

[9]   Uchil D,Pipalia D,Chawla M,Patel R,Maniar S,Narayani ,Junela A.Nonalcoholic fatty liver disease (NAFLD)-the hepatic component of metabolic syndrome. *J. Assoc. Physicians India* 2009; 57: 201-4.

[10] Wang CC,Lin SK,Tseng YF,Hsu CS,Tseng TC,Lin HH,Wang LY,Kao JH.Elevation of serum aminotransferase activity increases risk of carotid atherosclerosis in patients with non-alcoholic fatty liver disease. *J. Gastroenterol. Hepatol.* 2009: 24(8): 1411-6.

[11] Matheson PJ, Hurt RT, Franklin GA, McClain CJ, Garrison RN. Obesity-induced hepatic hypoperfusion primes for hepatic dysfunction after resuscitated hemorrhagic shock. *Surgery* 2009 ; 146(4):739-47.

[12] Feldstein AE,Charatcharoenwitthava P,Treeprasertsuk S,Benson JT,Enders FB, Angulo P.The natural history of nonalcoholic fatty liver disease in children: a follow/up study for up to 20 years. *Gut* 2009; 58(11): 1538-44.

[13] Kauffman RP,Baker TE,Baker V,Kauffman MM,Daniel Castracane V. Endocrine factors associated with non-alcoholic fatty liver disease in women with polycystic ovary syndrome: Do androgens play a role? Gynecol. *Endocrinol.* 2009; [Epub ahead of print].

[14] Rull A,Rodriguez F,Aragones G,Beltran R,Alonso-Villaverde C,Camps J,Joven J. Hepatic monocyte chemoattractant protein-1 is upregulated by dietary cholesterol and contributes to liver steatosis. *Cytokine* 2009;48(3):273-9.

[15] Marchesini G,Babini M.Nonalcoholic fatty liver disease and the metabolic syndrome. *Minerva Cardioangiol.* 2006;54(2):229-39.

Chronic Kidney Disease

Chronic kidney disease (CKD) is a progressive loss of renal function over a period of months or years. All individuals with a Glomerular Filtration Rate(GFR) <60 mL/min/1.73 m2 for 3 months are classified as having chronic kidney disease, irrespective of the presence or absence of kidney damage. The rationale for including these individuals is that reduction in kidney function to this level or lower represents loss of half or more of the adult level of normal kidney function, which may be associated with a number of complications. All individuals with kidney damage are classified as having chronic kidney disease, irrespective of the level of GFR. The rationale for including individuals with GFR 60 mL/min/1.73 m2 is that GFR may be sustained at normal or increased levels despite substantial kidney damage and that patients with kidney damage are at increased risk of the two major outcomes of chronic kidney disease: loss of kidney function and development of cardiovascular disease.The loss of protein in the urine is regarded as an independent marker for worsening of renal function and cardiovascular disease (CVD).Hence, British guidelines append the letter "P" to the stage of chronic kidney disease if there is significant protein loss. The metabolic effects of obesity are the most common risk factors for diabetes,hypertension and atherosclerosis , the leading causes of end-stage renal failure.

Chronic kidney disease increases the rate of CVD,development of end-stage renal disease, and can lead to premature death. Although, no direct causally link between obesity and CKD can be yet established , this appears highly likely.and CKD should be regarded as a major complication of overweight and obesity. Is still unclear if the association is independent or influenced by diabetes, hypertension, CVD, metabolic syndrome and high fructose intake [1].

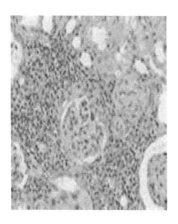

The most common causes of CKD are diabetic nephropathy, hypertension, and glomerulonephritis. Together, these cause represent approximately 75% of all adult cases. Certain geographic areas have a high incidence of HIV nephropathy. Historically, kidney disease has been classified according to the part of the renal anatomy that is involved, as vascular(bilateral renal artery stenosis, hemolytic-uremic syndrome, ischemic nephropathy) ,glomerular (primary : focal segmental glomerulo- sclerosis and IgA nephritis; secondary :diabetic nephropathy and lupus nephritis), tubointerstitial and obstructive

The prevalence of the metabolic syndrome in the United States is almost 47 million and rising as a result of the current obesity and diabetes epidemics [2].The Third National Health and Nutrition Examination Survey reported that CKD is also increasingly common, with an estimated 8 million people in the US with GFR <60 ml/min. Many aspects of the metabolic syndrome phenotype are associated with CKD,suggesting that individuals with visceral obesity are at increased risk for progressive loss of renal function. An increased waist-hip ratio conferred a greater risk of microalbuminuria and a greater risk of diminished estimated glomerular filtration rate(eGFR) .An Indian study performed in a population of 3.155 males and 2.097 females established that the mean age for low GFR subjects was 54 years.The survey population had a 2.25% prevalence of proteinuria.Age above 60 years,female gender,low educational status,increased waist circumference, hypertension and diabetes were associated with low eGFR. Similar factors were also associated with proteinuria [3].CKD risk in individuals with the metabolic syndrome may reflect the presence of known risk factors for CKD initiation and progression as hypertension and diabetes rather than an independent effect. One approach to identifying a distinction would be to compare the prevalence of CKD in metabolic syndrome cohorts who do or do not satisfy diagnostic criteria for diabetes. It is reasonable to view the renal risks and consequences of the metabolic syndrome and diabetes as indistinguishable [4].A significant study was performed on 5083 subjects with a glomerular filtration rate $\geq$ 60ml/min/ 1.73 m^2 without micro-or macroalbuminuria with the aim to analyze the association between BMI and elevated serum cystatin C. Elevated cystatin C was defined as $\geq$ 1.09 mg/L(or $\geq$ 99th percentile for participants, 20-39 years of age without diabetes, hypertension, micro-or macroalbuminuria or stage 3-5 chronic kidney disease). The odds ratio of elevated serum cystatin C was 1.46 for overweight, 2.36 for class I obesity and 2.82 for class II-III obesity. Therefore, this research showed a greater association between higher BMI and elevated serum cystatin C [5]. The Framingham study considered 2676 subjects (mean age 43 years) of whom 52% women free of stage 3 CKD. At baseline, 36% of the sample was overweight and 12% was obese.Two hundred-two (7.9%) of the sample developed stage 3 CKD during 18.5 years of follow-up.The results of this study showed that obese subjects had a 68% increased risk of developing stage 3 CKD. Furthermore, it was demonstrated that proteinuria occurred in 14.4% of the cases and overweight and obese subjects were at increased for the highest proteinuria.However, considering that the participants to this study were mainly white,these findings may not apply to different ethnic groups. In the mean time,the study showed that obesity is associated with an increased risk of developing stage 3 CKD but this relationship may be mediated through cardiovascular disease risk factors [6].The risk starts to increase at a body mass index of 25. In Japan, more strictly to residents of Okinawa and Iseki ,was also found that body mass index was an independent predictor of end-stage renal disease. But it is important to note that here the risk starts at a body mass index of 21 kg\m². Consequently BMI is not BMI across ethnicities. From the Framingham study we know that BMI is an independent predictor of reduction of estimated GFR: It is also known that obesity is not only an independent predictor of end-stage renal disease but is also correlated to albuminuria. The interest in obesity started three decades ago when, not surprisingly,in the USA a syndrome of focal segmental glomerulosclerosis with proteinuria and rapid progression into renal failure was found in morbidly obese individuals who had no primary renal disease. The syndrome, discovered in 1974, has meanwhile also been observed in Europe. Recent guidelines of the European Society of Hypertension (ESH)and the European Society of Cardiology (ESC) for the management of arterial hypertension (AH) have recognized the importance of renal function impairment on cardiovascular prognosis in patients with this condition. Chronic kidney disease is associated with increased risk of CVD and end-stage renal disease (ESRD), particularly among patients with AH. CKD, diagnosed according to estimated GFR, was found in 314 \ 749 considered patients with essential AH (42%). Patients with CKD were significantly more likely to be older, to have atherogenic dyslipidemia and a history of cardiovascular diseases (coronary heart disease, prior myocardial infarction, heart failure). To identify this high risk population, the systemic assessment of GFR and other CV factors should be done in every case of AH, especially in older and female patients [7].Only a few studies have evaluated the prevalence of CKD in type 2 diabetes in primary care, and few studies are available on hypertensive diabetics. An Italian national project involving general practitioners and nephrologists, retrieved demographic, laboratory and clinical data regarding 7582 hypertensive type 2 diabetics (3564 men; age 25-89 years) who were selected using the diagnostic Classification of Diseases ICD-9-CM for diabetes and hypertension. CKD prevalence was 26%, although renal disease was diagnosed by GPs in only 5.4% of cases. The prevalence of both LVH and major CV events was 8%. Adequate blood pression control was only achieved in 10.4% of patients.Patients whose GFR was <60 mL/min/1.73 m2 were older, prevalently female, had increased pulse pressure and higher prevalence of dyslipidaemia .Moreover, the prevalence of both LVH and major CV events was higher in patients with CKD as compared to patients with normal GFR.This study shows that CKD is highly prevalent in hypertensive type 2 diabetic patients,where it is a strong predictor of CV adverse outcome.However, awareness of CKD by GPs is low.Therefore,patients with hypertension and diabetes type II may be considered an high- risk population [8].The largest database has been presented on the NHANES Study(National Health and Nutrition Examination Study).In this Finnish study(FinnDIANE study)the presence of a metabolic syndrome was found in 38% of men and 40% of women with type I diabetes.This is not proving causality but it is very suggestive. Interestingly, there was interaction between glycaemic control reflected by haemoglobin A1C and the prevalence of the metabolic syndrome.Overall for patients with type I diabetes and the metabolic syndrome, the odds ratio for the presence of diabetic nephropathy was higher by a factor of 3.75.Obviously, obesity is associated with progression promoters such as hypertension, diabetes, potentially dyslipidemia. But there are also more fascinating causal links. It has been proposed by Luyckx and Brenner the association between low birth weight and renal dysfunction in humans. Anatomic measurements of infants, children, and adults show significant inverse correlation between LBW and nephron number.Nephron numbers are also lower in individuals with hypertension compared with normotension among white and Australian Aboriginal populations. The relationship between nephron number and hypertension among black individuals is still unclear, although the high incidence of LBW predicts low nephron number in this population as well. Because early postnatal growth also affects subsequent risk for higher BP or reduced renal function, postnatal nutrition, a potentially modifiable factor, in addition to intrauterine effects, has significant influence on long-term cardiovascular and renal health. Therefore,a maternal malnutrition and a disturbed prenatal environment, followed by postnatal catch up growth, could cause a lower number of nephrons, as is also reported for patients with essential hypertension [9].This constellation is associated with a greater risk of insulin resistance and obesity. For several years, the epidemiological data have shown an inverse relationship between birth-weight and the development in later life of cardiovascular disease and metabolic disorders. The term "small for gestational age" (SGA) describes a neonate whose birth-weight is two standard deviations (SD) below the reference mean, corrected for gestational age and gender. SGA is associated with increased risks of developing hypertension, insulin resistance and type2 diabetes. However, the association with an atherogenic lipid profile is less clear. In the meantime, in spite of the large body of data in the literature, the biological mechanisms underlying this association are still unclear. To explain the association, various hypotheses have been proposed, pointing to the role of a detrimental fetal environment or genetic susceptibility, or interaction between the two, and to the particular dynamic changes in adiposity that occur during catch-up growth. However, not only quantitative, but also qualitative, abnormalities of adipose tissue have been observed, suggesting a critical role of this organ in the development of metabolic complications. Recently, in women aged 40 who had undergone myocardial infarction it was found that their birth weight was lower and their post-natal catch up growth was higher. So, the cardiovascular, as well as the renal risk, begins in part in utero [10]. A second, and possibly complementary, explanation would be the high concentrations of the adipocyte hormone leptin. Were hypothesized the following actions : induction of TGF beta, oxidative stress, modulation of growth processes in the kidney, elevated sympathetic nerve tone,increased hypertension, proinflammatory responses and upregulation of TGF beta-receptors. So, there are many factors through which leptin might be injurious to the kidney. Wisse described the link between chronic inflammation of visceral adiposity and insulin resistance and pathologic features that characterize the metabolic syndrome [11,12,13,14]. The prevalence of chronic kidney disease was 39.17% (358 patients), and patients with metabolic factors had a significantly higher prevalence of chronic kidney disease than those without metabolic factors (40.90% vs. 17.65%, p < 0.01). The metabolic factors and microinflammatory biomarkers were significantly higher in patients with chronic kidney disease. Patients who had more abnormal metabolic factors also had higher levels of microinflammatory biomarkers, as well as higher risk of chronic kidney disease. Several analyses revealed that systolic blood pressure , serum triglyceride, low density lipoprotein, age, and duration of type 2 diabetes were independent risk factors of chronic kidney disease . The abnormality of metabolic factors in type 2 diabetes mellitus had a close relationship to the microinflammatory state and chronic kidney disease. Hypertension and hyperlipidemia were independent factors of chronic kidney disease in type 2 diabetes mellitus [15]. The role of specific mediators in the pathogenesis of the metabolic syndrome including leptin, IL-6, TNF-, adiponectin and acylation-stimulating protein, was discussed in the Wisse study [11].Until recently, adipocytes were viewed as the most likely source of soluble, metabolic syndrome mediators [16]. However,some published studies within the past year implicating macrophages, which infiltrate fat tissue, as the principal site of obesity-related cytokine synthesis [17,18,19]. It is possible to speculate that progressive kidney disease could be regulated by proinflammatory cytokines in the context of the metabolic syndrome. Other potential mechanisms include physical compression of kidney parenchyma by adipose tissue, reduced birth weight and nephron number, enhanced glucocorticoid activity, or altered uric acid metabolism [20].The symptoms of worsening kidney function are unspecific, and might include feeling generally unwell and experiencing a reduced appetite.Often, chronic kidney disease is diagnosed as a result of screening of people known to be at risk of kidney problems, such as those with high blood pressure or diabetes and those with a blood relative with chronic kidney disease. Chronic kidney disease may also be identified when it leads to one of its recognized complications, such as cardiovascular disease, anemia or pericarditis. Chronic kidney disease is identified by a blood test for creatinine. Higher levels of creatinine indicate a falling glomerular filtration rate and as a result a decreased capability of the kidneys to excrete waste products. Creatinine levels may be normal in the early stages of CKD, and the condition may be suspected through a testing on urine sample that may reveal the loss of protein or red blood cells into the urine. To fully investigate the underlying cause of kidney damage, various forms of medical imaging, blood tests and often renal biopsy are employed to find out if there is a reversible cause for the kidney dysfunction .Recent professional guidelines of NKF (National Kidney Foundation) classify the severity of chronic kidney disease in five stages, with stage 1 being the mildest and usually causing few symptoms and stage 5 being a severe illness with poor life expectancy, if untreated.

Stages of Chronic Kidney Disease-NKF (National Kidney Foundation)

Stage 1 Slightly diminished function; Kidney damage with normal or relatively high GFR (>90 mL/min/1.73 m^2). Kidney damage is defined as pathologic abnormalities or markers of damage, including abnormalities in blood or urine test or imaging studies

Stage 2 Mild reduction in GFR (60-89 mL/min/1.73 m^2) with kidney damage .Kidney damage is defined as pathologic abnormalities or markers of damage, including abnormalities in blood or urine test or imaging studies.

Stage 3 Moderate reduction in GFR (30-59 mL/min/1.73 m^2) British guidelines distinguish between stage 3A (GFR 45-59) and stage 3B (GFR 30-44) for purposes of screening and referral.

Stage 4 Severe reduction in GFR (15-29 mL/min/1.73 m^2) Preparation for renal replacement therapy

Stage 5 Established kidney failure (GFR <15 mL/min/1.73 m^2, or permanent renal replacement therapy (RRT)

Stage 5 CKD is synonymous with the now outdated terms end-stage renal disease (ESRD), chronic kidney failure (CKF) or chronic renal failure (CRF). There is no specific treatment unequivocally shown to slow the worsening of chronic kidney disease. If there is an underlying cause to CKD, such as vasculitis, this may be treated directly with treatments aiming to slow the damage. In more advanced stages, treatments may be required for anemia and bone disease. Severe CKD requires one of the forms of renal replacement therapy; this may be a form of dialysis, but ideally constitutes a kidney transplant.

Prognosis

The prognosis of patients with chronic kidney disease ,considered as epidemiological data, has shown that the overall mortality rate increases as kidney function decreases [21].The leading cause of death in patients with chronic kidney disease is cardiovascular disease, regardless of whether there is progression to stage 5 [22,23].Renal transplantation significantly increases the survival of patients with stage 5 CKD when compared to other therapeutic options; however in some cases, it is associated with an increased short-term mortality, due to complications of the surgery. Transplantation aside, high intensity home hemodialysis appears to be associated with improved survival and a greater quality of life, when compared to the conventional three times a week hemodialysis and peritoneal dialysis [26].

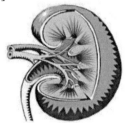

Although, renal replacement can maintain patients indefinitely and prolong their life, in some patients the quality of life may be severely affected (24,25).

Only 3.3% of subjects with renal impairment is aware of the disease. Primary prevention and management targeted at CKD risk factors must play a critical role in controlling rising CKD magnitude. Cost-benefit analysis of targeted screening programs is needed [27]. In conclusion the high mortality risk of chronic kidney disease and the strict link with obesity,diabetes and cardiovascular disease induce to provide urgent national programs of screening and prevention as well as intervention in improving chronic kidney disease outcomes, while reducing the cost of care [28].

References

[1] Ting SM,Nair H, Ching I, Taheri S,Dasgupta I.Overweight,obesity and chronic kidney disease. Nephron. *Clin. Pract.* 2009;112 (3): 121-7.

[2] Coresh J, Astor BC, Greene T, Eknoyan G, Levey AS: Prevalence of chronic kidney disease and decreased kidney function in the adult US population: Third National Health and Nutrition Examination Survey. *Am. J. Kidney Dis.* 2003; 41: 1–12.

[3] Singh NP,Ingle GK,Saini VK,Jami A,Beniwal P,Lai M,Meena GS. Prevalence of low glomerular filtration rate, proteinuria and associated risk factors in North India using Cockcroft-Gault and Modification of Diet in Renal Disease equation: an observational, cross-sectional study. *BMC Nephrol.* 2009; 10:4.

[4] Weisinger JR, Kempson RL, Eldridge FL, Swenson RS: The nephrotic syndrome: A complication of massive obesity. *Ann. Intern. Med.* 81: 440–447, 1974.

[5] Muntner P,Winston J,Uribarri J,Mann D,Fox CS. Overweight,obesity,and elevated serum cystatin C levels in adults in the United States. *Am. J. Med.* 2008;121(4):341-8.

[6] Foster MC,Hwang SJ,Larson MG,Lichtman JH.Parikh NI,Vasan RS,Levy D,Fox CS. Overweight ,obesity,and the development of stage 3 CKD :the Framingham hearth study. *Am. J. Kidney Dis.* 2008;52(1): 39-48.

[7] Grabysa R,Cholewa M. .Diminished glomerular filtration rate as a marker of chronic kidney disease in hypertensive patients. *Pol. Merkur Lekasski* 2008;24(144):478-91.

[8] Ravera M., Noberasco G,Re M,Filippi A,Gallina AM,Weiss U,Cannavo R, Ravera G,Cricelli C,Deferrari G.Chronic kidney disease and cardiovascular risk in hypertensive type 2 diabetics: a primary care perspective. *Nephrol. Dial Transplant.* 2009;24(5):1528-33.

[9] Luyckx VA, Brenner BM. The Clinical Importance of Nephron Mass. *J. Am. Soc. Nephrol.* 2010 Feb 11. [Epub ahead of print].

[10] Means T. Fetal origins of insulin resistance and the metabolic syndrome: A key role for adipose tissue? *Diabetes Metab.* 2009; [Epub ahead of print].

[11] Wisse BE: The inflammatory syndrome: the role of adipose tissue cytokines in metabolic disorders linked to obesity. *J. Am. Soc. Nephrol.* 2004;15: 2792–2800.

[12] Hirosumi J, Tuncman G, Chang L, Gorgun CZ, Uysal KT, Maeda K, Karin M, Hotamisligil GS: A central role for JNK in obesity and insulin resistance. *Nature* 2002;420: 333–336.

[13] Perreault M, Marette A: Targeted disruption of inducible nitric oxide synthase protects against obesity-linked insulin resistance in muscle. *Nat. Med.* 2001; 7: 1138–1143.

[14] Guebre-Egziabher F,Kalbacher E,Fouque D.Insulin resistance and inflammation in chronic kidney diseases. *Nephrol. Ther.* 2009; Suppl. 5: 346-52.

[15] Cao C,Wan X, Chen Y,Wu W.Metabolic factors and microinflammatory state promote kidney injury in type 2 diabetes mellitus patients. *Ren. Fail.* 2009; 31(6):470-4.

[16] Rajala MW, Scherer PE: Minireview: The adipocyte.At the crossroads of energy homeostasis, inflammation, and atherosclerosis. *Endocrinology* 2003;144: 3765–3773.

[17] Weisberg SP, McCann D, Desai M, Rosenbaum M, Leibel RL, Ferrante A W Jr: Obesity is associated with macrophage accumulation in adipose tissue. *J. Clin. Invest.* 2003;112: 1796–1808.

[18] Xu H, Barnes GT, Yang Q, Tan G, Yang D, Chou CJ, Sole J, Nichols A, Ross JS, Tartaglia LA, Chen H: Chronic inflammation in fat plays a crucial role in the development of obesity-related insulin resistance; therefore, many of these cytokines have been suggested to mediate renal disease pathophysiology. *J. Clin. Invest.* 2003;112: 1821–1830.

[19] Wolf G, Chen S, Han DC, Ziyadeh FN: Leptin and renal disease. *Am. J. Kidney Dis.* 2002; 39: 1–11.

[20] Masuzaki H, Yamamoto H, Kenyon CJ, Elmquist JK, Morton NM, Paterson JM, Shinyama H, Sharp MG, Fleming S, Mullins JJ, Seckl JR, Flier JS: Transgenic amplification of glucocorticoid action in adipose tissue causes high blood pressure in mice. *J. Clin. Invest.* 112: 83–90, 2003.

[21] Perazella MA, Khan S (March 2006). "Increased mortality in chronic kidney disease: a call to action". *Am. J. Med. Sci.* 331 (3): 150–3.

[22] Sarnak MJ, Levey AS, Schoolwerth AC, et al. Kidney disease as a risk factor for development of cardiovascular disease. *Circulation* 2003; 108 (17): 2154–69.

[23] Tonelli M , Wiebe N, Culleton B, et al. Chronic kidney disease and mortality risk: a systematic review. *J. Am. Soc. Nephrol.* 17 (7): 2034–47.).

[24] Heidenheim AP, Kooistra MP, Lindsay RM "Quality of life". *Contrib. Nephrol.* 2004; 145: 99–105.

[25] de Francisco AL, Piñera C ( ). "Challenges and future of renal replacement therapy". *Hemodial. Int.* 2006; 10 Suppl 1: S19–23.

[26] Pierratos A, McFarlane P, Chan CT "Quotidian dialysis--update 2005". *Curr. Opin. Nephrol. Hypertens* 2005;14 (2): 119–24.

[27] Singh NP,Ingle GK,Saini VK,Jami A,Beniwal P,Lai M,Meena GS. Prevalence of low glomerular filtration rate, proteinuria and associated risk factors in North India using Cockcroft-Gault and Modification of Diet in Renal Disease equation: an observational, cross-sectional study. *BMC Nephrol.* 2009; 10:4.

[28] Ramirez SP.Chronic kidney disease prevention in Singapore. *Clin. J. Am. Soc. Nephrol.* 2008;3(2):610-5.

PCOS and Gynaecological Cancer Risk

PCOS is accompanied by such conditions as oligo/anovulation, hyperandrogenism, lower cell sensitivity to insulin, type II diabetes, hyperlipidemia and obesity that are factors considered to predispose towards cancer [1,2]. Really, infertile women with anovulation and polycystic ovarian syndrome seem to have an increased lifetime risk for neoplasms of the reproductive tract, like endometrial, breast and ovary cancer .An interesting study evaluating long-term consequences of polycystic ovary syndrome during a 31 year follow- up estimated that the proportion of women with involuntary infertility was 17.5% in PCOS women compared with 1.3% in the control women. In addition, the same study reported that PCOS women were not at significantly increased risk of mortality or morbidity for breast carcinoma but were at increased risk of endometrial cancer [3]. Clinical and laboratory data such as anthropometric measurements,endogenous hormones and growth factors may explain the mechanisms which link tumorogenesis or tumor promotion to infertility [4].There is a possible correlation between PCOS and endometrial cancer, which emerges from clinical research focused on molecular changes in endometrium of patients with PCOS. While, correlation between PCOS and breast or ovary cancer is not so strong, in spite of single trials which are showing the link [5]. In conclusion, women with PCOS appear to be three time more likely to develop endometrial cancer but they are not at increased risk for breast cancer .There is insufficient evidence to implicate PCOS in the development of vaginal, vulval, cervical or ovarian cancer.

Ovarian Cancer

Although it is relatively uncommon, it is the 5th leading cause of cancer death in women. One of every seventy women will develop this cancer during her lifetime. It is the leading cause of death from gynecologic cancers. About 25,000 women in the US are diagnosed each year. About 14,000 die each year from the disease. Ovarian cancer can occur in adult women of any age, although women over age 60 have the highest rate High local steroid and growth factor concentrations are considered risk factors for ovary carcinoma and are frequently observed in PCOS women [6]. A few studies have addressed the possibility of an association between PCOS and epithelial ovarian cancer risk, and the results are conflicting but generally reassuring and similarly the few available data appear to exclude a strong association between PCOS and breast cancer [5]. Obesity seems to increase the woman' s risk of developing histological subtypes of ovarian cancer. The association seems to exist for clear cell carcinoma but not for invasive endometrioid or mucinous tumors.Although there was no association with invasive serous tumors overall. Olsen et al reported an increased risk of serous peritoneal tumors but not of serous tumors of the ovary and fallopian tube. Of the borderline subtypes, obesity was positively associated with serous but not mucinous tumors [7]. Ovarian cancer risk was found to increase 2.5 fold among women with PCOS. This association was found to be stronger among women who never used hormonal contraceptives and women who were in the first quartile of body mass index (13.3-18.5 kg / m² at age 18) [8].Furthermore, exploratory analyses suggested a positive association between BMI and ovarian cancer among women without a family history of ovarian cancer, but no relation with BMI was apparent among women with a positive family history of ovarian cancer [9].Although parity seems to be inversely related to risk of benign, borderline and invasive ovarian tumours , increasing numbers of births did not further decrease risk of any of the tumour types [10]. Additionally, some findings showed that a history of incomplete pregnancy, spontaneous or induced abortions, does not influence a woman's risk of epithelial ovarian cancer [11]. In some studies, researchers have found that prolonged use of the fertility drug clomiphene citrate, especially without achieving pregnancy, may increase the risk for developing ovarian tumors.   However, infertility also increases the risk of ovarian cancer, even without use of fertility drugs.Few studies have addressed the possibility of an association between polycystic ovaries and ovarian cancer, and the results are conflicting and generally reassuring [5]. Although PCOS has not generally been associated with a significant increase in the risk of ovarian cancer or colon cancer, it is important to remember that the use of oral contraceptives can also decrease the risk of ovarian cancer.

Breast Cancer

In 2001, the US population reached 277 million, with women representing 51.2% of the total population. According to the Women's Health USA 2003, females under 54 years of age accounted for more than 80 million. Community-based studies have estimated the prevalence of polycystic ovaries in the normal population to be in the order of 5-10% (4-8 million), indicating that they are extremely common.In 1998, Pierpoint et al. first reported that the standardised mortality ratio (SMR) calculated for 786 patients with PCOS compared with the normal population and found that the SMR for all neoplasms was 0.91(95% CI 0.60–1.32) and for breast cancer 1.48 (95% CI 0.79–2.54). In their cohort study, breast cancer was the leading cause of death [12]. Nevertheless, it is unclear if women with PCOS have an increased risk of breast cancer, partially because other factors like obesity and nulliparity are confounding variables.In fact, studies examining the relationship between PCOS and breast carcinoma have not always identified a significantly increased risk. It is believed that the proportion of women with a positive family history of breast cancer was significantly greater in women with PCOS compared with controls.Although other studies found similar percentages of women with a family history of breast cancer in PCOS and controls and no significant difference between the groups [2].Two long and broad streams of medical literature, from the 1950's to date, have established the existence of two unrelated abnormalities of androgen production in women with breast cancer. One is the genetically determined presence of subnormal production of adrenal androgens, DHEA and DHEAS, in women with premenopausal breast cancer and their sisters, who are at increased risk for breast cancer. The other is the excessive production of testosterone, of ovarian origin, in subsets of women with either premenopausal or postmenopausal breast cancer and women with atypical breast-duct hyperplasia, who are at increased risk for breast cancer; along with the hypertestosteronism, there is frequently chronic anovulation in the premenopausal patients [13,14].The combination of ovarian hypertestosteronism and chronic anovulation is characteristic of the polycystic ovary syndrome and is also frequently seen in women with abdominal obesity[15].Increased testosterone secretion by the ovaries is currently the only major hormonal abnormality shown to be associated with increased risk of both premenopausal and postmenopausal breast cancer[16].In addition, upper body type obesity is linked to hyperandrogenism as well as to hyperinsulinaemia which can increase the ovarian production of androgens. The increased prevalence of ER+ breast cancers in patients with higher levels of IGF-1, IGFBP-3(IGF-Binding Protein) or testosterone implicate these hormones in the etiology of hormone dependent breast cancer [17]. However, the risk of breast cancer associated with serum IGF-1 and IGFBP may depend upon menopausal status. In fact, serum IGFBP-1 was not associated with breast cancer risk in either pre- or postmenopausal women.In premenopausal women, elevated serum IGF-1 and IGFBP-3 seem to be associated with increased breast cancer risk, whereas elevated serum IGFBP-2 seems to be inversely associated with risk of postmenopausal breast cancer[18].Therefore, this observation leads to consider that the risk of breast cancer is not increased in women with polycystic ovary syndrome who have chronic estrogen exposure and androgen excess . Although in postmenopausal women who are estrogen deplete and have increased aromatase activity ,higher testosterone has been associated with greater breast cancer risk This consideration could suggest to avoid the testosterone therapy in estrogen deplete women because of the potential risk of enhanced aromatization to estrogen [19].Insulin-like growth factors and estrogens are essential hormones regulating the growth and differentiation of mammary cells and at higher levels are strong mitogens for breast cancer. Furthermore , a possible synergy between IGF and steroid hormones, as estrogen and androgen, in relation to breast cancer risk has been suggested [20]. Because an association between PCOS and breast cancer is plausible, it is imperative to be vigilant about breast disease in the follow up care of all women with PCOS. The problem is that women with PCOS tend to have multiple hormones that are seriously out of balance with each other. For example, prolonged lack of ovulation with consequent continued secretion of estrogen unopposed by progesterone may enhance the development and growth of endometrial cancer, especially in young women. "Estrogen dominance" is also one of the risk factors for breast cancer. However, the overall risk of developing ovarian cancer as a result of PCOS is not much higher than other women. So,women with PCOS could be at a higher risk of developing breast cancer. The reason is because the risk of breast cancer increases with estrogen levels, which tend to be higher among women with Polycystic Ovarian Syndrome. Women with PCOS are also more likely to be overweight or obese, which raises the risk of breast cancer. Having regular mammograms and doing self breast exams are two preventative steps that women with PCOS can take to help ensure early detection of breast cancer. The evidence of the adverse effects of obesity, especially abdominal obesity, is overwhelming and indisputable. Obesity substantially increases the risk of several major cancers in women, including post-menopausal breast cancer. Although the link between excess abdominal fat and cancer is not clearly understood, scientists believe that the higher levels of insulin and glucose in the blood stream, a hallmark of Insulin Resistance and an underlying cause of PCOS somehow stimulate cancer cell growth. In women after menopause, excessive abdominal fat doubles the risk of breast cancer, regardless of overall weight.Scientists believe that the components of Insulin Resistance and Polycystic Ovarian Syndrome - namely hyperinsulinemia, dyslipidemia, hypertension and atherosclerosis - actually favor the growth of breast cancer cells, creating an environment ripe for the development of this disease. Clinical and epidemiological evidence suggests that both breast cancer and PCOS are polygenic and multifactorial in origin, meaning there are a variety of genes and factors that result in these conditions. While studies are still on-going, preliminary data suggests that increased levels of insulin in the blood increase the formation of breast cancer cells. Because an association between PCOS and breast cancer is plausible, it is imperative to be vigilant about breast disease in the follow up care of all women with PCOS.Nutritional and lifestyle modifications that improve insulin sensitivity may not only decrease a tendency to atherosclerosis but also reduce breast cancer risk in women. A realistic exercise program, nutritional guidance and a support system could help to change unhealthy lifestyle choices.

Endometrial Hyperplasia and Endometrial Cancer

There is increasing evidence that the endocrinologic and metabolic abnormalities of PCOS may have complex effects on the endometrium contributing to the infertility and endometrial disorders observed in women with this syndrome. It has been demonstrated in numerous studies that women who did not achieved a pregnancy have two to three times the risk of developing the endometrial cancer compared to women who have had a successful pregnancy. Many women who are unable to achieve a pregnancy are anovulatory. Anovulatory cycles result in chronic estrogen exposure to the endometrial lining and in increased risk of developing endometrial cancer.[14,21]. Many women who cannot become pregnant are anovulatory, meaning they don't ovulate on a regular cycle or sometimes they don't ovulate at all. PCOS is one of the most common causes of anovulation. Without progesterone which causes the endometrium to shed each month as a menstrual period, the endometrium may grow too much and undergo atypical cell changes. This is a precancerous condition called endometrial hyperplasia(EH). The primary presenting symptom of EH is abnormal uterine bleeding. Approximately 70% of women with abnormal uterine bleeding are diagnosed with benign findings and 15% are diagnosed with carcinoma [22].If the thickened endometrium is not treated, over a long period of time it can develop into endometrial cancer.Fortunately, the use of oral contraceptives can help regulate hormone levels, thereby lowering the risk of developing this cancer.Scientists believe it : the chronic exposure to estrogen of the endometrial lining increases the risk of developing endometrial cancer

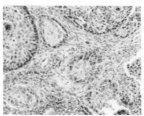

Endometrial carcinoma

Thus, elevated estrogen without the opposing effects of progesterone in the absence of ovulation, hyperinsulinemia,elevated free IGF-I,androgens, and obesity all, likely contribute to endometrial dysfunction, infertility, increased miscarriage rate, endometrial hyperplasia, and endometrial cancer, common in women with PCOS [23]. Lack of ovulation or late ovulation play a crucial role in endometrial cyclic transformation and its disorders[24].The prolonged endometrial proliferation phase is a characteristic feature of women suffering from PCOS and PCOS is one of the most common causes of anovulation [25]. Polycystic ovary syndrome is often associated with weight problems. Another troubling statistic is that women who are 21 to 50 pounds overweight run 3 times the risk of endometrial cancer, while women who are more than 50 pounds overweight have a ten-fold higher risk. It is well known that the peripheral conversion of adrenal androstenedione to estrone results in chronic exposure of the endometrium to circulating estrogens increasing the risk of endometrial cancer [26].On the other hand, estrogen producing ovarian tumors are also associated with an increased risk of endometrial cancer. Women who do not undergo menopause until 52 years of age are at a twofold increased risk of developing endometrial cancer. Anovulatory cycles in the perimenopausal years again result in a prolonged exposure of the endometrium to progesterone-deficient menstrual cycles, thus increasing the risk of endometrial cancer. Diabetes mellitus also increases the woman's risk of developing endometrial cancer by greater than two fold. The menopausal use of estrogen replacement therapy, without progestins,increases the risk of endometrial cancer four to eight fold [27] Tamoxifen , the antiestrogen commonly used in the treatment of breast cancer, is also associated with a two to three fold increased risk for the development of endometrial cancer [28,29].The spectrum of pathological findings in patients treated with tamoxifen suggests that this drug promotes endometrial growth and that endometrial polyps may be an important intermediate step in endometrial carcinogenesis [30].Therefore, prominent risk factors for carcinoma are unopposed estrogen therapy, obesity, diabetes, early menarche, and late menopause [24,31].In conclusion, epidemiological studies, laboratory data and theoretical grounds suggest the increased potential for endometrial hyperplasia and malignancy in women with anovulation PCOS - related. Although data available in the literature do not consent an exact estimate of the relative risk of endometrial carcinoma in PCOS women.

Pathogenesis

There is a clear relationship between the amount of estrogen and progesterone secreted by the ovary, from puberty to menopause, and the development of hyperplastic endometrium of all types and finally endometrial carcinoma [27,32,33].The classical risk increase for endometrial cancer is associated with oligomenorrhea or polimenorrhea combined with corpus luteum deficiency or anovulation. The prolonged anovulation with consequent continued secretion of estrogen unopposed by progesterone may enhance the development and growth of this malignancy, particularly in young women [34,35,36].Progesterone deficiency seems to be the key factor leading to endometrial disorders. Corpus luteum deficiency can represent the most frequent endogenous endocrine pattern but treatment with estrogen or estrogen and progestogen can also induce progesterone deficiency in pre and postmenopausal women. One main factor is the level of SHBG determined by the amount of free, biologically active estradiol. It is believed that endometrial hyperplasia arises when estrogen, unopposed by progesterone, stimulates endometrial cell growth by binding to estrogen receptors in the nuclei of endometrial cells [26,28,32]. Exposure of these estrogen-induced proliferating cells to progesterone prompts the shedding of endometrial tissue both by reducing the number of estrogen receptors and by increasing the rate of conversion of estradiol to estrone, a less potent estrogen, through an increase in the activity of estradiol dehydrogenase [26,28,37] Diabetes mellitus also increases a woman's risk of developing endometrial cancer by greater than two fold.[38] .Several studies have appreciated the higher incidence of endometrial adenocarcinoma in the presence of anovulatory conditions and unopposed estrogen. Polycystic ovary syndrome is the most common cause of oligoovulation and anovulation in infertile women. Prolonged endometrial exposure to estrogen and unopposed by the inhibitory effects of progesterone in these patients makes them susceptible to endometrial hyperplasia. [39].However, age and endometrial thickness (ET) were recognized as independent risk factors for EH. The chances for EH in infertile women with PCOS will increase by age, obesity and ET more than 7mm. Multiple mechanisms may be responsible for the increased risk of endometrial cancer in the context of PCOS. To be sure, endometrial carcinoma need not be associated with abnormally high estrogen or insulin levels. Yet, the chronic anovulatory or oligo-ovulatory state of PCOS is characterized by high estrogen and insulin but little or no progestogen activity, with resultant endometrial hyperplasia. The fact that tonically elevated insulin up-regulates estrogen-producing aromatase enzyme systems in endometrial glands and stroma ,brings additive and deleterious results for the woman who is both hyperinsulinemic and anovulatory[40,41] Research has implicated these two derangements as fundamental in classic PCOS.[42]. Thus, for a woman who has not had hysterectomy and who has insulin resistance and chronic anovulation , endometrial hyperplasia represents a common end-point of two distinct pathophysiologic processes. Anectodal cases of low-grade endometrial stromal sarcoma and carcinosarcoma have been also reported in association with prolonged unopposed estrogen stimulation,and in particular with PCOS. .A low level of SHBG is for instance induced by high body weight. Therefore,the amount of overweight correlates with increased risk of hyperplasia and carcinoma [39]. Obesity could lead to the development of endometrial hyperplasia by increasing the concentration of circulating estrogens and stimulation of the endometrium growth. This could happen in several ways: by decreasing levels of circulating SHBG or by increasing the conversion of androstenedione to estrone that occurs with increased adipose tissue [26,43]. It was observed that the risks of both complex hyperplasia and hyperplasia with atypia decreased in proportion to the number of deliveries, at least among women younger than age 52 years. The reduction in risk was particularly great for women who had three or more children on the order of 70 percent and 90 percent decreased risks for complex hyperplasia and hyperplasia with atypia, respectively.This finding contradicts that previously believed on the etiology of endometrial hyperplasia that examined an association with parity. Studies examining the association of parity with endometrial cancer have consistently found an inverse relation between risk and number of births, with an even greater reduction in risk among women younger than 50 or 55 years of age [24,44,45,46].There was a suggestion of a decrease in risk of endometrial hyperplasia with atypia among current smokers. Smoking may decrease the rate of conversion of androgens to estrogens by blocking the aromatase enzyme [47] Smoking is also associated with earlier menopause and lower body fat, both of which are associated with a reduced risk of endometrial hyperplasia and could be the underlying basis for the association. Smoking has been associated with a reduced risk of endometrial cancer in most studies, with the reduction in risk being especially strong among postmenopausal women [44]. In a study of women without endometrial hyperplasia or endometrial cancer, Lambe et al.observed decreasing levels of free estradiol and increasing levels of sex hormone-binding globulin in the postmenopausal period associated with increasing parity. This hormonal milieu of low estradiol and high sex hormone-binding globulin would be expected to not stimulate endometrial cell growth [48]. Premenopausal women who are obese could be at additional risk, since they are more likely to have periods of anovulation and therefore lower progesterone levels which increases their risk of endometrial proliferation and inadequate menstrual shedding of the endometrium[49].Androgen receptors and steroid receptor co-activators are over-expressed in the endometrium of women with PCOS. In addition, to being responsive to the steroid hormones estradiol, progesterone and androgens, the endometrium is also a target for insulin, the receptor for which is cyclically regulated in normo-ovulatory women. In addition, insulin-like growth factors (IGF s) and their binding proteins are regulated in and act on endometrial cells,and hyperinsulinemia down-regulates hepatic IGFBP-1,resulting in elevated free IGF-1 in the circulation. Likely, elevated estrogen, without the opposing effects of progesterone in the absence of ovulation, elevated free IGF-1, androgens and obesity all, contribute to endometrial dysfunction, infertility, increased miscarriage rate, endometrial hyperplasia and endometrial carcinoma common in women with PCOS [23].

Classification of Endometrial Hyperplasia

Endometrial hyperplasia (EH) is a precursor to endometrial carcinoma, the most common malignancy of the female reproductive tract.[50].EH is an important cause of abnormal uterine bleeding, a result of a variety of disordered glandular and stromal growth patterns [51,52]. In 1985, Kurman et al clarified the classification system for endometrial hyperplasia, proposing 2 broad categories :simple and complex. Simple hyperplasia (SH) is characterized by benign proliferation of endometrial glands, which are irregular and perhaps dilated, but which lack back-to-back crowding or cellular atypia Complex hyperplasia (CH) is characterized by grossly irregular endometrium and abnormal vasculature. It exhibits proliferation of endometrial glands with irregular outlines, architectural complexity, and back-to-back crowding but no atypia. Presence or absence of atypia characterizes subdivisions of these 2 categories by degree of nuclear atypia and loss of polarity. Atypia can be found in both complex and simple hyperplastic lesions.In their sentinel article on the classification of endometrial hyperplasia,

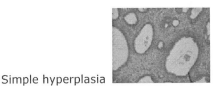
Simple hyperplasia

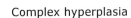
Complex hyperplasia

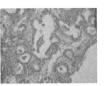

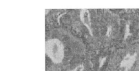
Atypical hyperplasia

Kurman et al describe the behavior of the 4 categories of endometrial hyperplasia in 170 patients. They found that, during a mean follow-up of 11.4 years, disease regressed in 69% of patients with simple atypical hyperplasia, 57% of patients with complex atypical hyperplasia, and 58% of patients with hyperplasia with cellular atypia Disease progressed to carcinoma in 8% of patients with simple atypical hyperplasia, 29% of patients with complex atypical hyperplasia, and 23% of patients with hyperplasia and cellular atypia. The average age for patients with atypia was 35 or younger in 40 women ; 38% of them [53]. Emerging data indicate the long-term risk among women with simple hyperplasia (SH) or complex (CH) is less than 5% but the risk among women with AH (atypical hyperplasia) is approximately 30% [22]. In a similar study involving 77 women with hyperplasia, 79% of cases with simple hyperplasia regressed over the 3 years of follow-up, as did the 1 case of simple hyperplasia with atypia, 94% of cases with complex hyperplasia, and 55% of cases with complex hyperplasia with atypia. Only 1 patient experienced progression to endometrial carcinoma; she initially had complex atypical hyperplasia.[54].In conclusion, there are four types of endometrial hyperplasia: simple endometrial hyperplasia (SH), complex endometrial hyperplasia (CH), simple endometrial hyperplasia with atypia (SAH), and complex endometrial hyperplasia with atypia (CAH) as established by World Health Organization , although the two forms of atypical hyperplasia(AH) are often collapsed into one category. These differ in terms of how abnormal the cells are and how likely it is that the condition will become cancer. In practice, the term of endometrial hyperpsia (EH) refers to endometrial abnormalities that range from mild proliferation to incipient carcinoma. [55,56]. Emerging data indicated that long-term risk among women with SC or CH is less than 5%,but the risk among women with AH is approximately 30% [57] Among women observed for at least 1 year after receiving a biopsy-based EH diagnosis, EIN (endometrial intraepithelial neoplasia) and AH were both found to have similarly increased risks of progression to carcinoma [58].

Simple	Benign proliferation of endometrial glands that are irregular and perhaps dilated but do not display back-to-back crowding or cellular atypia
Complex	Proliferation of endometrial glands with irregular outlines, architectural complexity, and back-to-back crowding but no atypia
Atypical	Varying degrees of nuclear atypia and loss of polarity Found in both simple and complex hyperplastic lesions

Untreated, atypical endometrial hyperplasia progresses to adenocarcinoma in 23% of patients, persists as hyperplasia in 19%, and regresses in 58%. Another study was conducted retrospectively in 116 women who had simple,complex or mixed, simple with focal complex endometrial hyperplasia; 87 without atypia and 29 with atypia This investigation found an incidence of endometrial carcinoma in 27.6% of the patients with atypia and 3.4% in those without atypia [59] Finally, endometrial hyperplasia per se is a non invasive proliferation of the lining of the uterus that results in a spectrum of glandular alterations; although hyperplasia in which there are atypical changes in cells is considered a precancerous lesion.

Diagnosis

Transvaginal Ultrasound

In practice, the routine evaluation of a woman suspected of having PCOS includes a fasting insulin measurement and a transvaginal ultrasonography (TVS).Measurement of fasting plasma insulin has been proposed as a sensitive and cost-effective method of screening for hyperinsulinemia. This targeted evaluation can identify those patients with relative hyperinsulinemia and increased risk for endometrial hyperplasia. An important aim of sonography is to document enlarged, polycystic,or otherwise abnormal ovaries, information about intrauterine contour and endometrial thickness also derives from this evaluation [60].In cases of PCOS in chronically anovulatory women of reproductive age, when the endometrial thickness is >10 mm. a biopsy is mandatory. While, in postmenopausal women with abnormal uterine bleeding, TVS is the less invasive procedure for detecting carcinoma than blind biopsy; although, endometrial thickness < 4 mm in postmenopausal women can miss malignancies [61].In 1997, a significant study estimated that transvaginal ultrasonography is a noninvasive procedure that may be used to detect endometrial disease showing that with a threshold value of 5 mm for endometrial thickness, transvaginal ultrasonography had a positive predictive value of 9 percent for detecting any abnormality, with 90 percent sensitivity, 48 percent specificity, and a negative predictive value of 99 percent. With this threshold, a biopsy would be indicated in more than half the women, only 4 percent of whom had serious disease. Therefore,these observations led to consider that transvaginal ultrasonography has a poor positive predictive value but a high negative predictive value for detecting serious endometrial disease in asymptomatic postmenopausal women [62].However, current knowledge showed as transvaginal sonography is rarely non diagnostic In the meantime, it was shown that transvaginal sonography (TVS)combined with saline contrast, sonohysterography (SCSH), is superior to TVS used alone for detection of intracavitary abnormalities showing higher sensitivity(TVS 0.94,SCSH 0.97) and; specificity(TVS 0.56,SCSH 0.62) than TVS [63].Therefore, this procedure is a simple,minimally invasive and cost/effective tool enhancing the diagnostic accuracy of TVS and can be an effective screening test prior to hysteroscopy [64]. It was also shown that the transvaginal sonography combined with Pipelle endometrial biopsy and hysteroscopy is as effective as hysteroscopy and curettage [65,66].Normalization of insulin metabolism and ovulation can lead to reduce the risk of endometrial carcinoma. Furthermore, early detection of endometrial hyperplasia in the setting of PCOS may reduce the risk of gynecologic malignancy, and may consent the preservation of reproductive potential.

Sampling of Endometrial Cells

Endometrial Biopsy

Endometrial assessment by means of biopsy or sampling of endometrial cells is a minimally invasive alternative to dilatation and curettage or hysteroscopy.The use of this technique is believed to reduce the cost of the diagnostic workup for abnormal uterine bleeding without reducing accuracy. A meta-analysis including 7914 women showed that the detection rate for endometrial carcinoma was higher in postmenopausal women compared with premenopausal women. In both postmenopausal and premenopausal women, the Pipelle was the best device, with detection rates of 99. 6% and 91%, respectively. Considering this evaluation, endometrial biopsy with the Pipelle seems to be superior to other endometrial techniques in the detection of endometrial carcinoma and atypical hyperplasia [66].In a laboratory study 62.234 cytological samples were examined. Of 138 cases identified as endometrial adenocarcinoma,126 were confirmed hystologically; while twelve were showed to be false positives [67]. A recent study investigated about the role of the cervical smear in the diagnosis of endometrial cancer in 543 women with postmenopausal bleeding. A precancerous or cancerous lesion was present in 11.7% of them. So,adding the results of the cervical smear to endometrial thickness is possible to detect incidental endometrial cancers that are missed by TVS ($\leq$5mm);while, the presence in women with postmenopausal bleeding of normal endometrial cells is not predictive of endometrial cancer [68]. Hence, the presence of benign looking endometrial cells with postmenopausal bleeding always indicated a careful work up to exclude endometrial pathology [69]. Brush biopsy seems an available method to detect endometrial carcinoma and its precursor In fact, when correlated with the final diagnosis, the Tao brush has 95.5% sensitivity . Together with Pipelle it seems to have a positive predictive value of 100% and negative predictive value of 98% [70]. In addition, endometrial brush biopsy may help to monitor endometrial conditions during the follow-up [71]. Some authors draw attention to endometrial fluid detected by transvaginal ultrasound.

They evaluated 128 asymptomatic postmenopausal women with uterine bleeding and 29 asymptomatic postmenopausal women with transvaginal ultrasound, curettage and histopathological exam of the specimens. This investigations led to establish that the presence of endometrial fluid is a good marker for pathological changes of the endometrium in postmenopausal women if the thickness is greater than 4 mm.If the endometrial thickness is 4 mm or less,the presence of endometrial fluid is not an indication for further invasive investigation[72,66].Endometrial biopsy or DandC are utilized to detect endometrial hyperplasia or endometrial cancer and are performed in patients who are at significant risk or who have symptoms as irregular bleeding which could be consistent with endometrial cancer. Approximately 90 percent of women with endometrial cancer have vaginal bleeding or discharge as their only presenting complaint. Endometrial cancer most often occurs in women in the sixth and seventh decade of life. Those with abnormal perimenopausal or postmenopausal bleeding should always be investigated. In these cases at high risk, a direct biopsy by hysteroscopy may be performed. Hysteroscopy proves to be a safe and effective method in the diagnosis of abnormal uterine bleeding.

Treatment

Many gynecologists proceed to hysterectomy when hyperplasia with cellular atypia is found on an endometrial biopsy or curettage specimen, Until recently, hysterectomy was the only alternative for patients with atypical endometrial hyperplasia,the immediate precursor lesion to endometrial cancer, but in recent years a number of organ-sparing treatment possibilities have emerged. Conservative therapies are particularly useful for younger patients who wish to preserve fertility, and for women who do not desire or cannot undergo hysterectomy. In the meantime, in women who wish to preserve fertility, management of endometrial hyperplasia can be a challenge. Fortunately, we now have sound data indicating that conservative treatment can be used for certain patients.With proper monitoring, oral progestin therapy is a reasonable alternative to hysterectomy for treatment of hyperplasia [73].

Conservative therapy

- Progestogens (oral , intramuscolar, vaginal cream micronized, LNG device)
- Aromatase inhibitors
- GnRH analogues
- Thermal balloon ablation.
- Laser therapy
- Resectoscopic surgery

It is important to remember that untreated, atypical endometrial hyperplasia progresses to adenocarcinoma in 23% of patients, persists as hyperplasia in 19%, and regresses in

58%.Several studies found that progestin was associated with regression in 90% of women with hyperplasia arising from unopposed estrogen therapy.Because endometrial hyperplasia is estrogen dependent, progestins are often used to induce regression.Progestin appears to decrease glandular cellularity in these lesions by triggering apoptosis [74]. In addition, medroxyprogesterone acetate (MPA) could significantly inhibit angiogenesis in the myometrium immediately underlying complex endometrial hyperplasia [75] Progestin administration may be performed by different ways: oral, intramuscular, micronized progesterone vaginal cream, levonorgestrel intrauterine device [76]. If a lower dose progestin regimen fails to clear hyperplasia with atypia, the patient may be given a choice between high dose progestin given continuously over a period of three months or hysterectomy. Failure of the high dose progestin treatment course to completely resolve the hyperplasia with atypia, it is a clear indication for hysterectomy. Resolution of the hyperplasia on the repeated DandC offers the patient the opportunity to try and conceive.However, she will require close medical supervision with repeated biopsies to monitor the endometrium until pregnancy. The DandC after completion of progesterone treatment should be delayed about a month following completion of the progesterone course of treatment in order not to miss a treatment failure. In pre-menopausal women,high dose progestin treatment with close monitoring is an accepted alternative to hysterectomy in cases of hyperplasia with atypia. In the post-menopausal woman with endometrial hyperplasia with atypia, hysterectomy is recommended.With proper monitoring ,oral therapy could be a reasonable alternative to hysterectomy for treatment of hyperplasia Patients on this regimen should undergo endometrial sampling every 2 to 3 months during therapy until regression to no hyperplasia is evident. Thereafter, sampling should be every 6 to 12 months because recurrence is possible. Endometrial hyperplasia in patients with a history of breast cancer presents a therapeutic dilemma. In fact, in these women the usual conservative treatment with high-dose progestin is contraindicated. While,anastrozole,an aromatase inhibitor used as adjuvant therapy for breast cancer, may have protective effects on the endometrium. Therefore, aromatase inhibitor such anastrozole may be beneficial in resolving EH in breast cancer patients [77].Another study investigated the effects of 12 months-anastrozole in 11 obese postmenopausal women with high operative risk,in order to treat endometrial hyperplasia (4 cases of simple EH,5 cases of complex EH and 2 of atypical EH).The results showed a good tolerance profile and the atrophical endometrium during treatment and an additional mean follow-up of 10.2 months [78]. Other medical alternatives are Gonadotropin-releasing hormone (GnRH)agonists and Levonorgestrel/releasing intrauterine device. Gonadotropin-releasing hormone (GnRH) analogues suppress the hypothalamic pituitary-ovarian axis, thereby inhibiting estrogen production and, potentially, causing the regression of endometrial hyperplasia. GnRH analogues also appear to have a direct antiproliferative effect on endometrial cells [79,80]. GnRH analogues appear to be an effective treatment for hyperplasia without atypia, whether simple or complex. At this time, a standardized treatment protocol cannot be recommended without additional data. However, using a GnRH analogue for 6 months with sampling every 3 months,this is a reasonable option in patients without atypia. The combination of progestin and GnRH agonists increases effectiveness ,thagainst atypical hyperplasia, and therefore offers promise for patients desiring conservative therapy [81]. Further studies are needed before GnRH analogues can be recommended for clinical use in patients with atypical hyperplasia.. Progesterone treatment may also be given with an intra-uterine system (IUD) containing progestin (levonorgestrel IUS) .A recent study affirmed that oral progestogens appear to induce a lower disease regression rate than Levonorgestrel-releasing intrauterine system in the treatment of endometrial hyperplasia. However,there was no statistical difference in simple hyperplasia [82]. Levonorgestrel intrauterine system (LNG-IUS) could be the best choice for young women with endometrial hyperplasia. It act on endometrium inducing secretory or atrophic glands with decidualized stroma.[83,84]. After LNG-IUS removal a pregnancy can be reached following ovulation induction [85].In practice,LNG-IUS seems to be an effective and safe method for treating non-atypical EH. Whether LNG-IUS could provide safe and cost-effective alternative to hysterectomy for atypical EH warrants further evaluation. Therefore, it is important to monitor such patients closely long after completion of a successful course of treatment.

Alternative treatments

Recently, there have been several encouraging reports of resolution of hyperplasia following endometrial ablation by hot water balloon, laser or resectoscopic endometrial resection..The gold standard techniques(laser,transcervical resection of endometrium and rollerball) require visualization of the uterus with a hysteroscope and,although safe, require skilled surgeons. In some cases, even atypical hyperplasia was successfully eliminated.However, at the present time, larger studies are needed to determine the overall success of such treatment modalities before we can accept them as routine alternatives in women who refuse progesterone therapy or hysterectomy.

Ablation

Second-generation endometrial ablation procedures are the following:

Balloon Endometrial Ablation [86,87]: involves the use of a balloon at the tip of a catheter tube that is filled with fluid and inflated until it conforms to the walls of the uterus. A probe in the balloon heats the fluid to destroy the endometrial lining. After eight minutes the fluid is drained out and the balloon is removed. Hysteroscopic guidance is not required for this procedure.

- Electric Wand Ablation: (Nova Sure System) involves inserting a slender wand up through the cervix.[88] A triangular mesh-like device is passed through the wand and expands to fit the uterus. Electrical energy is passed through it for about 90seconds and the mesh and wand are then withdrawn. Hysteroscopic guidance is not required for this procedure.
- Freezing (Cryoablation): involves placing a liquid nitrogen probe into the uterus to destroy tissue by freezing. Ultrasound is used to guide the procedure.

- Hydro-Therm-Ablator [HTA] system. Involves the use of hot saline to destroy the uterine lining. This device is a closed loop system designed to ablate the endometrial lining of the uterus by recirculating heated saline within the uterus.This is not a "blind" procedure but uses hysteroscopy so that the surgeon can view the uterus.
- Endometrial laser ablation (ELA) uses a distention media delivered into the uterus.After the uterus has been distended, a laser is used to destroy the lining of the uterus. This is not a blind procedure, but uses hysteroscopy so that the surgeon can view the uterus [89].

In practice,there are mainly two different systems with similar efficacy : the endometrial ablation devices-a hot water balloon ablation system (ThermaChoice, Gynecare; Johnson and Johnson, Somerville, NJ) and the bipolar,radiofrequency, impedance-controlled endometrial ablation system(NovaSure Endometrial Ablation Device; Novacept, Palo Alto, CA) [90].

In 2001 Minassian and Mira reported the use of thermal balloon ablation of the endometrium in a patient with complex endometrial hyperplasia with atypia [91] .Traditionally endometrial hyperplasia has been treated with progestins. Unfortunately, quite often hyperplasias are resistant to treatment, or they recur after therapy. A study compared traditional progestin administration with thermal balloon endometrial ablation in the treatment of non-atypic endometrial hyperplasia in 34 women. Endometrial biopsy samples were taken 6 and 12 months after the treatment; if any signs of hyperplasia were detected, hysterectomy was performed. In patients treated with thermal ablation, the hyperplasias persisted at 6 or 12 months in 4 out of 17 patients, whereas the rate was 6 out of 17 patients in the progestin treatment. A total of 14 of the 34 patients (41%) have been hysterectomized so far. These preliminary results suggested that thermal balloon endometrial ablation therapy could be as effective as traditional progestin administration in the treatment of non-atypic endometrial hyperplasia. The hysterectomy rate during the follow-up period was, however, considerably high, and, therefore, hysterectomy might be considered even a first-choice treatment for endometrial hyperplasia.[92].

Laser Therapy

Firstly, Vilos and Ettler reported a case in which a patient with complex atypical hyperplasia underwent laser intrauterine thermal therapy. After 13 months of surveillance with transvaginal sonography, there was no evidence of disease [93].

Resectoscopic Surgery

Resectoscopic surgery has been investigated in the treatment of atypical endometrial hyperplasia. Vilos et al in 2002 successfully treated 8 patients using hysteroscopic endometrial resection [94]. Later,a larger study involving 73 women with hyperplasia without atypia showed complete regression in 71 of the 73 patients over an average of 34 months of follow-up [95,

96,97] Resectoscopic surgery may be an alternative to hysterectomy in high-risk women with atypical endometrial hyperplasia [97].

Concurrent Endometrial Carcinoma

There is much interest in conservative therapies for atypical endometrial hyperplasia, but with such a high incidence of endometrial carcinoma in cases of atypical endometrial hyperplasia diagnosed by endometrial biopsy, it would seem prudent to exercise caution when considering any conservative therapy. The Gynecologic Oncology Group (GOG) recently reported a rate of 42.6% in a large prospective study in the USA This study investigates the rate of endometrial carcinoma found at hysterectomy in women with a biopsy diagnosis of atypical endometrial hyperplasia. It was suggested that when women have a biopsy diagnosis of AEH, clinicians and patients should take into account the considerable rate of concurrent carcinoma (American Cancer Society)[98]. A retrospective study identified a similar rate of 45.9% at the John Radcliffe (Headington, Oxford, UK) [99].An italian prospective study evaluated the correlation between hysteroscopic diagnosis and pathologic finding on hysterectomy specimens.In the 11 cases showing infiltrating carcinoma, hysteroscopic view was consistent with endometrial malignancy in 9 patients and with endometrial hyperplasia in 2 patients. From this estimate emerged that sensitivity, specificity, negative and positive predictive values of hysteroscopy to foresee a diagnosis of infiltrating carcinoma were 84.6%, 100%, 87.5%, and 100%, respectively.

Therefore,hysteroscopic view seems to be a sensitive and specific method to identify among patients with a diagnosis of atypical hyperplasia on endometrial biopsy those with a coexisting infiltrating carcinoma [100].A significantly better positive predictive value (PPV) to foresee hyperplasia was found in postmenopausal women compared with premenopausal patients [101].A recent investigation evaluated the prevalence of concurrent endometrial carcinoma in 126 women diagnosed with atypical endometrial hyperplasia (AEH) by endometrial biopsy. All underwent to hysterectomy. The incidence of endometrial carcinoma was considerably high (13/126, 10.3%).Eleven of 13 cases were confined to the endometrium and the remaining two were located at the adenomyosis without myometrial invasion. All patients with endometrial carcinoma displayed coexisting atypical complex hyperplasia following hysterectomy [102]. In conclusion, when women have a biopsy diagnosis of AEH, it is important to take into account the considerable rate (10.3%)of concurrent carcinoma.

References

[1]   Coulam CB,Annegers JF,Kranz JS. Chronic anovulation syndrome and associated neoplasia. *Obstet. Gynecol.* 1983;61:403-407.

[2]   Balen A Polycystic ovary syndrome and cancer. *Human Reproduction Update* 2001; Vol.7, No.6 pp.522-525.

[3] Wild S, Pierpoint T,Jacobs H,NcKeigue P. Long-term consequences of polycystic ovary syndrome:results of a 31 year follow-up study. *Hum. Fertil.* (Camb) 2000; 3(2): 101-105.

[4] Meirow D,Schenker JG. The link between female infertility and cancer: epidemiology and possible aetiologies. *Hum. Reprod.Update* 1996;2(1): 63-75.

[5] Gadducci A,Gargini A,Palla E, Fanucchi A,Genazzani AR. Polycystic ovary sindrome and gynecological cancers:is there a link. Gynecol.Endocrinol. 2005;20(4):200-8.

[6] 6.Spritzer PM,Morsch DM,Wiltgen D. Polycystic ovary syndrome associated neoplams. *Arq. Bras. Endocrinol. Metab.* 2005; 49(5): 805-10.

[7] Olsen CM,Nagle CM,Whiteman DC,Purdie DM,Green AC,Webb PM. Body size and risk of epithelial ovarian and related cancer : a population-based case-control study. *Int. J. Cancer* 2008;123(2): 450-6.

[8] Schildkraut JM,Schwingl PJ,Bastos E,Evanoff A,Hughes C. Epithelial ovarian cancer risk among women with polycystic ovary syndrome. *Obstet.Gynecol.* 1996; 88(4Pt1) 554-7.

[9] Leitzmann MF,Koebnick C, Danforth KN,Brinton LA,Moore SC,Hollenbeck AR, Schatzkin A,Lacey JV Jr. Body mass index and risk of ovarian cancer. *Cancer* 2009; 115(4): 812-22.

[10] Jordan SJ,Green AC,Whiteman DC, Webb PM. Risk factors for benign, borderline and invasive mucinous ovarian tumours :epidemiological evidence of a neoplastic continuum? *Gynecol. Oncol.* 2007;107(2): 223-30.

[11] Dick ML,Siskind V,Purdie DM,Green AC. Incomplete pregnancy and risk of ovarian cancer:results from two Australian case-control studies and systematic review. *Cancer Causes Control* 2009;20(9): 1571-85.

[12] Pierpoint T,McKeigue PM, Isaacs AJ,Wild SH,Jacobs HS. Mortality of women with polycystic ovary syndrome at long-term follow-up. *J. Clin. Epidemiol.* 1998; 51(7): 581-6.

[13] Grattarola R. Ovariectomy alone or in combination with dexamethasone in patients with advanced cancer and high levels of testosterone secretion. *J. Natl. Cancer. Inst.* 1976; 56: 11-16.

[14] Secreto G,Zumoff B. Abnormal production of androgens in women with breast cancer. *Anticancer Res.* 1994; 14(5B): 2113-7.

[15] Leon Speroff and Marc A. Fritz. Anovulation and the polycystic ovary. *Clinical Gynecology Endocrinology and Infertility*. 2005;7th ed. p: 465-98.

[16] Stoll BA, Secreto G. New hormone-related markers of high risk to breast cancer. *Ann. Oncol.* 1992; 3(6): 435- 8.

[17] Kahàn Z,Gardi J,Nyari T,Foldesi I,Hajnal –Papp R,Ormandi K,Lazar G,Schally AV. Elevated levels of circulating insulin-like growth factor-1,IGF-binding globulin-3 and testosterone predict hormone dependent breast cancer in postmenopausal women: a case-control study. *Int. J. Oncol.* 2006; 29(1): 193-200.

[18] Krajcik RA,Borofsky ND, Massardo S,Orentreich N. Insulin-like growth factor 1(IGF-1),IGF- binding proteins, and breast cancer. *Cancer Epidemiol. Biomarkers Prev.* 2002;11(12):1566-73.

[19] Somboonporn W,Davis SR. Postmenopausal testosterone therapy and breast cancer risk. *Maturitas* 2004; 49(4): 267-75.

[20] Tingthanatikul Y, Choktanasiri W, Rochanawutanon M, Weerakeit S. Prevalence and clinical predictors of endometrial hyperplasia in anovulatory women pre-senting with amenorrhea. *Gynecol. Endocrinol.* 2006; 22:101-105.

[21] Giudice LC, Endometrium in PCOS: Implantation and predisposition to endocrine CA, *Best Pract. Res. Clin. Endocrinol. Metab.* 2006 Jun;20(2):235-44.

[22] Lacey JV Jr, Chia VM.Endometrial hyperplasia and the risk of progression to carcinoma. Maturitas 2009; 63(1):39-44.

[23] Ricci E, Moroni S, Parazzini F, et al. Risk factors for endometrial hyperplasia: results from a case-control study. *Int. J. Gynecol. Cancer*. 2002; 12:257–260.

[24] Rudnicka E., Wierzba W, Radowicki S. Evaluation of endometrial histologic morphology in patients with polycystic ovary syndrome. *Ginekol. Pol.* 2009 Feb ;80 (2):103-6.

[25] MacDonald PC, Edman CD, Hemsell DL, et al. Effect of obesity on conversion of plasma androstenedione to estrone in postmenopausal women with and without endometrial cancer. *Am. J. Obstet. Gynecol.* (1978) 130:448–55.

[26] Anderson JN, Peck EJJ, Clark JH. Estrogen-induced uterine responses and growth: relationship to receptor estrogen binding by uterine nuclei. *Endocrinology* 1975; 96:160–7.

[27] King RJ,Whitehead MI,Campbell S.Effects of estrogen and progestin treatment on endometria from postmenopausal women. *Cancer Res.* 1979; 39: 1094-101.

[28] The Writing Group for the PEPI Trial. Effects of hormone replacement therapy on endometrial histology in postmenopausal women: The Postmenopausal Estrogen/Progestin Interventions (PEPI) Trial. *JAMA* (1996) 275:370–5.

[29] Ismail S M Pathology of endometrium treated with tamoxifen. *J. Clin. Pathol.* 1994 ;47 (9):827-33.

[30] Widra EA, Dunton CJ, McHugh M, et al. Endometrial hyperplasia and the risk of carcinoma. *Int. J. Gynecol. Cancer* (1995) 5:233–5.

[31] Gusberg SB. Hormone-dependence of endometrial cancer. *Obstet. Gynecol.* 1967; 30:287–93.

[32] Kreiger N, Marrett LD, Clarke EA, et al. Risk factors for adenomatous endometrial hyperplasia: a case-control study. *Am. J. Epidemiol.* (1986) 123:291–300.

[33] Chamlian DL, Taylor HB. Endometrial hyperplasia in young women. *Obstet. Gynecol.* 1970;36: 659-66.

[34] Gallup DG, Stock RJ: Adenocarcinoma of the endometrium in women 40 years of age or younger. *Obstet. Gynecol.* 1984; 64:417-420.

[35] Cairns JD, Noble AJ, Bryant ME:Carcinoma of endometrium and polycystic ovaries in a 22 year-old patient. *Can. Med. Assoc. J.* 1967; 96:1473-1476.

[36] Tseng L, Gurpide E. Induction of endometrial estradiol dehydrogenase by progestins. *Endocrinology* 1975; 97:825–33.

[37] Hull MG: Epidemiology of infertilty and polycystic ovary syndrome: endocrinological and demographic studies. *Gynecol. Endocrinol.* 1987; 1:235-245.

[38] Schindler AE. Progesteron deficiency and endometrial cancer risk. *Maturitas* 2009;62(4):334-7.

[39] Chang JR, Nakamura RM, Judd HL, et al: Insulin resistance in nonobese patients with polycystic ovary syndrome. *J. Clin. Endocrinol. Metab.* 1983; 57:356-359 .

[40] Nagamani M, Hannigan EV, Dinh TV, et al: Hyperinsulinemia and stromal luteinization of the ovaries in postmenopausal women with endometrial cancer. *J. Clin. Endocrinol. Metab.* 1988; 67:144-148.

[41] Randolph JF Jr, Kipersztok S, Ayers JW, et al: The effect of insulin on aromatase activity in isolated human endometrial glands and stroma. *Am. J. Obstet. Gynecol.* 1987; 157:1534-1539.

[42] Kaye SA, Folsom AR, Soler JT, et al. Association of body mass and fat distribution with sex hormone concentrations in postmenopausal women. *Int. J. Epidemiol.* (1991) 20:151–6.

[43] Cook LS, Weiss NS, Doherty JA, et al, Endometrial cancer. Cancer epidemiology and prevention. 3rd ed.

[44] Schottenfeld D, Fraumeni JF Jr, eds. (2006) New York, NY: Oxford University Press. 1027–43.

[45] Brinton LA, Sakoda LC, Lissowska J, et al. Reproductive risk factors for endometrial cancer among Polish women. *Br. J. Cancer* (2007) 96:1450–6.

[46] Chubak J, Tworoger SS, Yasui Y, et al. Associations between reproductive and menstrual factors and postmenopausal sex hormone concentrations. *Cancer Epidemiol. Biomarkers Prev.* (2004) 13:1296–301.

[47] Tankó LB, Christiansen C. An update on the antiestrogenic effect of smoking: a literature review with implications for researchers and practitioners. *Menopause* (2004) 11:104–9.

[48] Lambe M, Wuu J, Weiderpass E, et al. Childbearing at older age and endometrial cancer risk (Sweden). *Cancer Causes Control* 1999; 10:43–9.

[49] Sherman BM, Korenman SG. Measurement of serum LH, FSH, estradiol and progesterone in disorders of the human menstrual cycle: the inadequate luteal phase. *J. Clin. Endocrinol. Metab.* (1974) 39:145–9.

[50] Jemal A,Murray T,Samuels A, et al. Cancer statistics, 2003. *CA Cancer J. Clin.* 2003;53:5–26.

[51] Farquhar CM, Lethaby A, Sowter M, et al. An evaluation of risk factors for endometrial hyperplasia in premenopausal women with abnormal menstrual bleeding. *Am. J. Obstet. Gynecol.* (1999) 181:525–9.

[52] Weber AM, Belinson JL, Piedmonte MR. Risk factors for endometrial hyperplasia and cancer among women with abnormal bleeding. *Obstet. Gynecol.* (1999) 93:594–8.

[53] Kurman RJ,Kaminski PF, Norris HJ. The behavior of endometrial hyperplasia: a long-term study of "untreated"hyperplasia in 170 patients. *Cancer.* 1985;56:403–412.

[54] Tabata T,Yamawaki T, Yabana T, et al. Natural history of endometrial hyperplasia: study of 77 patients. *Arch. Gynecol. Obstet.* 2001; 265:85–88.

[55] Mazur MT.Endometrial hyperplasia/adenocarcinoma a conventional approach .*Ann. Diagn. Pathol.* 2005;9: 174-81.

[56] Montgomery BE, Daum GS, Dunton CJ. Endometrial hyperplasia :a review. Obstet review. *Obstet. Gynecol. Surv.* 2004; 59:368-78.

[57] Lacey JV, Chia VM. Endometrial hyperplasia and the risk of progression to carcinoma. *Maturitas* 2009;63(1): 39-44.

[58] Lacey JV, Mutter GL,Nucci MR,Ronnett BM,Ioffe BB,Glass AG,Richesson DA,Chatterjee N,Langholz B,Sherman ME Risk of subsequent endometrial carcinoma associated with endometrial intraepithelial neoplasia classification of endometrial biopsies. *Cancer* 2008;113(8): 2073-81.

[59] Ho SP,Tan KT,Pang MW,Ho TH. Endometrial hyperplasia and the risk of endometrial carcinoma. *Singapore Med. J.* 1997; 38(1): 11-5.

[60] Cheung AP. Ultrasound and menstrual history in predicting endometrial hyperplasia in polycystic ovary syndrome. *Obstet. Gynecol.* 2001;98:325-31.

[61] Litta P,Merlin F,Saccardi C,Pozzan C,Sacco G,Fracas M,Capobianco G,Dessole S. Role of hysteroscopy with endometrial biopsy to rule out endometrial cancer in postmenopausal

women with abnormal bleeding. Maturitas 2005;50(2): 117-23 N. *Engl. J. Med.* 1997; 337 (25):1792-8.

[62] Langer R D, J J Pierce J J, O'Hanlan K A, Johnson S R, Espeland M A, Trabal J F, Barnabei V M, Merino M J, Scully R E Transvaginal ultrasonography compared with endometrial biopsy for the detection of endometrial disease. Postmenopausal Estrogen/Progestin Interventions Trial. *N. Engl. J. Med.* 1997 ; 337 (25):1792-8.

[63] Kazandi M, Aksehirli S,Cirpan T,Akercan F. Transvaginal sonography. combined with saline contrast sonohysterography to evaluate the uterine cavity in patients with abnormal uterine bleeding and postmenopausal endometrium more than 5mm. *Eur. J. Gynaecol. Oncol.* 2003; 24(2): 185-90.

[64] Mathew M,Gowri V,Rizvi SG. Saline infusion sonohysterography : an effective tool for evaluation of the endometrial cavity in women with abnormal uterine bleeding. *Acta Obstet. Gynecol. Scand.* 2010; 89(1): 140-2.

[65] Davidson KG,Dubinsky TJ. Ultrasonographic evaluation of the endometrium in postmenopausal vaginal bleeding. *Radiol. Clin. North Am.* 2003;41(4): 769-80.

[66] Dijkhuizen F P, Mol B W, Brölmann H A, Heintz A P The accuracy of endometrial sampling in the diagnosis of patients with endometrial carcinoma and hyperplasia: a meta-analysis. *Cancer.* 2000 : 89 (8):1765-72.

[67] Mazur MT, Kurman RJ. Mazur MT, Kurman RJ. Diagnosis of endometrial biopsies and curettings: a practical approach. 2005 New York, NY: Springer Publishing Company.

[68] van Doom HC,Opmeer BC,Kooi GS,Ewing-Graham PC,Krultwagen RF, Mol BW. Value of cervical cytology in diagnosing endometrial carcinoma in women with postmenopausal bleeding. *Acta Cytol.* 2009; 53(3): 277-82.

[69] Kaur J,Dey P,Saha SC,Rajwanshi A,Njhawan R,Radhika S,Gupta N. Cervical cytology in patients with postmenopausal bleeding. *Diagn. Cytopathol.* 2009; Epub ahead of print.

[70] Del Priore G,Williams R,Harbatkin CB,Wan LS,Mittal K,Yang GC. Endometrial brush biopsy for the diagnosis of endometrial cancer. *J. Reprod. Med.* 2001; 46(5):439-43

[71] Belowska A .Endometrial brush biopsy in monitoring endometrial cytology during hormone replacement therapy. *Ginekol. Pol.* 2004;75(6):475-81.

[72] Curcic A,Durdevic S,Mihaldzic'Tubic S,Miadenovic'Segedi L,Maksimovic M. Ultrasound detection of endometrial fluid in postmenopausal women. *Med. Pregl.* 2009; 62(7-8): 337-41.

[73] Childs AJ, Check WE, Hoskins WJ. Conservative management of endometrial hyperplasia: New strategies and experimental options. *OBG Management* 2003; 15(9): 15-26.

[74] Amezcua CA,Lu JJ,Felix JC, et al. Apoptosis may be an early event of progestin therapy for endometrial hyperplasia. *Gynecol. Oncol.* 2000;79:169–176.

[75] Abulafia O,Triest WE,Adcock JT, et al. The effect of medroxyprogesterone acetate on angiogenesis in complex endometrial hyperplasia. *Gynecol. Oncol.* 1999;72:193–198.

[76] Affinito P,DiCarlo C,DiMauro P, et al. Endometrial hyperplasia: efficacy of a new treatment with a vaginal cream containing natural micronized progesterone. *Maturitas.* 1995;20:191–198.

[77] Stilwill SE,Cooper BC. Resolution of endometrial hyperplasia with adjuvant anastrozole trearment in postmenopausal breast cancer:a case report. *J. Reprod. Med.* 2007; 52(10): 979-80.

Metabolic Syndrome in PCOS Women 275

[78] Agorastos T,Vaitsi V,Pantazis K,Efstathiadis E,Vavilis D,Bontis JN. Aromatase inhibitor anastrozole for treating endometrial hyperplasia in obese postmenopausal women. *Eur. J. Obstet. Gynecol. Reprod. Biol.* 2005; 118(2): 239-40.

[79] Agorastos T,Bontis J,Vakiani TO, et al. Treatment of endometrial hyperplasia with gonadotropin-releasing hormone agonists: pathological, clinical, morphometric, and DNA-cytometric data. *Gynecol. Oncol.* 1997;65:102–114.

[80] Grimbizis G,Tsalikis T,Tzioufa V, et al. Regression of endometrial hyperplasia after treatment with gonadotrophin-releasing hormone analogue triptorelin: a prospective study. *Hum. Reprod.* 1999;14:479–484.

[81] Perez-Medina T,Bajo J,Folgueira G, et al. Atypical endometrial hyperplasia treatment with progesterone and gonadotropin-releasing hormone analogues: long-term follow-up. *Gynecol. Oncol.* 1999;73:299–304.

[82] Gallos ID,Shehmar M,Thangaratinam S,Papapostolou TK,Coomarasamy A,Gupta JK.Oral progestogens vs levonorgestrel-releasing intrauterine system for endometrial hyperplasia: a systematic review and metaanalysis. Am.J.Obstet.Gynecol. 2010 Oct 8 [Epub ahead of print].

[83] Gupta HP,Singh U,Sinha S. Laevonorgestrel intrauterine system –a revolutionary untrauterine device. *J. Indian Med. ASSoc.* 2007;105(7): 382-5.

[84] Perino A,Quartararo P,Catinella E, et al. Treatment of endometrial hyperplasia with levonorgestrel releasing intrauterine devices. *Acta Eur. Fertil.* 1987;18:137–140.

[85] Qi X,ZhaoW,Duan Y,Li Y.Successful pregnancy following insertion of a levonorgestrel-releasing intrauterine system in two infertile patients with complex atypical endometrial hyperplasia. *Gynecol..Obstet. Invest.* 2008;65(4): 266-8.

[86] William S. Alford, D.O., and Michael P. Hopkins, M.D. Endometrial Rollerball Ablation. *J. Reproductive Medicine* 1996; 41:251-254.

[87] Furst, S. N., Phillipson, T., and Jorgensen, J. C. (2007). Ten year follow-up of endometrial ablation. *Acte Obstetrician ET Gynecological Scandinavica*, 2007; 86 (3), 334-338.

[88] Gallinat, A. . NovaSure impedance-controlled system for endometrial ablation: Three-year follow-up of 107 patients. *American Journal of Obstetrics and Gynecology*, 2004; 191 (5) 1585-1589.

[89] Gallinat, A. (2007). An impedance-controlled system for endometrial ablation: Five-year follow-up of 107 patients. *Journal of Reproductive Medicine*, 2007; 52 (6), 467-472.

[90] Bongers, Marlies Y.; Bourdrez, Petra; Mol, Ben W. J.; Heintz, A Peter; Brölmann, Hans A. M. Randomized, Controlled Trial of Bipolar Radiofrequency Endometrial Ablation and Balloon Endometrial Ablation. *Obst. and Gynecol. Survey*: 2005; 60(2): 93-94.

[91] Minassian VA,Mira JL. Balloon thermoablation in a woman with complex endometrial hyperplasia with atypia: a case report. *J. Reprod. Med.* 2001;46:933–936.

[92] Järvelä IY, Santala M Treatment of non-atypic endometrial hyperplasia using thermal balloon endometrial ablation therapy. *Gynecol. Obstet. Invest.* 2005;59(4):202-6.

[93] Vilos GA,Ettler HC. Atypical complex endometrial hyperplasia treated with the GyneLase system. *J. Am. Assoc. Gynecol. Laparosc.* 2002;9:73–78.

[94] Vilos GA,Harding PG,Ettler HC. Resectoscopic surgery in 10 women with abnormal uterine bleeding and atypical endometrial hyperplasia. *J. Am. Assoc. Gynecol. Laparosc.* 2002;9:138–144.

[95] Cianferoni L,Giannini A, Franchini M. Hysteroscopic resection of endometrial hyperplasia. *J. Am. Assoc. Gynecol. Laparosc.* 1999;6:151–154.

[96] Janicek MF, Rosenshein NB. Invasive endometrial cancer in uteri resected for atypical endometrial hyperplasia. *Gynecol. Oncol.* 1994; 52:373-8.

[97] Edris F, Vilos GA, Al-Mubarak A, Ettler HC, Hollett-Caines J, Abu-Rafea B.Resectoscopic surgery may be an alternative to hysterectomy in high-risk women with atypical endometrial hyperplasia. *J. Minim. Invasive Gynecol.* 2007 ;14(1):68-73.

[98] Trimble CL, Kauderer J, Zaino R, et al. Concurrent endometrial carcinoma in women with a biopsy diagnosis of atypical endometrial hyperplasia: a Gynecologic Oncology Group study. *Cancer* 2006; 106:812–19.

[99] Pennant S, Manek S, Kehoe SEndometrial atypical hyperplasia and subsequent diagnosis of endometrial cancer: a retrospective audit and literature review. *J. Obstet. Gynaecol.* 2008 ;28(6): 632-3.

[100] Garuti G, Mirra M, Luerti M.Hysteroscopic view in atypical endometrial hyperplasias: A correlation with pathologic findings on hysterectomy specimens. *J. Minim. Invasive Gynecol.* 2006 ;13(4):325-30.

[101] Garuti G, Cellani F, Garzia D, Colonnelli M, Luerti M.Accuracy of hysteroscopic diagnosis of endometrial hyperplasia: a retrospective study of 323 patients. *J. Minim. Invasive Gynecol.* 2005 ;12(3):247-53.

[102] Hahn HS, Chun YK, Kwon YI, Kim TJ, Lee KH, Shim JU, Mok JE, Lim KT Concurrent endometrial carcinoma following hysterectomy for atypical endometrial hyperplasia. *Eur. J. Obstet. Gynecol. Reprod. Biol.* 2010 ;150(1):80-3.

Conclusion

Rosa Sabatini

*Expert Family Planning Service. Department of Obstetrics and Gynecology Policlinico-University of Bari. Piazza Giulio Cesare 11.70124 Bari. Italy

Polycystic ovary syndrome is the most common endocrine disorder affecting 5-10% of women in their childbearing age, about 1 out of 15 women worldwide. In former times, the syndrome was considered as a reproductive disorder showing hyperandrogenism, chronic anovulation and infertility ; while it is now well accepted that PCOS represents a multifaceted syndrome with important metabolic and health long-term consequences. Affected individuals typically come to clinical attention for infrequent menses, acne, infertility, and/or hirsutism but they are more likely to be insulin resistant and overweight or obese.Therefore, key factors of this syndrome are hyperandrogenism and hyperinsulinemia. Great controversy exists as to which state precedes the other. Although current data seem to suggest a primary role of hyperinsulinemia, a primary defect in the hypothalamic-pituitary-adrenal axis could also be considered . Several affected women present abdominal adiposity with a level of peripheral insulin resistance (IR), similar to that present in women with type 2 diabetes (NIDDM), in association with an increased incidence of impaired glucose tolerance (IGT). Although NIDDM occurs commonly among women with polycystic ovary syndrome, the prevalence and natural history of its precursor, impaired glucose tolerance,is less well known. Current knowledge supports that the increased risk of glucose intolerance and type 2 diabetes mellitus are independent of body mass index (BMI). In spite of this, a lot of research has consistently demonstrated that the first line of treatment for this condition is weight loss. Therefore, weight loss and dietary changes appear to affect the abnormal hormonal status of these women. PCOS has also been associated with an increased prevalence of lipid-related abnormalities, including reduced high-density lipoprotein (HDL) cholesterol and increased low-density lipoprotein (LDL) cholesterol and triglyceride concentrations. Although obesity is often associated with metabolic disorders, lean women with PCOS have also been found to have hyperinsulinemia and dyslipidemia.Available data suggest that rates of hypertension, gestational diabetes, and pregnancy-induced hypertension may likewise be increased in these women, although the extent to which obesity mediates these risks is unclear. Obesity, atherogenic dyslipidemia, hypertension, impaired fasting glucose/impaired glucose tolerance, hyperinsulinemia and vascular abnormalities are all common metabolic abnormalities present in PCOS and together characterize the metabolic syndrome (MS). The presence of the metabolic syndrome in PCOS suggests a greater degree of insulin resistance compared to PCOS without the metabolic syndrome. Therefore, in addition to reproductive and hyperandrogenic concerns, PCOS is also associated with a number of metabolic perturbations that ultimately may contribute to an excess risk for type 2-diabetes, cardiovascular events and estrogen-related cancers. A growing body of evidence suggests the association of PCOS with hypertension , markers of subclinical atherosclerosis and vascular dysfunction (Legro 2001, Solomon 2001,Palmert 2002,Christian 2003, Talbott 2004, Apridonidze 2005). Hence, PCOS is one of the leading causes of infertility, but the reproductive aspects are secondary to metabolic derangements associated with this condition which may lead to a range of diseases with attendant morbidity and mortality risks. The pathogenic link between the MS and PCOS is most likely the insulin resistance. Lifestyle modification and pharmacological therapy with insulin-sensitizing agents have proven benefit in the treatment of the metabolic syndrome.Hyperinsulinemia has been found to correlate with an increased cardiovascular risk whether they are obese or not (Mather 2000).It has been supposed that obese women with PCOS could have a subclinical cardiovascular disease; however, it is well known that dyslipidemia, occurring in younger age, translates into atherosclerosis and cardiovascular disease later in life(Meyer 2005).Cardiovascular risk factors seem to be related to metabolic alterations such as dyslipidemia, hypertension, endothelial dysfunction and low grade chronic inflammation,that are present even at early age in PCOS women. Pathogenetic mechanisms of these impairments have been not yet been completely clarified . Nevertheless, IR appears to play a critical role such as the key factor linking hypertension, glucose intolerance, obesity and lipid abnormalities to coronary artery disease (Orio 2008). Recent data demonstrate that insulin resistance is present in PCOS adolescents, however, its prevalence has not been determined. Currently, insulin-resistance and beta-cell-dysfunction are recognized as the major risk factors for the development of type 2 diabetes. The defects in pancreatic beta-cell function are heritable. There are post-binding defects in insulin receptor signaling,with selective resistance to insulin's metabolic actions. Intrinsic and environmental abnormalities interact to produce peripheral insulin resistance in PCOS. A susceptibility gene region for PCOS is located on chromosome 19p13.2. The susceptibility allele is also associated with the metabolic phenotype (Dunaif 2006) Long-term studies, evaluating the glucose-insulin system in women affected by PCOS, have shown an higher incidence of glucose intolerance, including both impaired glucose tolerance and type 2 diabetes, compared to age and weight matched control populations.The risk of glucose intolerance among PCOS subjects seems to be approximately 5 to10 fold higher than normal and appears not limited to a single ethnic group. Moreover, the onset of glucose intolerance in PCOS women has been reported to occur at an earlier age than in the normal population.

However, other risk factors such as obesity, positive family history of type 2 diabetes and hyperandrogenism may contribute to increasing diabetes risk in PCOS (Pelusi 2004). Systemic insulin resistance has been implicated as one possible factor that links visceral obesity to adverse metabolic consequences; however, the mechanism whereby adipose tissue causes alterations in insulin sensitivity remains unclear. Infection and inflammation are commonly associated with insulin resistance, and visceral obesity is associated with a chronic, low-grade inflammatory state, suggesting that inflammation may be a potential mechanism, whereby obesity leads to insulin resistance.Insulin resistance, hyperleptinaemia and low plasma levels of adiponectin are also widely related to features of the MS. PCOS women with abnormalities of glucose metabolism tend to have a greater body mass index, higher fasting glucose and 2-h post-load glucose levels than those with normal glucose tolerance .Therefore , the prevalence of glucose intolerance significantly increases with BMI (Weerakiet 2001).The functional capacity of the adipose tissue varies among subjects explaining the incomplete overlapping among the metabolic syndrome and obesity. Along with the increasing prevalence of obesity,the number of people with prediabetes is worldwide increased . The diagnostic criteria for prediabetes include impaired fasting glucose,impaired glucose tolerance and MS.The presence of two or more of these three criteria renders a person at high risk for future diabetes.The treatment approach is twofold: glycemic control and control of cardiovascular risk factors,mainly hypertension and hyperlipidemia. Intensive lifestyle modification is the mainstay of treatment in low-risk patients. Hence, adipose tissue is now recognized as an immune organ that secretes many immunomodulatory factors and seems to be a significant source of inflammatory signals known to cause insulin resistance. Therefore, proinflammatory cytokines and hormones released by adipose tissue can induce the chronic inflammatory profile associated with visceral obesity. Chronic inflammation may represent a triggering factor in the origin of the metabolic syndrome.Stimuli such as overnutrition, physical inactivity and aging would result in cytokine hypersecretion and eventually lead to insulin resistance and diabetes, in genetically or metabolically predisposed subjects The prevalence and magnitude of childhood obesity have dramatically increased in recent years. Metabolic consequences of obesity including insulin resistance,type 2 diabetes mellitus, hyperlipidemia, hypertension and non-alcoholic fatty liver infiltration, are rapidly emerging in the pediatric population. Looking for effective strategies to identify and treat these obesity related comorbidities in children are crucial for the prevention of future CVD and poor health outcomes. Obesity is a serious health concern for children and adolescents and disproportionately affects certain minority youth populations. The metabolic syndrome,of course, is driven by the epidemic of obesity (Dunaif 2006). In conclusion, the prevalence of IGT and NIDDM in women with PCOS is substantially higher than expected when compared with age-and weight-matched populations of women without PCOS. Furthermore, the conversion from IGT to NIDDM is accelerated in PCOS. As in adults, adolescents with PCOS are at increased risk for IGT and DM and the fasting glucose concentration does not reliably predict the glucose concentration at 2 h after an oral glucose challenge, particularly among those with IGT, the subgroup at highest risk for subsequent development of NIDDM. Therefore, the women with PCOS should periodically have an OGTT and must be closely monitored for deterioration in glucose tolerance (Ehrmann 1999).There is an impressive correlation between the degree of hypersinsulinemia and hyperandrogenism.At higher concentrations,insulin receptors are blocked or deficient in numbers and it is to be expected that insulin would bind to the Type 1 IGF receptors.In view of the known actions of IGF-1 in augmenting the thecal androgen response to LH, activation of Type 1 IGF receptors by insulin would lead to increased androgen production in thecal cells. It is evident that not all women with hyperinsulinemia have hyperandrogenism and type 2 diabetes because an additional genetic factor leading to ovarian susceptibility is likely required. Hyperandrogenism and insulin resistance are often associated with acanthosis nigricans, which is dependent on the presence and severity of hyperinsulinemia. Metabolic syndrome is also closely associated with the liver steatosis, mostly benign and reversible liver disease. Nonalcoholic fatty liver disease and its subset nonalcoholic steatohepatitis represent the liver manifestations of insulin resistance. Nonalcoholic fatty liver disease (NAFLD) is now considered to be the most common liver disease in the United States and involves a spectrum of progressive histopathologic changes. Common risk factors associated with NAFLD include obesity, diabetes, and hyperlipidemia. Although most patients with NAFLD have simple hepatic steatosis, a significant number develop nonalcoholic steatohepatitis, which may progress to fibrosis, cirrhosis, or end-stage liver disease. The metabolic effects of obesity are the most common risk factors for diabetes,hypertension and atherosclerosis,the leading causes of end-stage renal failure. Chronic kidney disease (CKD) increases the rate of cardiovascular disease, development of end-stage renal disease,and can lead to premature death.Although,no direst causally link between obesity and CKD can be established yet, this appears highly likely.and CKD should be regarded as a major complication of overweight and obesity. Endothelial dysfunction and increased arterial stiffness occur early in the pathogenesis of diabetic vasculopathy.They are both independent predictors of cardiovascular risk.The metabolic syndrome and type 2 diabetes mellitus are both becoming more prevalent, and both increase the risk of cardiovascular disease. Many patients are not receiving appropriate treatment for the type of dyslipidemia that commonly occurs in these disorders of high serum triglyceride levels, low serum high-density lipoprotein cholesterol (HDL-C)levels,and a preponderance of small,dense,low density lipoprotein cholesterol (LDL-C) levels. Infertile women with anovulation and polycystic ovarian syndrome seem to have an increased lifetime risk for neoplasms of the reproductive tract ,like endometrial, breast and ovary cancer. Few studies have addressed the possibility of an association between polycystic ovaries and ovarian or breast cancer,and the results are conflicting and generally reassuring. Anovulatory cycles result in chronic estrogen exposure to the endometrial lining and in increased risk of developing endometrial cancer and its precursor : endometrial hyperplasia..Thus, elevated estrogen, without the opposing effects of progesterone in the absence of ovulation, hyperinsulinemia, elevated free IGF-I , androgens, and obesity, all likely contribute to endometrial dysfunction, infertility, increased miscarriage rate, endometrial hyperplasia, and endometrial cancer, common in women with PCOS. Almost 50% to 70% of all women with PCOS have some degree of insulin resistance,and this hormone insensitivity probably contributes to hyperandrogenism that is responsible for the signs and symptoms of PCOS. Even though uncertainty exists, early detection and treatment of insulin resistance in this population could ultimately reduce the incidence or severity of diabetes mellitus, dyslipidemia, hypertension, and cardiovascular disease. The high prevalence of multiple cardiovascular risk factors among women with PCOS, at a relatively young age, highlights the public health relevance of this condition. It is important to screen and diagnose adolescent PCOS in order to prevent the development of future infertility, type II diabetes mellitus, cardiovascular disease, and even endometrial cancer.Lifestyle modification is of the greatest benefit for adolescents in terms of management, with the condition that full support is available from both the clinicians and their families. Indeed, PCOS has been described as the female specific manifestation of the metabolic syndrome, a clustering of metabolic risk factors that has gained increasing attention as an independent predictor of cardiovascular events. Future studies are needed to further delineate the racial/ethnic differences in PCOS-associated clinical features and cardiovascular risk factors together with the impact of lifestyle changes or pharmacologic intervention on these factors.Finally,careful longitudinal studies are needed to examine the long-term cardiovascular outcomes and underlying mechanisms in these women and to develop strategies to prevent future cardiovascular events. Cumulating evidence showed how the hyperandrogenic manifestations and the long-term health risks associated with PCOS may have a negative impact on psychosocial well-being. Indeed, the diagnosis of PCOS has been found to be associated with feelings of frustration , anxiety and depression.These problems in socioemotional well-being, particularly symptoms of depression, could very conceivably contribute to an exacerbation of the effects of medical illness. Thus, in patients with PCOS, disease-related changes in appearance, particularly hirsutism, acne and obesity, irregular or absent menstrual periods, infertility and psychological distress appear to have a considerable effect on the quality of life. In addition, these problems may impact self-esteem and life satisfaction influencing the adherence to tretment-program. Therefore, psychological status of the PCOS women deserve more attention in clinical practice Because of its contribution to the growing prevalence of type 2 diabetes, and the associated increased CVD risk, the recognition of Metabolic Syndrome and its consequences are critical in the course of morbidity and mortality risk assessment .Data have emerged regarding the link between cardiovascular risk and abdominal obesity, specifically the significance of intra-abdominal adiposity as an important risk factor for cardiovascular disease. Finally, PCOS is a hormonal disorder that involves multiple tissues and organ systems within the body, and is believed to be fundamentally caused by insensitivity to the insulin. It can be diagnosed in all phases of life , in girls as young as 8-9 years of age, up through post-menopause. Asymptomatic women with PCOS may have impaired endothelial function at an early age suggesting an increased risk for early onset of cardiovascular disease.Endothelial dysfunction in PCOS does not depend on obesity,and its determinants vary among lean,overweight and obese women. In conclusion, in spite of the various studies which have been investigated the aetiology, pathogenesis and genetic aspects of polycystic ovary syndrome, this endocrinological disorder remains enigmatic. Current data lead to theorize that perhaps insulin resistance could be the underlying cause of PCOS. In addition, 26% of Americans age 20 and older, and 40% of Americans age 65 and older, have impaired fasting glucose, a pre-diabetes condition that increases the risk for diabetes. Historically, type 2 diabetes usually developed after the age of 40, but it is now also increasing in children. Given the current epidemic of obesity, experts are now estimating that over a third of all people born in 2002 will eventually develop diabetes. Furthermore, the dramatic increase in diabetes is occurring worldwide as American lifestyles become global. Evidence strongly suggests that healthy lifestyles can prevent most cases of type 2 diabetes. People with pre-diabetes can substantially lower their risk by losing weight through diet and exercise. Patients with diabetes have higher mortality rates than nondiabetics regardless of sex, age, or other factors. Heart disease and stroke are the leading causes of death in these patients. All lifestyle and medical efforts should be made to reduce the risk for these conditions. In industrial societies, the prevalence of overweight, diabetes,dyslipidemia, and hypertension is steadily increasing. Women with PCOS may gain particular benefit from early screening for cardiovascular risk factors and cardioprotective measures directed toward improving endothelial function, including diet, physical exercise, and possibly insulin sensitizers or androgen-lowering agents. Nonetheless, the better approach could be based on prevention of overweight and obesity in childhood and adolescence, screening programs of type 2 diabetes and its precursor,impaired glucose tolerance, and early treatment of PCOS women ,in order to avoid the long-term health consequences and to permit long-term compliance, are mandatory.

Index

A

abortion, 124, 134, 137, 142

abortion rate, 124, 134, 137

absorption, 170

accuracy, 33, 64, 198, 200, 205, 265, 274

achondroplasia, 159, 164

acid, 68, 70, 98, 126, 146, 159, 160, 161, 169, 184, 189, 192, 194, 197, 207, 209, 212, 215, 220, 225, 233

acne, 7, 9, 39, 51, 91, 111, 112, 116, 144, 145, 146, 147, 150, 151, 152, 153, 165, 182, 227, 277

acne vulgaris, 147

ACTH, 45, 46, 48, 63, 70, 85, 91

activity level, 45, 228

acylation, 252

adenocarcinoma, 156, 159, 261, 264, 265, 266, 273

adenomyosis, 270

adenosine, 172, 222

adenovirus, 210

adhesion, 221, 233

adipocyte, 85, 118, 192, 193, 212, 220, 225, 252, 255

adiponectin, 41, 106, 107, 120, 140, 169, 175, 185, 191, 193, 194, 197, 207, 209, 212, 213, 221, 226, 252, 279

adipose, 82, 84, 85, 86, 87, 106, 107, 174, 186, 191, 192, 193, 194, 197, 198, 200, 201, 209, 212, 215, 222, 245, 252, 255, 261, 279

adipose tissue, 82, 84, 85, 86, 106, 107, 174, 191, 192, 193, 194, 197, 198, 200, 201, 209, 212, 215, 222, 245, 252, 255, 261, 279

adiposity, 40, 52, 54, 55, 64, 67, 75, 169, 184, 195, 201, 202, 205, 216, 220, 228, 232, 252, 277

adjustment, 12, 124, 207, 229

adolescent female, 201

adolescents, 9, 12, 39, 46, 50, 57, 60, 114, 115, 116, 119, 121, 147, 163, 185, 195, 196, 201, 202, 203, 204, 205, 207, 208, 209, 278

adrenal gland, 43, 44, 67, 70, 151, 153

adrenal glands, 43, 67, 151

adrenal hyperplasia, 153, 154

adult obesity, 121

adulthood, 40, 52, 145, 203, 205, 216, 230

advantages, 27, 190

adverse event, 123

aetiology, 9, 18, 39, 59, 61, 281

affective disorder, 166, 168

African Americans, 149, 156, 204, 222, 226

aggregation, 88, 222, 226

agonist, 32, 41, 43, 46, 49, 54, 63, 65, 66, 67, 70, 73, 77, 97, 129, 136, 155

alanine, 246

Alaska, 238

Alaska Natives, 238

albumin, 192

albuminuria, 251

alcohol use, 218

aldosterone, 65, 234

algorithm, 124

allele, 64, 92, 94, 102, 106, 108, 109, 212, 278

alopecia, 37, 39, 112, 144, 145, 146, 148, 149, 151, 152, 153, 154, 155

alpha activity, 82

ALT, 245

alternative treatments, 128

amenorrhea, 10, 15, 24, 28, 39, 69, 94, 99, 112, 114, 115, 116, 118, 126, 144, 271

American Heart Association, 216, 217, 242

amplitude, 16, 55, 56, 58, 64, 77

amyloidosis, 235

anatomy, 26

androgen, 9, 16, 19, 21, 23, 24, 26, 30, 36, 39, 40, 41, 43, 44, 45, 46, 47, 51, 52, 53, 54, 55, 56, 57, 58, 59, 61, 62, 64, 67, 69, 70, 71, 72, 73, 76, 77, 80, 82, 83, 86, 87, 88, 89, 91, 92, 93, 95, 100, 103, 105, 112, 115, 118, 120, 125, 137, 144, 145, 146, 147, 148, 150, 151, 152, 153, 154, 157, 158, 178, 182, 189, 195, 209, 228, 247, 258, 280

androgenic alopecia, 113, 144

androgens, 7, 9, 13, 16, 20, 21, 38, 40, 41, 43, 45, 53, 54, 56, 57, 58, 59, 61, 62, 66, 69, 77, 81, 82, 84, 92, 95, 100, 112, 116, 118, 120, 126, 143, 145, 148, 150, 152, 153, 165, 169, 174, 189, 190, 192, 195, 247, 249, 258, 260, 262, 271, 280

anemia, 236, 253

angina, 195, 214, 217

angiogenesis, 267, 274

angiography, 221

anticoagulant, 136, 233

antioxidant, 227, 239

antiphospholipid syndrome, 142

anxiety, 165, 168, 281

anxiety disorder, 167

apnea, 113, 217, 221, 222, 223, 225, 226

apoptosis, 72, 97, 100, 267

appetite, 118, 215, 253

arginine, 64, 94, 108

arrest, 21, 30, 95

arrhenoblastoma, 153

arson, 130, 132

arterial hypertension, 184, 186, 243, 251

arteries, 231, 234

artery, 117, 179, 214, 221, 227, 234, 242, 246

Asia, 202, 245, 248

Asian Americans, 238

assessment, 21, 22, 24, 26, 30, 45, 75, 145, 149, 155, 173, 182, 218, 224, 225, 245, 251, 265

asthma, 214

asymptomatic, 25, 27, 36, 89, 227, 246, 265, 266

atherogenesis, 183, 232

atherosclerosis, 118, 162, 179, 184, 194, 208, 210, 215, 222, 226, 227, 232, 237, 238, 240, 241, 242, 246, 248, 249, 255, 259, 278

atherosclerotic plaque, 231

atherosclerotic vascular disease, 179, 234

ATP, 182, 231

autoimmune diseases, 160

autosomal dominant, 70, 89, 158

B

back pain, 214

bacteria, 146

bacteriophage, 147

bacterium, 145

base pair, 93

basement membrane, 186

basic research, 39

behaviors, 218

Beijing, 100

beneficial effect, 142, 234, 240

benign, 45, 156, 157, 158, 159, 164, 243, 257, 259, 262, 265, 271, 280

benzoyl peroxide, 146

bias, 124

binding globulin, 43, 48, 77, 82, 100, 101, 115, 120, 183, 262, 271

bioassay, 60, 67

biochemistry, 139

biological activity, 95

biomarkers, 252

biopsy, 149, 160, 245, 253, 263, 264, 265, 269, 270, 274, 276

biosynthesis, 64, 69, 70, 73, 76, 78, 91, 103

birth control, 146

birth rate, 123, 136

birth weight, 40, 42, 44, 45, 47, 51, 58, 61, 92, 101, 105, 140, 196, 251

births, 124, 135, 139, 257, 262

birthweight, 44, 54, 125

black women, 50, 238

bleeding, 140, 259, 262, 264, 265, 273, 274, 275

blood clot, 137

blood flow, 20, 22, 25, 31, 193, 234, 235, 242, 246

blood pressure, 117, 127, 141, 180, 184, 190, 205, 218, 221, 227, 236, 238, 239, 241

blood stream, 112, 166, 236, 259

blood supply, 23

blood vessels, 237

body composition, 44, 120, 121, 178, 191, 192, 228

body dissatisfaction, 166

body fat, 49, 52, 55, 88, 118, 120, 140, 189, 190, 195, 198, 199, 200, 214, 228, 262

body image, 168

body mass index (BMI), 9, 20, 22, 40, 41, 45, 46, 48, 50, 51, 55, 64, 72, 86, 102, 104, 106, 107, 115, 119, 116, 119, 121, 122, 132, 133, 135, 138, 139, 140, 141, 167, 169, 172, 183, 184, 186, 188, 190, 191, 198, 199, 200, 201, 202, 206, 208, 210, 213,

214, 215, 216, 218, 220, 221, 222, 224, 226, 227, 240, 244, 245, 250, 251, 257, 277
body weight, 21, 23, 78, 117, 121, 185, 190, 192, 193, 195, 198, 200, 204, 213, 218, 227, 261
bone, 41, 44, 50, 193, 254
bone age, 44, 50
bone marrow, 193
brain, 112, 219, 223
breakdown, 137, 192
breast cancer, 256, 257, 260, 267, 271, 274, 280
breast carcinoma, 256, 258
breathing, 217, 218, 219, 220, 223, 224, 225
Britain, 36
brothers, 89, 90
Butcher, 208

C

calcification, 117, 227
calcium, 166, 185
caloric intake, 215
caloric restriction, 211
calorie, 122, 212
cancer, 10, 154, 156, 158, 167, 213, 214, 231, 256, 257, 259, 260, 261, 263, 265, 266, 267, 270, 271, 272, 273, 274, 276, 280
cancer cells, 259
candidates, 56, 125, 134, 161
capillary, 193, 234
carbohydrate, 79, 103, 104, 172, 179, 189, 193, 210
carbohydrate metabolism, 79, 103, 210
carbon, 223, 231, 242
carbon dioxide, 223, 231, 242
carcinogenesis, 260
carcinoma, 13, 154, 247, 257, 259, 260, 261, 263, 264, 265, 270, 272, 273
cardiac catheterization, 231
cardiomyopathy, 235
cardiovascular disease, 11, 13, 50, 79, 101, 103, 113, 117, 121, 141, 154, 162, 171, 180, 184, 186, 187, 195, 196, 199, 203, 205, 213, 214, 216, 219, 220, 224, 225, 227, 232, 233, 235, 239, 241, 242, 245, 249, 250, 254, 255, 278
cardiovascular function, 232
cardiovascular morbidity, 206, 221, 227, 234
cardiovascular risk, 10, 141, 171, 180, 182, 185, 186, 189, 190, 192, 197, 198, 199, 206, 208, 221, 226, 227, 232, 233, 239, 242, 243, 246, 255, 278
cardiovascular system, 183, 236, 237, 238
Caribbean, 36, 38, 81, 115, 177

carotid arteries, 229
catheter, 268
Caucasians, 36, 198, 226
causality, 251
causation, 159, 201
cauterization, 62
central nervous system, 14
central obesity, 9, 85, 118, 139, 141, 199, 228, 245
central sleep apnea, 218, 225
cerebrovascular disease, 232
cervix, 139, 268
chaos, 239
chemokines, 193, 234
chemotherapy, 160
childhood, 25, 32, 41, 42, 44, 45, 47, 50, 52, 53, 54, 96, 121, 158, 201, 202, 203, 204, 205, 207, 208, 209, 279
China, 196, 198, 206, 245
Chinese women, 21, 93, 99
cholesterol, 69, 70, 73, 89, 91, 180, 182, 184, 195, 205, 210, 215, 221, 228, 233, 236, 238, 247, 249, 277
chorionic gonadotropin, 68, 98
chromatography, 85
chromosome, 70, 73, 90, 94, 103, 108, 278
chronic diseases, 196, 243
chronic kidney failure, 253
chronic obstructive pulmonary disease, 215
chronic renal failure, 214, 253
cigarette smoking, 218
circulation, 262
cirrhosis, 243, 244, 247, 280
class, 101, 104, 124, 174, 198, 214, 250
cleavage, 73, 91, 145
clinical presentation, 113, 158
clinical symptoms, 20
clinical syndrome, 80, 156, 182
clinical trials, 21, 137, 171
cloning, 79
clustering, 88, 89, 90, 182, 221, 281
coding, 68, 91, 96, 97
codon, 64, 94
cognitive dysfunction, 218
colon, 236, 257
colon cancer, 236, 257
common symptoms, 63
community, 36, 166, 180, 245
compatibility, 23
compensatory effect, 86
complaints, 113

complement, 69
complexity, 262, 264
compliance, 122, 130, 234, 241, 282
complications, 9, 12, 19, 122, 131, 133, 138, 139, 140, 141, 143, 167, 194, 197, 203, 207, 214, 238, 249, 252, 254
composition, 75, 88, 120, 191
compounds, 161, 174, 211
compression, 253
computed tomography, 200
concordance, 78
conference, 17, 18, 25
confounding variables, 257
congenital adrenal hyperplasia, 40, 43, 53, 87, 150, 152
congestive heart failure, 243
consensus, 10, 17, 18, 20, 22, 23, 29, 30, 32, 52, 111, 137, 184, 219
consent, 144, 223, 260, 265
consumption, 196, 197
contour, 264
contraceptives, 12, 144, 146, 147, 154, 178, 257, 260
control group, 42, 63, 123, 134, 138, 139, 140, 183, 184, 211, 231
controlled trials, 129, 133, 142
controversies, 11, 14
COPD, 215
coronary artery disease, 117, 217, 221, 224, 231, 232, 236, 239, 278
coronary heart disease, 10, 194, 228, 232, 251
corpus luteum, 61, 95, 99, 261
correlation, 20, 21, 44, 63, 64, 68, 72, 77, 86, 98, 115, 120, 157, 165, 172, 184, 191, 199, 209, 212, 227, 251, 256, 270, 276, 280
correlations, 48, 96, 209
cortex, 58, 70, 87, 95
corticosteroid cream, 161
corticosteroids, 158, 189
cortisol, 48, 55, 63, 84, 85, 87, 88, 92, 112, 154, 165, 219, 220
cost, 124, 138, 216, 242, 254, 264, 265, 268
counsel, 128, 227
craving, 189
creatinine, 253
critical analysis, 82
cross-sectional study, 243, 254, 256
crown, 150, 153
CT scan, 200
culture, 62, 65, 67, 73, 152

CVD, 117, 219, 235, 249, 251, 279
cycles, 23, 24, 32, 36, 56, 64, 84, 88, 94, 115, 122, 137, 150, 152, 259, 260, 280
cycling, 21, 61, 148, 237
cyst, 137
cytochrome, 49, 63, 70, 73, 78, 82, 91, 145, 150, 178
cytokines, 107, 193, 194, 198, 201, 222, 233, 253, 255, 279
cytology, 274
cytoplasm, 97
cytosine, 145

D

database, 251
death rate, 238
deaths, 216, 244
deciliter, 138
defects, 24, 79, 80, 83, 84, 87, 99, 103, 125, 146, 159, 175, 177, 178, 189, 209, 214, 220, 240, 278
deficiencies, 84, 86, 135
deficiency, 39, 61, 95, 114, 118, 126, 146, 147, 172, 261, 272
degradation, 169, 189, 234
demographic characteristics, 219
Denmark, 51
dephosphorylation, 192
deposition, 114, 160, 164
deposits, 237
depression, 146, 165, 168, 169, 214, 218, 281
deprivation, 218
derivatives, 215
dermatologist, 146, 162
dermis, 160
desensitization, 64
detection, 27, 138, 259, 265, 274, 281
developed countries, 196, 216, 243
developing countries, 196, 202, 235
diabetes, 11, 13, 41, 50, 53, 74, 82, 101, 102, 105, 106, 112, 113, 115, 124, 133, 138, 139, 140, 143, 154, 156, 157, 158, 159, 161, 163, 165, 166, 169, 171, 174, 176, 177, 178, 179, 180, 187, 190, 191, 195, 196, 197, 203, 205, 211, 214, 219, 220, 224, 226, 230, 232, 233, 238, 242, 243, 244, 248, 249, 250, 254, 256, 260, 277
diabetic nephropathy, 251
diabetic patients, 170, 233, 246, 251
diagnostic criteria, 10, 16, 18, 22, 23, 29, 36, 52, 75, 96, 186, 191, 197, 250, 279
diagnostic parameters, 180

dialysis, 254, 256
diastolic blood pressure, 138, 184, 206, 227
diastolic pressure, 237
diet, 113, 122, 138, 161, 166, 172, 174, 178, 179, 195, 196, 202, 203, 212, 214, 215, 237, 238, 282
dietary supplementation, 161
dieting, 201
dilatation and curettage, 265
dilation, 185
direct cost, 216
direct costs, 216
discordance, 88
disease progression, 248
disorder, 7, 9, 14, 15, 17, 19, 22, 25, 27, 38, 58, 67, 69, 72, 74, 79, 80, 92, 103, 111, 112, 114, 126, 136, 138, 145, 149, 151, 154, 155, 165, 171, 173, 185, 209, 217, 222, 233, 243, 244, 277
disposition, 145
dissatisfaction, 167
distress, 167
disturbances, 11, 30, 32, 47, 60, 113, 122, 152, 157, 165, 166, 171, 189, 234
divergence, 55, 201, 205
dizygotic, 88
dizygotic twins, 88
DNA, 89, 91, 212, 275
doctors, 167
dominance, 71, 114, 258
dosage, 65, 174
dose-response relationship, 65
double blind study, 133
double-blind trial, 126, 132
drugs, 124, 131, 133, 153, 154, 156, 166, 174, 257
dyslipidemia, 42, 43, 45, 47, 89, 117, 171, 176, 185, 190, 201, 219, 226, 228, 232, 233, 243, 245, 248, 251, 259, 278
dysmenorrhea, 153
dysplasia, 159, 164

E

East Asia, 94, 98, 152
Easter, 208
eating disorders, 116, 118, 167, 168
economic consequences, 216
economic status, 196
ectopic pregnancy, 137
editors, 29
EGF, 71
egg, 112

elective abortion, 136
electrical resistance, 200
electrocautery, 124
elongation, 160
EMG, 223
emotional distress, 167, 168
encoding, 64, 73, 91, 94, 102, 105, 108
encouragement, 12
endocrine, 9, 13, 22, 28, 38, 41, 45, 51, 58, 71, 78, 83, 106, 111, 119, 121, 123, 138, 143, 144, 150, 152, 156, 158, 159, 169, 175, 178, 187, 193, 194, 215, 229, 261, 272, 277
endocrine disorders, 10, 144
endocrinology, 13, 29, 55, 88, 165
endometrial biopsy, 265, 266, 270, 273, 274
endometrial carcinoma, 154, 260, 261, 262, 263, 264, 265, 270, 273, 274, 276
endometrial hyperplasia, 259, 260, 261, 262, 263, 264, 266, 269, 270, 271, 272, 273, 274, 275, 276, 280
endometrial polyps, 260
endothelial cells, 193
endothelial dysfunction, 182, 220, 227, 232, 233, 242, 278
endothelium, 233
endotoxemia, 210
end-stage renal disease, 249, 251, 253, 280
energy density, 217
England, 87
environmental factors, 47, 61, 66, 88, 173, 209
enzymes, 69, 70, 86, 93, 145, 150, 215, 234
epidemic, 140, 161, 190, 195, 198, 202, 205, 217, 221, 279
epidemiology, 13, 37, 83, 201, 207, 271, 273
epidermis, 160
epilepsy, 37, 38
epithelial cells, 108
epithelial ovarian cancer, 257
equilibrium, 197
equipment, 200
erythropoietin, 222
ester, 234
estrogen, 38, 56, 61, 113, 114, 115, 120, 125, 134, 142, 148, 152, 165, 174, 189, 258, 259, 260, 261, 267, 272, 278
ethnic background, 10
ethnic groups, 36, 50, 152, 157, 199, 238, 250
ethnic minority, 203
ethnicity, 38, 172, 203, 204, 245

etiology, 7, 9, 17, 37, 108, 116, 135, 137, 145, 147, 154, 248, 258, 262

exaggeration, 112

examinations, 185

exclusion, 18, 39, 47

excretion, 84, 85

exercise, 12, 113, 118, 138, 161, 203, 237, 238, 244, 259, 270, 282

experiences, 27

exploration, 26

exposure, 9, 40, 42, 43, 52, 53, 57, 58, 88, 131, 229, 258, 259, 260, 261, 280

extracellular matrix, 186

extraction, 75

F

FAI, 182, 247

false positive, 265

family history, 75, 114, 170, 172, 218, 232, 246, 257, 258, 279

family members, 89

fasting, 20, 48, 76, 89, 102, 118, 119, 120, 138, 139, 157, 171, 174, 177, 182, 186, 193, 197, 205, 209, 219, 220, 225, 227, 247, 264, 278

fasting glucose, 48, 119, 120, 138, 171, 177, 182, 197, 209, 221, 231, 247, 278

fat, 13, 40, 44, 84, 107, 114, 117, 118, 140, 152, 169, 174, 178, 185, 189, 190, 192, 198, 199, 200, 206, 208, 214, 215, 229, 243, 252, 255, 259, 273

fatty acids, 173, 207, 209, 215

FDA, 203

feedback, 46, 58, 59, 65

feedback inhibition, 58

feelings, 281

female pattern baldness, 148

fertility, 9, 20, 24, 27, 29, 37, 119, 121, 122, 132, 133, 139, 150, 174, 257, 266

fertilization, 107, 123, 132, 137

fetal abnormalities, 124

fetal demise, 139

fetal growth, 43

fetus, 88, 139

fibrinogen, 180, 182, 234

fibrinolysis, 83, 171, 178, 185, 186, 240

fibroblast growth factor, 159, 164

fibroblast proliferation, 159

fibroblasts, 76, 177, 193

fibroids, 114

fibrosis, 243, 244, 280

fibrous cap, 234

filtration, 250, 254, 255, 256

first degree relative, 88, 90, 172, 175

fish, 161

fish oil, 161

fitness, 221

fluid, 265, 268, 274

focal segmental glomerulosclerosis, 251

folate, 137

folic acid, 119, 122

follicle, 16, 21, 24, 26, 28, 31, 52, 56, 60, 63, 64, 67, 69, 72, 73, 82, 94, 98, 99, 100, 112, 115, 124, 141, 148, 152, 209, 240

follicle stimulating hormone, 56, 63, 94, 98, 99, 112

follicles, 11, 16, 20, 21, 22, 24, 30, 32, 62, 66, 71, 72, 74, 92, 94, 99, 112, 118, 122, 141, 149

follicular fluid, 72, 73, 74, 95, 118, 127

food intake, 118, 209

Ford, 241

formula, 21, 198, 200, 219

France, 29, 37

freezing, 268

frequencies, 96

friction, 159

fructose, 249

functional activation, 161

G

gastroesophageal reflux, 214

gene expression, 56, 70, 73, 101, 194, 211, 222

gene promoter, 108

gene therapy, 234

general practitioner, 251

genes, 58, 70, 72, 73, 74, 79, 88, 91, 92, 93, 96, 99, 101, 102, 107, 109, 150, 177, 211, 222, 259

genetic defect, 173, 189

genetic disease, 89, 164

genetic factors, 50, 108, 145, 222

genetic marker, 91

genetic syndromes, 209

genetics, 109, 215, 226

genome, 226

genotype, 89, 96, 99, 101, 105, 106, 135, 211

Germany, 156, 168

gestation, 40, 44, 52, 58, 61, 135, 138, 139

gestational age, 41, 42, 44, 48, 54, 138, 252

gestational diabetes, 123, 133, 138, 140, 143, 144, 169, 175, 278

gland, 78, 112, 118, 144, 145

glucagon, 170

gluconeogenesis, 85

glucose, 10, 13, 14, 24, 38, 41, 45, 48, 49, 74, 79, 81, 82, 85, 92, 99, 102, 103, 104, 112, 113, 115, 117, 123, 134, 138, 141, 142, 143, 153, 155, 162, 165, 166, 169, 171, 174, 175, 176, 177, 178, 179, 180, 181, 182, 183, 185, 186, 187, 189, 191, 194, 197, 200, 205, 210, 212, 219, 220, 224, 225, 230, 232, 233, 236, 239, 244, 259, 277

glucose regulation, 170

glucose tolerance, 10, 13, 14, 41, 48, 75, 113, 115, 126, 134, 138, 141, 142, 155, 165, 169, 171, 174, 175, 176, 177, 178, 182, 183, 189, 191, 194, 197, 200, 210, 212, 231, 232, 239, 277

glucose tolerance test, 41, 48, 75, 115, 134, 138, 141, 142, 171, 183, 211, 212

glucose-induced insulin secretion, 170

glycan, 174

glycans, 160

glycerol, 192

glycogen, 103, 161

glycoproteins, 122

gonadotropin-releasing hormone (GnRH), 16, 65, 67, 125

gonads, 43, 70, 96

gout, 179, 214

grading, 153

gradings, 199

Greece, 36

grouping, 238

growth factor, 16, 28, 39, 69, 71, 73, 74, 82, 96, 102, 112, 118, 153, 159, 162, 164, 222, 233, 242, 256, 257, 258, 262, 271

growth hormone, 43, 77, 118, 193

guidance, 259, 268

guidelines, 24, 180, 184, 186, 245, 248, 249, 251

H

hair, 42, 51, 92, 111, 112, 120, 144, 148, 149, 151, 152, 153, 154, 155, 158, 165

hair follicle, 92, 112, 148, 150, 152, 154

hair loss, 148, 149, 151, 155, 165

haplotypes, 92, 99, 105

headache, 114

health care costs, 216

health care system, 138

health problems, 187, 205

heart attack, 195, 230, 236, 238

heart disease, 176, 179, 214, 231, 235, 236, 237, 238, 240

heart failure, 214, 215, 217, 221, 225, 235, 242, 243, 251

heart rate, 223, 231, 241

height, 21, 42, 43, 44, 48, 50, 54, 125, 206

hemodialysis, 214, 254

hemoglobin, 139

hemorrhage, 234

hepatitis, 245

heredity, 145

heterogeneity, 10, 39, 55, 58, 123, 180, 189

high blood cholesterol, 214

high blood pressure, 184, 195, 205, 214, 219, 221, 224, 227, 235, 238, 253, 255

hirsutism, 7, 9, 15, 24, 30, 36, 37, 39, 45, 47, 51, 63, 81, 85, 87, 88, 91, 93, 102, 105, 112, 113, 114, 127, 139, 144, 145, 146, 150, 151, 152, 153, 154, 155, 165, 166, 168, 174, 182, 227, 277

Hispanics, 36, 50, 157, 163, 204

histology, 62, 244, 272

homeostasis, 86, 104, 118, 169, 184, 189, 197, 209, 215, 255

homocysteine, 127, 132, 135, 165, 168, 229, 234

human chorionic gonadotropin, 67, 99

Hunter, 155

hybrid, 77

hygiene, 146

hyperactivity, 63

hyperandrogenism, 10, 16, 17, 18, 19, 20, 23, 26, 27, 35, 36, 37, 38, 39, 40, 41, 42, 43, 44, 45, 46, 47, 51, 53, 54, 55, 57, 58, 60, 61, 62, 63, 65, 66, 67, 70, 72, 73, 74, 76, 77, 79, 80, 81, 87, 91, 93, 103, 105, 107, 108, 111, 112, 115, 120, 126, 140, 144, 145, 146, 152, 160, 169, 175, 176, 178, 182, 229, 256, 258, 277

hyperbilirubinemia, 139

hypercholesterolemia, 179, 184

hyperglycaemia, 184, 233, 246

hyperglycemia, 82, 184, 244

hyperinsulinemia, 9, 16, 40, 43, 44, 45, 47, 64, 74, 77, 80, 92, 103, 106, 113, 115, 117, 120, 137, 142, 144, 153, 156, 158, 159, 161, 163, 169, 174, 175, 176, 178, 179, 182, 187, 200, 209, 229, 239, 241, 259, 260, 262, 264, 277

hyperinsulinism, 20, 42, 43, 47, 61, 79, 129, 175

hyperlipidemia, 179, 197, 202, 203, 243, 244, 252, 256, 279

hyperlipoproteinemia, 179, 185

hyperplasia, 63, 145, 258, 260, 261, 262, 263, 264, 265, 266, 268, 269, 270, 272, 273, 274, 276, 280
hyperprolactinemia, 152
hypersensitivity, 145
hypertension, 45, 86, 117, 130, 133, 139, 140, 159, 171, 179, 180, 184, 186, 190, 196, 197, 202, 203, 205, 214, 216, 220, 224, 226, 228, 232, 235, 237, 238, 239, 240, 241, 245, 249, 250, 259, 278
hypertrichosis, 151, 154
hypertriglyceridemia, 179, 184
hypertrophy, 23, 30, 236
hyperuricemia, 179, 180, 182, 184
hypogonadism, 25, 32, 126
hypothalamus, 39, 52, 59, 118, 122, 197, 209, 216
hypothesis, 23, 24, 41, 49, 55, 57, 58, 61, 66, 69, 76, 79, 89, 101, 115, 135, 172
hypoxia, 218, 220, 224
hypoxia-inducible factor, 222
hysterectomy, 261, 266, 267, 268, 269, 270, 276

I

iatrogenic, 139
ideal, 122
idiopathic, 25, 36, 37, 42, 63, 145, 152, 159
IGFs, 72
imbalances, 166
immigrants, 36
immune reaction, 145
immune system, 191, 194
immunomodulatory, 198, 279
impairments, 220, 232, 278
in utero, 40, 62, 252
in vivo, 64, 68, 94, 98, 165
incidence, 37, 44, 47, 49, 88, 115, 123, 133, 134, 137, 149, 167, 170, 173, 206, 210, 224, 232, 243, 252, 261, 264, 270, 277
India, 248, 254, 256
Indians, 163, 238
induction, 12, 59, 118, 122, 131, 132, 133, 137, 142, 210, 252, 268
induction methods, 127
industrialized countries, 244
infancy, 10, 62, 96
infants, 41, 48, 139, 251
infarction, 236, 252
infertility, 10, 15, 19, 27, 28, 64, 84, 86, 88, 94, 111, 112, 114, 119, 121, 130, 132, 133, 134, 137, 141, 143, 154, 165, 166, 168, 173, 190, 214, 256, 257, 259, 260, 262, 271, 277

inflammation, 96, 107, 108, 141, 144, 145, 146, 182, 186, 194, 197, 200, 201, 210, 215, 218, 219, 220, 224, 225, 229, 232, 234, 240, 247, 252, 255, 278
inflammatory disease, 215, 233
inflammatory mediators, 183, 222
infusion model, 75
inheritance, 88, 89, 90, 151, 158, 222
inherited disorder, 151
inhibition, 16, 28, 46, 52, 56, 57, 61, 65, 76, 78, 93, 108, 146, 228
inhibitor, 117, 125, 135, 142, 184, 185, 186, 228, 239, 267, 275
initiation, 44, 96, 138, 219, 250
inositol, 126, 131, 132, 174
insertion, 275
insulin dependent diabetes, 10
insulin sensitivity, 40, 48, 61, 75, 77, 81, 83, 85, 101, 103, 105, 107, 109, 119, 120, 127, 161, 163, 169, 174, 175, 176, 183, 189, 194, 195, 197, 201, 210, 220, 226, 228, 244, 259, 279
insulin signaling, 104, 105, 126, 194
intensive care unit, 130, 133
intercellular adhesion molecule, 183
interface, 137
intertrigo, 214
intervention, 9, 138, 139, 147, 174, 184, 248, 254, 281
intima, 185, 227, 240, 246
inversion, 23, 31
iron, 114
irritability, 218
IRS, 76, 101, 104, 105, 108, 172, 174
isoleucine, 64, 94

J

Japan, 196, 198, 202, 245, 251
Japanese women, 36, 212
joints, 156
Jordan, 271

K

keratinocyte, 147, 159
kidney, 85, 113, 214, 215, 249, 250, 253, 254, 255, 256, 280
kinase activity, 76, 108
kinetics, 64, 68, 94, 98
knees, 156

L

laboratory tests, 149
lactation, 118
laser ablation, 269
later life, 45, 252
LDL, 69, 89, 180, 182, 183, 195, 210, 228, 233, 236, 239, 277
leptin, 72, 74, 118, 120, 121, 173, 185, 191, 192, 193, 197, 209, 239, 252
lesions, 145, 156, 157, 159, 161, 164, 210, 222, 231, 263, 264, 267
life expectancy, 213, 216, 253
life satisfaction, 281
lifestyle changes, 45, 212, 281
lifetime, 167, 237, 256, 280
ligand, 174
lipid metabolism, 197, 215, 234
lipids, 41, 173, 183, 201, 211, 215, 240
lipolysis, 209
lipoproteins, 215, 230, 233, 240
liver, 82, 85, 86, 113, 118, 146, 192, 194, 197, 203, 214, 215, 236, 243, 244, 247, 248, 249, 279
liver cells, 118
liver damage, 146
liver disease, 113, 214, 215, 243, 244, 247, 248, 249, 280
liver enzymes, 246
liver failure, 248
liver function tests, 244
liver transplant, 247
liver transplantation, 247
localization, 92, 93
locus, 61, 89, 96, 106, 151
longitudinal study, 45, 74, 169
low birthweight, 53
low-density lipoprotein, 119, 183, 185, 228, 233, 242, 277
low-grade inflammation, 107, 140, 186, 191, 229
lumen, 234
lupus, 160
luteinizing hormone, 16, 28, 52, 58, 59, 60, 62, 65, 67, 68, 69, 73, 74, 80, 82, 97, 98, 112, 115, 168, 177, 183, 195, 201, 209
lymphedema, 214
lymphocytes, 234
lymphoma, 214

M

Mackintosh, 241
macrophages, 108, 193, 194, 217, 234, 252
macrosomia, 143
magnetic resonance, 200, 219
magnetic resonance imaging, 200, 219
majority, 36, 88, 134, 138, 150, 154, 166, 170, 199, 226, 248
malignancy, 156, 157, 158, 159, 260, 261, 262, 265, 270
malnutrition, 252
management, 11, 12, 13, 30, 115, 116, 122, 132, 133, 140, 142, 147, 149, 154, 155, 174, 185, 234, 238, 245, 251, 254, 266, 274, 281
manufacturing, 215
markers, 42, 47, 78, 97, 121, 141, 144, 146, 170, 180, 182, 185, 186, 191, 192, 195, 219, 227, 244, 271, 278
marrow, 193
mass spectrometry, 85
maternal smoking, 196
matrix, 183, 186, 234
matrix metalloproteinase, 184
MCP, 183, 241, 247
mechanical ventilation, 198
media, 185, 196, 206, 227, 240, 246, 269
median, 50, 212
medication, 125, 150
Mediterranean, 152
melanin, 160
membranes, 139
memory, 218, 219
menarche, 44, 50, 55, 113, 114, 115, 260
menopause, 148, 149, 218, 259, 260, 261, 281
menstruation, 9, 116, 118
mental health, 167, 168, 169, 235
mental illness, 166
messenger ribonucleic acid, 99
meta-analysis, 99, 124, 131, 140, 142, 144, 217, 265, 274
metabolic disorder, 11, 49, 75, 117, 118, 141, 186, 195, 201, 210, 252, 255, 277
metabolic disturbances, 106, 118, 163, 171, 174, 228
metabolic dysfunction, 41, 187, 194, 220
metabolic pathways, 218, 224
metabolic syndrome, 10, 45, 54, 84, 86, 117, 120, 121, 139, 146, 178, 179, 180, 182, 186, 187, 188, 190, 191, 192, 194, 195, 197, 199, 200, 201, 205,

208, 211, 214, 215, 216, 217, 218, 220, 224, 225, 227, 232, 233, 235, 238, 240, 241, 242, 243, 244, 247, 248, 249, 250, 255, 278

metabolism, 55, 69, 76, 79, 80, 84, 85, 87, 91, 92, 101, 103, 124, 145, 147, 149, 152, 165, 172, 174, 177, 194, 195, 197, 200, 209, 216, 219, 220, 224, 225, 228, 234, 243, 253, 265, 279

metabolites, 85, 173, 215

metabolizing, 150

metformin, 11, 30, 44, 78, 81, 82, 83, 96, 100, 101, 123, 131, 132, 133, 134, 138, 140, 142, 144, 166, 174, 176, 178, 195, 197, 201, 212, 213, 228, 240

mice, 40, 52, 96, 99, 146, 164, 255

micrograms, 47

migration, 233, 241

mineralocorticoid, 86

miniaturization, 149

minorities, 238

minority groups, 50

miscarriage, 123, 133, 142, 143, 260, 262, 280

mitosis, 72

modification, 19, 25, 123, 144, 197, 213, 234, 278

molecular biology, 98, 105

molecular weight, 211

molecules, 193, 221, 234

monitoring, 146, 223, 266, 267, 274

monoclonal antibody, 161, 165

monocyte chemoattractant protein, 193, 221, 249

monolayer, 73

monozygotic twins, 88

mood disorder, 167

Moon, 196

morbidity, 50, 133, 180, 216, 218, 221, 232, 256, 278

morphology, 18, 21, 23, 24, 29, 32, 47, 71, 72, 134, 139, 170, 231, 272

morphometric, 275

mortality rate, 213, 235, 243, 254, 282

mortality risk, 213, 254, 256, 278

Moses, 82, 165

MRI, 26, 200, 219

mRNA, 71, 95, 99

mucosa, 156

muscle mass, 152

muscles, 218

mutant, 161, 165

mutation, 64, 94, 99, 107, 135, 164

myocardial infarction, 151, 179, 186, 195, 202, 214, 235, 239, 251

myocardium, 235, 241

N

National Health Service, 242

National Institutes of Health, 17, 18, 19, 25, 196

Native Americans, 149, 157, 163

natural selection, 215

necrosis, 107, 108, 207

negative feedback, 56, 85, 234

negative mood, 165

negative relation, 203

neoplasm, 156

nephron, 251

nephrotic syndrome, 255

nerve, 252

Netherlands, 18

neurons, 216

neutrophils, 108, 160

New England, 142, 162, 225

nicotinic acid, 157, 158

nitric oxide, 231, 233, 255

nitric oxide synthase, 255

nitrogen, 268

nodules, 145

non-insulin dependent diabetes, 9, 80, 137, 162, 171, 173, 178

nonsmokers, 213

non-smokers, 237

norepinephrine, 193, 230

normal children, 188

normal distribution, 149

North America, 37, 89, 105, 208

nuclei, 261, 272

nulliparity, 257

nutrition, 10, 49, 51, 190, 252

O

obstruction, 218, 223

obstructive sleep apnea, 180, 213, 214, 218, 219, 222, 223, 224, 225, 226

occlusion, 234

Oceania, 202

oil, 112, 161

oligomenorrhea, 15, 18, 36, 39, 40, 47, 64, 114, 116, 261

oocyte, 97, 127

oophorectomy, 77

oral antibiotic, 146

oral antibiotics, 146

organ, 194, 198, 241, 244, 252, 266, 279

osteoarthritis, 213, 214

outpatients, 243

ovarian cancer, 256, 257, 258, 271

ovarian tumor, 152, 257, 260

ovaries, 10, 13, 15, 16, 18, 19, 20, 21, 23, 24, 26, 27, 28, 29, 30, 31, 32, 35, 36, 37, 38, 39, 40, 47, 53, 58, 59, 61, 62, 69, 72, 73, 74, 75, 79, 81, 82, 83, 89, 92, 93, 94, 100, 105, 107, 108, 111, 112, 115, 116, 118, 120, 122, 136, 141, 143, 153, 175, 176, 182, 231, 236, 242, 257, 264, 272, 280

overnutrition, 198, 279

overproduction, 7, 9, 152

overweight, 9, 22, 44, 50, 81, 86, 106, 117, 119, 128, 139, 162, 163, 165, 172, 185, 190, 191, 195, 196, 199, 201, 202, 203, 204, 206, 208, 209, 214, 216, 218, 222, 230, 238, 243, 244, 249, 250, 259, 260, 261, 277

ovulation, 11, 16, 25, 27, 30, 46, 52, 56, 57, 59, 62, 78, 82, 83, 86, 95, 101, 107, 112, 114, 118, 121, 131, 132, 133, 137, 142, 174, 189, 258, 260, 262, 265, 268, 280

oxidation, 194, 197, 233

oxidative stress, 102, 219, 220, 228, 233, 239, 252

oxygen, 218, 219, 223, 226

P

Pacific, 36, 199, 238, 245, 248

pain, 166, 231

palate, 218

pancreas, 95, 112, 187, 189, 192

pancreatic cancer, 214

pandemic, 245

panic disorder, 167

parallel, 65, 245

paraneoplastic syndrome, 164

parenchyma, 253

parity, 257, 262

pathogenesis, 11, 14, 18, 25, 27, 39, 46, 57, 62, 63, 72, 76, 81, 88, 91, 93, 94, 101, 105, 106, 126, 145, 147, 165, 174, 175, 185, 194, 195, 210, 219, 220, 230, 232, 233, 238, 244, 252, 280

pathology, 90, 265

pathophysiology, 11, 15, 32, 37, 38, 56, 58, 83, 90, 141, 182, 189, 190, 215, 221, 255

pathways, 105, 210, 224, 233

PCR, 64, 94

pelvic ultrasound, 37, 47, 115, 231

pelvis, 30

penetrance, 89, 151

peptides, 71, 95, 122

percentile, 50, 205, 250

perfusion, 246

pericarditis, 253

perinatal, 53, 60, 121, 133, 138

permeability, 233

permit, 21, 24, 45, 172, 234, 282

phenotype, 10, 29, 35, 47, 58, 69, 72, 73, 89, 91, 97, 98, 102, 106, 107, 120, 173, 206, 208, 215, 235, 250, 278

phenytoin, 161

Philippines, 245

phosphorylation, 76, 78, 81, 101, 103, 172, 177, 192, 233

physical activity, 49, 51, 202, 204, 209, 215

physical exercise, 282

physiology, 97, 107, 193, 217

pigmentation, 152, 156

pilot study, 67, 143, 247

pioglitazone, 131

pituitary gland, 59, 112

placebo, 30, 83, 123, 134, 174, 212, 213

placenta, 118, 137

plaque, 215, 229

plasma cells, 160

plasma levels, 108, 109, 197, 220, 279

plasmapheresis, 161

plasminogen, 117, 135, 142, 184, 228, 239

platelets, 234

plethysmography, 234

PM, 31, 87, 178, 201, 208, 225, 241, 242, 248, 271

PMS, 114

point mutation, 68, 94, 97

polarity, 263, 264

policy makers, 216

polycystic ovarian syndrome, 13, 18, 29, 30, 32, 33, 38, 45, 60, 61, 66, 67, 69, 73, 80, 87, 92, 118, 121, 128, 131, 132, 142, 143, 145, 152, 168, 171, 173, 175, 176, 177, 178, 192, 203, 256, 280

polymorphism, 12, 51, 55, 73, 89, 91, 93, 97, 100, 101, 102, 104, 105, 107, 108, 109, 145

polymorphisms, 47, 51, 91, 92, 95, 98, 101, 102, 105, 106, 107, 108, 135, 142, 145, 211, 213

polypeptide, 96, 170

positive correlation, 42, 44, 76, 86, 183, 191, 209, 228

positive relationship, 20, 228

postmenopausal women, 152, 153, 154, 227, 258, 261, 264, 265, 267, 270, 271, 272, 273, 274, 275

precocious puberty, 43
prediction models, 124
preeclampsia, 133, 139
pregnancy, 41, 74, 83, 86, 104, 118, 122, 131, 132, 133, 134, 137, 139, 140, 142, 143, 144, 148, 153, 178, 190, 196, 214, 215, 236, 257, 259, 267, 271, 275, 278
premature adrenarche, 45, 47
premature death, 249, 280
prematurity, 44, 54
preschool, 206
preterm delivery, 139
prevention, 11, 203, 216, 242, 254, 256, 273, 279
primate, 40, 52
probability, 88
proband, 88
probands, 89
probe, 21, 61, 212, 268
productivity, 216
progesterone, 12, 16, 43, 46, 56, 57, 59, 61, 65, 70, 72, 78, 114, 125, 131, 134, 142, 146, 174, 189, 209, 247, 258, 259, 260, 261, 267, 268, 273, 274, 275, 280
progestins, 154, 260, 267, 269, 272
prognosis, 246, 251, 254
programming, 42, 53, 61
pro-inflammatory, 194, 215
project, 251
prolactin, 60, 115, 150, 154
proliferation, 16, 28, 97, 145, 159, 260, 262, 263, 264
promoter, 91, 92, 93, 97, 107, 108
prostate cancer, 214
proteases, 72
protective mechanisms, 232
protective role, 150
protein kinase C, 93
proteins, 72, 74, 96, 99, 101, 105, 150, 209, 234, 235, 262, 271
proteinuria, 250, 254, 256
proteolytic enzyme, 234
prothrombin, 135
psoriasis, 160
psychiatric illness, 215
psychological distress, 165, 281
psychological problems, 166
psychological well-being, 144
pubarche, 42, 43, 44, 45, 46, 47, 49, 53, 54, 55, 58, 61, 91, 93, 112, 114
pubertal development, 41, 43, 49, 51, 55, 77

puberty, 10, 32, 41, 42, 44, 47, 49, 50, 51, 53, 54, 55, 57, 58, 61, 62, 66, 77, 99, 114, 118, 151, 152, 158, 188, 189, 191, 201, 261
public health, 50, 184, 196, 199, 207, 217, 219, 281
public schools, 157
pulmonary embolism, 214

Q

quality of life, 9, 144, 166, 168, 216, 218, 235, 243, 254, 281
quartile, 257

R

race, 163, 172, 203, 204
racial differences, 50, 55, 222
reactive oxygen, 182, 222
reactivity, 164, 228
receptor sites, 64
receptors, 69, 72, 77, 82, 107, 109, 118, 134, 142, 145, 150, 159, 162, 187, 192, 193, 252, 261, 280
recession, 150
recognition, 10, 24, 74, 138, 144, 224, 281
recommendations, iv, 138, 234
recurrence, 150, 267
red blood cells, 253
regeneration, 85
regression, 129, 159, 267, 269
reinforcement, 84, 86
rejection, 166
relatives, 53, 89, 171, 222
relevance, 60, 281
reliability, 31, 206
REM, 218
remission, 163
renal dysfunction, 236, 251
renal failure, 249, 251, 280
renal replacement therapy, 254, 256
renin, 228, 234
repair, 160, 164
replacement, 212, 231, 260, 272, 274
reproduction, 61, 95, 100, 108, 119, 121, 122, 130, 132, 139
reproductive age, 36, 89, 100, 112, 152, 165, 184, 264
reproductive organs, 118
resection, 62, 67, 82, 268, 269, 275
residues, 172

resistance, 10, 17, 19, 25, 41, 45, 48, 74, 77, 80, 81, 86, 89, 95, 102, 105, 107, 112, 115, 116, 117, 118, 120, 121, 132, 140, 152, 153, 158, 159, 161, 162, 165, 167, 169, 172, 174, 175, 176, 180, 182, 185, 187, 188, 189, 190, 191, 194, 195, 197, 201, 209, 215, 219, 220, 225, 228, 232, 233, 239, 241, 242, 244, 247, 252, 255, 272, 278

resolution, 20, 122, 146, 161, 268

responsiveness, 48, 66, 215

retinol, 70

risk assessment, 281

risk factors, 44, 47, 117, 135, 138, 163, 170, 176, 179, 180, 183, 184, 185, 186, 195, 201, 202, 205, 215, 220, 226, 227, 236, 237, 239, 240, 242, 243, 245, 248, 249, 250, 254, 256, 257, 258, 260, 261, 273, 278

risk profile, 11, 189, 229

robust design, 21

rodents, 194, 219, 220

rosiglitazone, 131, 211, 213

S

salts, 161

Samoa, 196

scleroderma, 160

screening, 20, 99, 138, 143, 183, 184, 241, 253, 254, 264, 282

sebum, 147

secrete, 62, 63, 193

secretion, 9, 16, 28, 38, 44, 45, 48, 49, 52, 53, 54, 55, 56, 57, 58, 59, 60, 61, 62, 64, 67, 68, 69, 70, 71, 72, 75, 78, 80, 81, 82, 83, 85, 90, 95, 98, 101, 102, 103, 104, 105, 109, 138, 163, 169, 172, 176, 177, 178, 189, 192, 230, 240, 258, 261, 271

sedatives, 223

sedentary behavior, 204

sedentary lifestyle, 214

segregation, 89

self-esteem, 146, 281

self-monitoring, 138

self-worth, 167

semen, 126

sensing, 215

sensitivity, 20, 46, 48, 51, 56, 57, 58, 60, 64, 75, 78, 91, 119, 123, 161, 169, 174, 177, 182, 191, 192, 194, 195, 211, 221, 228, 256, 264, 265, 270

sensitization, 17

sequencing, 96

serine, 76, 78, 103, 172, 177

serum, 13, 28, 30, 42, 48, 52, 59, 60, 62, 64, 67, 68, 78, 82, 83, 84, 87, 94, 98, 100, 101, 106, 118, 125, 132, 139, 141, 154, 159, 174, 177, 178, 182, 185, 186, 189, 192, 206, 209, 212, 227, 233, 240, 246, 248, 250, 255, 258, 273, 280

SES, 196, 203, 204

sex, 16, 28, 41, 43, 46, 48, 52, 57, 59, 77, 82, 88, 89, 90, 91, 100, 101, 115, 120, 123, 152, 177, 180, 183, 186, 206, 218, 247, 262, 273, 282

sex hormones, 91, 186

sex ratio, 123

sex steroid, 16, 28, 41, 43, 46, 52, 57, 59, 77, 177

sexual development, 50

sexual dimorphism, 87

shock, 246, 248

siblings, 92

side effects, 130, 136, 146

signal detection model, 244

signal transduction, 76, 101, 174

signaling pathway, 72, 99, 194

signalling, 75, 79, 105, 159, 197

signals, 50, 112, 118, 197, 216, 279

signs, 10, 15, 16, 18, 22, 24, 26, 43, 45, 50, 112, 115, 144, 148, 151, 153, 154, 156, 158, 269, 280

Sinai, 92

Singapore, 199, 256, 273

single-nucleotide polymorphism, 211, 213

skeletal muscle, 82, 177, 194, 215

skin, 85, 112, 144, 145, 147, 151, 155, 157, 158, 159, 161, 162, 164, 166, 193, 200, 217

skin grafting, 160

skin tags, 158

sleep apnea, 217, 219, 221, 222, 223, 224, 225, 226

sleep disturbance, 218, 225

sleeping pills, 222

smoking, 147, 182, 215, 219, 237, 238, 273

smooth muscle, 234

smooth muscle cells, 234

snoring, 218, 224

SNP, 92, 93, 102, 106, 211

social anxiety, 167

social consequences, 216

social development, 125

social phobia, 167

socioeconomic status, 203

sodium, 165

South Asia, 36, 38

Spain, 36, 38

species, 182, 194, 216, 222, 233

speculation, 218

sperm, 123
spontaneous abortion, 125, 133, 134, 142
Spring, 217
stabilization, 113, 115
standard deviation, 218, 252
statistics, 242, 273
stenosis, 221
steroids, 39, 42, 56, 62, 65, 83, 87, 189
stillbirth, 138
stimulus, 39, 56, 62, 190
storage, 196, 215
stratification, 217, 224
streams, 258
stressors, 236
stroke, 50, 179, 195, 196, 214, 219, 224, 225, 230, 236, 242, 282
stroma, 11, 16, 21, 22, 23, 26, 32, 82, 261, 268, 272
strong interaction, 219, 220
structural gene, 70
subgroups, 23, 39, 124, 191, 210, 214, 218, 245
subjectivity, 22, 25
sub-Saharan Africa, 152
substitutions, 68, 98
substrates, 76, 101
success rate, 128
suicide, 146, 167
suicide attempts, 167
Sun, 33, 55, 100, 142
supervision, 267
suppression, 56, 63, 77, 112, 189
surveillance, 269
survey, 36, 38, 81, 168, 203, 204, 208, 250
survival, 214, 217, 246, 247, 254
susceptibility, 91, 95, 101, 102, 105, 106, 107, 120, 171, 174, 211, 215, 222, 252, 278
Sweden, 83, 273
swelling, 141
sympathetic nervous system, 241
symptomatic treatment, 11
symptoms, 7, 9, 16, 18, 20, 30, 69, 88, 91, 101, 102, 112, 115, 116, 133, 137, 144, 150, 152, 153, 165, 169, 217, 236, 253, 266, 280
synthesis, 17, 39, 47, 54, 55, 56, 57, 65, 69, 71, 76, 78, 93, 95, 118, 120, 161, 189, 194, 252
systolic blood pressure, 83, 104, 142, 178, 206, 230, 252
systolic pressure, 237

T

T cell, 194
T lymphocytes, 234
tachycardia, 230
tamoxifen, 123, 260, 272
tandem repeats, 101, 105
teens, 203, 204
temperature, 215
testing, 24, 32, 54, 63, 65, 66, 67, 70, 96, 112, 244, 253
testosterone, 16, 21, 40, 41, 46, 47, 51, 52, 61, 64, 69, 73, 82, 83, 85, 91, 95, 112, 115, 118, 120, 126, 134, 139, 144, 146, 150, 152, 154, 165, 169, 174, 178, 182, 186, 189, 191, 209, 228, 247, 258, 271
tetracycline antibiotics, 146
TGF, 65, 71, 96, 159, 241, 252
therapeutic intervention, 234
therapy, 11, 44, 45, 77, 83, 96, 100, 104, 113, 115, 118, 122, 134, 138, 142, 144, 146, 147, 151, 153, 154, 155, 161, 165, 174, 178, 211, 221, 224, 228, 234, 240, 242, 244, 258, 260, 266, 267, 268, 269, 270, 271, 272, 274, 275, 278
thiazolidinediones, 174, 194, 197
thinning, 148, 149, 234
thoughts, 90, 99, 166
threonine, 64, 76, 78, 94, 103
thrombin, 185, 186
thrombosis, 136, 214
thrombus, 234
thymine, 145
thyroid, 64, 94, 141, 165
tissue, 21, 75, 78, 81, 85, 174, 191, 192, 193, 194, 197, 200, 209, 219, 223, 252, 261, 268, 279
TNF, 76, 107, 108, 173, 182, 194, 207, 209, 221, 252
TNF-alpha, 76, 173, 182, 194, 209, 221
total cholesterol, 183, 185, 230, 236
toxicity, 215
traits, 39, 106
tranquilizers, 222
transaminases, 244
transcription, 70, 91, 92, 174, 222
transcription factors, 174, 222
transformation, 260
transforming growth factor, 64, 71, 73, 95
transient ischemic attack, 225
transmembrane region, 164
transmission, 101
transplantation, 151, 155, 160, 247, 254
transport, 79, 82, 172

trauma, 198
trial, 30, 83, 125, 130, 131, 136, 143
triggers, 218, 224
triglycerides, 42, 127, 146, 180, 182, 184, 205, 215, 221, 228, 233, 236
tryptophan, 64, 94
TSH, 64, 94, 115, 154
tumor, 113, 141, 153, 159, 173, 182, 193, 207, 256
tumor necrosis factor, 141, 173, 182, 193, 207
tumors, 40, 43, 113, 153, 154, 164, 257
tumours, 257, 271
turnover, 197
twins, 88
type 2 diabetes, 13, 14, 19, 40, 75, 83, 101, 102, 103, 104, 105, 106, 113, 117, 138, 155, 161, 163, 164, 169, 172, 174, 176, 177, 179, 180, 182, 186, 187, 189, 191, 194, 197, 199, 200, 201, 202, 210, 213, 214, 215, 219, 220, 224, 225, 229, 232, 233, 242, 245, 248, 251, 255, 277
tyrosine, 76, 81, 101, 103, 108, 159, 164
Tyrosine, 76
tyrosine hydroxylase, 101

U

ultrasonography, 21, 22, 23, 26, 27, 30, 31, 33, 94, 139, 154, 229, 245, 264, 274
ultrasound, 13, 18, 20, 21, 22, 23, 26, 27, 29, 30, 31, 32, 33, 37, 39, 41, 59, 79, 126, 136, 141, 182, 245, 265
umbilical cord, 41, 53
underlying mechanisms, 248, 281
undernutrition, 196
uniform, 22, 181
urban life, 196
uric acid, 184, 222, 253
uric acid levels, 184
urine, 85, 86, 141, 154, 159, 249, 253
uterus, 156, 264, 268, 269
uvula, 218

V

vaccine, 146
valuation, 272
valvular heart disease, 235
vanadium, 161

variations, 60, 75, 88, 94, 145
vascular endothelial growth factor (VEGF), 226, 232
vasculature, 262
vasculitis, 253
vasoconstriction, 234
vasodilation, 234
vasodilator, 231
vein, 214
velocity, 231, 234, 241
vessels, 162, 237
video, 223
visceral adiposity, 252
viscosity, 185, 187
visualization, 268
vitamins, 166
vitiligo, 164
VLDL, 182, 233
vulnerability, 218

W

walking, 237
waste, 253
weight control, 12, 210
weight gain, 44, 54, 111, 118, 120, 138, 139, 141, 167, 195, 196, 209, 215
weight loss, 11, 78, 81, 103, 113, 118, 119, 122, 130, 161, 174, 194, 211, 213, 228, 238, 240, 244, 277
weight management, 212
weight reduction, 119, 122, 169, 189, 216
weight status, 207
wellness, 185
Western countries, 248
withdrawal, 140

X

X chromosome, 151
X-ray, 120, 140, 190, 200

Y

young adults, 87, 208, 230
young women, 10, 38, 167, 169, 172, 178, 185, 187, 229, 258, 261, 268, 272